Allergies for the Otolaryngologist

Guest Editors

B.J. FERGUSON, MD
SUMAN GOLLA, MD

OTOLARYNGOLOGIC CLINICS OF NORTH AMERICA

www.oto.theclinics.com

June 2011 • Volume 44 • Number 3

SAUNDERS an imprint of ELSEVIER, Inc.

W.B. SAUNDERS COMPANY
A Division of Elsevier Inc.

1600 John F. Kennedy Boulevard • Suite 1800 • Philadelphia, Pennsylvania 19103-2899

http://www.theclinics.com

OTOLARYNGOLOGIC CLINICS OF NORTH AMERICA Volume 44, Number 3
June 2011 ISSN 0030-6665, ISBN-13: 978-1-4557-1051-5

Editor: Joanne Husovski

Developmental Editor: Donald Mumford

Otolaryngologic Clinics of North America (ISSN 0030-6665) is published bimonthly by Elsevier, Inc., 360 Park Avenue South, New York, NY 10010-1710. Months of issue are February, April, June, August, October, and December. Business and Editorial Offices: 1600 John F. Kennedy Blvd., Suite 1800, Philadelphia, PA 19103-2899. Customer Service Office: 6277 Sea Harbor Drive, Orlando, FL 32887-4800. Periodicals postage paid at New York, NY and additional mailing offices. Subscription prices is $310.00 per year (US individuals), $590.00 per year (US institutions), $149.00 per year (US student/resident), $409.00 per year (Canadian individuals), $741.00 per year (Canadian institutions), $459.00 per year (international individuals), $741.00 per year (international institutions), $230.00 per year (international & Canadian student/resident). Foreign air speed delivery is included in all *Clinics*' subscription prices. All prices are subject to change without notice. **POSTMASTER:** Send address changes to *Otolaryngologic Clinics of North America*, Elsevier Health Sciences Division, Subscription Customer Service, 3251 Riverport Lane, Maryland Heights, MO 63043. **Telephone: 1-800-654-2452 (U.S. and Canada); 314-447-8871 (outside U.S. and Canada). Fax: 314-447-8029. E-mail: journalscustomerservice-usa@elsevier.com (for print support); journalsonlinesupport-usa@elsevier.com (for online support).**

Reprints. For copies of 100 or more of articles in this publication, please contact the Commercial Reprints Department, Elsevier Inc., 360 Park Avenue South, New York, NY 10010-1710. Tel.: 212-633-3812; Fax: 212-462-1935; E-mail: reprints@elsevier.com.

Otolaryngologic Clinics of North America is also published in Spanish by McGraw-Hill Interamericana Editores S.A., P.O. Box 5-237, 06500 Mexico D.F., Mexico.

Otolaryngologic Clinics of North America is covered in *MEDLINE/PubMed (Index Medicus), Current Contents/Clinical Medicine, Excerpta Medica, BIOSIS, Science Citation Index,* and *ISI/BIOMED.*

Printed and bound by CPI Group (UK) Ltd, Croydon, CR0 4YY

Transferred to Digital Print 2011

Contributors

GUEST EDITORS

B.J. FERGUSON, MD
Director, Division of Sino-Nasal Disorders and Allergy, Department of Otolaryngology, University of Pittsburgh School of Medicine, UPMC Mercy, Pittsburgh, Pennsylvania

SUMAN GOLLA, MD
Associate Professor of Otolaryngology, University of Pittsburgh School of Medicine; Director of UPMC St Margaret, UPMC Mercy, Pittsburgh, Pennsylvania

AUTHORS

SAMER AL-KHUDARI, MD
Resident, Department of Otolaryngology Head and Neck Surgery, Henry Ford Health Systems, Detroit, Michigan

KAREN H. CALHOUN, MD, FACS
Professor, Department of Otolaryngology–Head and Neck Surgery, The Ohio State University Medical Center, Gahanna, Ohio

NIPUN CHHABRA, MD
Department of Otolaryngology–Head and Neck Surgery, Case Western Reserve University & University Hospitals Case Medical Center, Cleveland, Ohio

MICHAEL A. DEMARCANTONIO, MD
Department of Otolaryngology–Head and Neck Surgery, Eastern Virginia Medical School, Norfolk, Virginia

M. JENNIFER DEREBERY, MD, FACS
Clinical Professor of Otolaryngology, Clinical Studies Department, University of South Carolina Keck School of Medicine, House Ear Institute, Los Angeles, California

CHARLES S. EBERT Jr, MD, MPH
Assistant Professor, Division of Rhinology, Allergy, and Sinus Surgery, Department of Otolaryngology–Head and Neck Surgery, University of North Carolina School of Medicine at Chapel Hill, Chapel Hill, North Carolina

BERRILYN J. FERGUSON, MD
Division of Sinonasal Disorders and Allergy, Department of Otolaryngology, University of Pittsburgh Medical Center, Pittsburgh, Pennsylvania

CHRISTINE FRANZESE, MD, FAAOA
Associate Professor, Residency Program Director, Department of Otolaryngology and Communicative Sciences, University of Mississippi Medical Center, Jackson, Mississippi

BRUCE R. GORDON, MA, MD, FACS, FAAOA
Chief of Otolaryngology, Cape Cod Hospital, Hyannis; Associate Staff, Massachusetts Eye and Ear Infirmary; Instructor, Laryngology and Otology, Harvard Medical School, Boston, Massachusetts

JOSEPH K. HAN, MD
Associate Professor, Director of Allergy and Rhinology and Endoscopic Sinus and Skull Base Surgery, Department of Otolaryngology–Head and Neck Surgery, Eastern Virginia Medical School, Norfolk, Virginia

STEVEN M. HOUSER, MD, FAAOA
Associate Professor, Department of Otolaryngology–Head and Neck Surgery, MetroHealth Medical Center, Case Western Reserve University, Cleveland, Ohio

DAVID S. HURST, MD, PhD
Associate Clinical Instructor, Tufts University, Department of Otolaryngology/Head and Neck Surgery, Boston, Massachusetts

JOHN H. KROUSE, MD, PhD
Professor and Chairperson, Department of Otolaryngology-Head and Neck Surgery, Temple University School of Medicine, Philadelphia, Pennsylvania

YEKATERINA A. KOSHKAREVA, MD
Resident Physician, Department of Otolaryngology-Head and Neck Surgery, Temple University School of Medicine, Philadelphia, Pennsylvania

BRYAN LEATHERMAN, MD, FAAOA
Coastal Ear, Nose and Throat Associates, Coastal Sinus and Allergy Center, Gulfport, Mississippi

SANDRA Y. LIN, MD, AAOA
Associate Professor, Department of Otolaryngology–Head & Neck Surgery, Johns Hopkins School of Medicine, Baltimore, Maryland

ELIZABETH J. MAHONEY, MD
Assistant Professor of Otolaryngology, Department of Otolaryngology–Head and Neck Surgery, Boston University Medical Center, Boston, Massachusetts

THUY-ANH N. MELVIN, MD
Johns Hopkins Department of Otolaryngology–Head and Neck Surgery, Baltimore, Maryland

JAMES W. MIMS, MD
Assistant Professor of Otolaryngology, Department of Otolaryngology, Wake Forest University School of Medicine, Winston-Salem, North Carolina

RICHARD R. ORLANDI, MD
Associate Professor, Division of Otolaryngology–Head and Neck Surgery, University of Utah, Salt Lake City, Utah

J. DAVID OSGUTHORPE, MD
Professor, Department of Otolaryngology–Head and Neck Surgery, Medical University of South Carolina, Charleston, South Carolina

MICHAEL J. PARKER, MD
Assistant Clinical Professor, Department of Otolaryngology and Communication Sciences, SUNY Upstate Medical University Syracuse, NY

ALPEN A. PATEL, MD
Department of Otolaryngology, Towson Medical Center, Lutherville, Maryland

HAROLD C. PILLSBURY III, MD
Thomas J. Dark Distinguished Professor of Otolaryngology–Head and Neck Surgery; Chair, Department of Otolaryngology–Head and Neck Surgery, University of North Carolina School of Medicine at Chapel Hill, Chapel Hill, North Carolina

WILLIAM R. REISACHER, MD, FACS, FAAOA
Assistant Professor of Otorhinolaryngology, Director, Department of Otorhinolaryngology, The Allergy Center, Weill Cornell Medical College, NewYork Presbyterian Hospital, New York, New York

MATTHEW W. RYAN, MD
Assistant Professor, Department of Otolaryngology, The University of Texas Southwestern Medical Center, Dallas, Texas

MINKA SCHOFIELD, MD
Assistant Professor, The Eye and Ear Institute, Department of Otolaryngology–Head and Neck Surgery, The Ohio State University Medical Center, Columbus, Ohio

RYAN J. SOOSE, MD
Director, Division of Sleep Surgery, Assistant Professor, Department of Otolaryngology, University of Pittsburgh School of Medicine, Pittsburgh, Pennsylvania

MATTHEW E. SPECTOR, MD
Resident Physician, Department of Otolaryngology, University of Michigan, Ann Arbor, Michigan

ROBERT J. STACHLER, MD, FACS, FAAOA
Senior Staff, Henry Ford Medical Group, Department of Otolaryngology, Head and Neck Surgery; Clinical Associate Professor, Wayne State University, Detroit, Michigan

MARIA C. VELING, MD
Associate Professor, Division of Otolaryngology, Department of Otolaryngology, University of Kentucky, Lexington, Kentucky

KEVIN F. WILSON, MD
Assistant Professor, Division of Otolaryngology–Head and Neck Surgery, University of Utah, Salt Lake City, Utah

KRISTIN WOODBURY, DO
Fellow in Sinonasal Disorders and Allergy, Department of Otolaryngology, University of Pittsburgh Medical Center, Pittsburgh, Pennsylvania

Contents

their ability to appropriately make correct decisions for prompt and efficient management of their patients with allergic or nonallergic diseases of the head and neck.

Immunology of Allergy 591

Minka Schofield and Karen H. Calhoun

Knowledge of the immune system is advancing rapidly. This review provides an update on the allergy players—the cells and major mediators—and the form and function of each; discusses how these cells and mediators weave together in the elegant but destructive dance of allergy; and details how specific immunotherapy can cure allergy.

Physical Findings in Allergy 603

Kristin Woodbury and Berrilyn J. Ferguson

Allergies are typically diagnosed based on detailed history elicited from a patient. Confirmation of the diagnosis by allergy skin or in vitro testing is sometimes also helpful. The authors discuss several physical examination features, specifically in the head and neck region, that are often suggestive of allergy presence.

Diagnosis of Inhalant Allergies: Patient History and Testing 611

Christine Franzese

In the United States, roughly 20% to 25% of the general adult population is afflicted by some form of chronic allergic respiratory disease, making allergy one of the most commonly diagnosed disorders. Among children, allergic disease is more common, with some sources estimating that it affects up to 40% of children. The focus of this article involves making the diagnosis of the most familiar and best understood of the hypersensitivity reactions, type 1 hypersensitivity, also termed immediate hypersensitivity. Although type 1 hypersensitivity can be caused by ingestion of food antigens or pharmaceuticals, this article focuses on IgE-mediated allergic disease caused primarily by inhalant allergens.

Role of Allergy in Sleep-Disordered Breathing 625

Ryan J. Soose

Sleep-related symptoms are extremely common in patients with allergic rhinitis. Sleep impairment is likely a major contributor to the overall disease morbidity, direct and indirect health care costs, and the loss of work productivity associated with allergic rhinitis. The association between allergic rhinitis and sleep, and the subsequent impact on disease-specific and general health quality of life measures, is well documented in large epidemiologic studies as well as controlled clinical trials. This article focuses on sleep disruption caused by allergic rhinitis, and the therapeutic and surgical options available to tackle the problem.

The Role of Allergy in Otitis Media with Effusion 637

David S. Hurst

The role of allergy in chronic otitis media with effusion (OME) is controversial. New evidence from cellular biology and immunology explain the

formation and bone erosion. Although its differentiation from other forms of chronic polypoid rhinosinusitis with eosinophilic mucin is sometimes problematic, type 1 hypersensitivity is a component of the disease process. Medical and surgical management can be augmented by immunotherapy directed toward the patient's specific allergen sensitivities. The primary rationale for immunotherapy is to control the allergic diathesis that may be contributing to the patient's chronic sinus inflammation.

Allergy Treatment: Environmental Control Strategies 711

William R. Reisacher

This article aims to help physicians and allergy care providers understand: the role of environmental control in the treatment of allergic disease; the concept of "the inflammatory load"; current published studies on environmental control; factors that influence levels of indoor and outdoor allergens; different methods to decrease patients' exposure to indoor and outdoor allergens; problems related to nonallergic symptom triggers; special considerations for school and workplace avoidance; role of environmental control in the prevention of allergic disease; various products available on the market to assist in avoidance; and how to plan with the patient to implement environmental control strategies.

Pharmacotherapy for Allergic Rhinitis 727

Thuy-Anh N. Melvin and Alpen A. Patel

Allergic rhinitis affects millions of Americans and the numbers continue to increase. Fortunately, there exists a wide array of pharmacotherapeutic options with relatively safe side effect profiles for the management of the varying subtypes. Additionally, there are newer agents on the horizon. The efficacies of intranasal corticosteroids, antihistamines, combination topical therapy, leukotriene inhibitors, mast cell stabilizers, anticholinergics, mucolytics, decongestants, and anti-IgE are reviewed.

Immunotherapy – Traditional 741

Yekaterina A. Koshkareva and John H. Krouse

Immunotherapy is an excellent treatment option for a selected subset of patients with inhalant allergies. It consists of intentional serial exposures to allergens, which modulate the immune system and induce immune tolerance through down-regulating the allergic response, resulting in an overall decrease in symptoms. Immunotherapy has been shown to have long-term efficacy in the management of inhalant allergies, as reflected by diminished frequency and duration of symptoms and improved quality of life. The therapy is considered safe, with side effects limited mostly to minor local reactions, and only occasional cases of systemic adverse reactions.

Sublingual Immunotherapy 753

Sandra Y. Lin and Bryan Leatherman

Sublingual immunotherapy (SLIT) has been shown to be safe and efficacious in treating allergic rhinitis. It has been used in Europe for more

than 20 years, and interest in the United States is increasing. SLIT has been shown to elicit immunologic changes similar to subcutaneous injection immunotherapy. SLIT may prevent new sensitizations, improve asthma control, and decrease asthma development in allergic individuals. Although differences in antigen quantification and standardization make European dosing schemes difficult to translate in the United States, several new studies suggest the range for effective dosing. Further studies will help clarify optimal dosing.

The Allergic March: Can We Prevent Allergies and Asthma? **765**

Bruce R. Gordon

The allergic march is a progression of atopic disease from eczema to asthma, and then to allergic rhinoconjunctivitis. It appears to be caused by a regional allergic response with breakdown of the local epithelial barrier that initiates systemic allergic inflammation. Genetic and environmental factors predispose to developing the allergic march. There are data to support 4 possible interventions to prevent the allergic march from progressing to asthma: (1) supplements of dietary probiotics, (2) exclusive breast feeding during the first few months of life, or, alternatively (3) use of extensively hydrolyzed infant formulas, (4) treatment with inhalant allergen immunotherapy by either subcutaneous or sublingual methods.

The Surgical Management of Allergic Rhinitis **779**

Nipun Chhabra and Steven M. Houser

In their discussion of the treatment of allergic rhinitis, the authors present key features of the disease and its management, allergen responses, the role of the inferior turbinate, and reviews of outcomes with submucosal resection, total inferior turbinectomy, cryosurgery, laser cautery, radical turbinectomy, submucous turbinectomy, submucous electrocautery, and microdebriber turbinoplasty. The authors discuss radiofrequency ablation and coblation outcomes and complications, along with the role of endoscopic sinus surgery in allergic rhinitis and emphasize the need for Otolaryngologists to be facile with a variety of procedures for best outcomes.

Inhalant Allergies in Children **797**

James W. Mims and Maria C. Veling

Children with chronic or recurrent upper respiratory inflammatory disease (rhinitis) should be considered for inhalant allergies. Risk factors for inhalant allergies in children include a first-degree relative with allergies, food allergy in infancy, and atopic dermatitis. Although inhalant allergies are rare in infancy, inhalant allergies are common in older children and impair quality of life and productivity. Differentiating between viral and allergic rhinitis can be challenging in children, but the child's age, history, and risk factors can provide helpful information. Allergic rhinitis is a risk factor for asthma, and if one is present, medical consideration of the other is warranted.

Food Allergy in Adults and Children 815

Elizabeth J. Mahoney, Maria C. Veling, and James W. Mims

Food allergy is defined as an adverse health effect arising from a specific immune response that occurs reproducibly on exposure to a given food and is distinct from food intolerance. Clinical manifestations of food allergy are varied and involve many systems including respiratory, cutaneous, and gastrointestinal. The double-blinded placebo-controlled oral food challenge remains the gold standard for the diagnosis of IgE-mediated food allergy. Areas of ongoing research include improved understanding of determinants for the development of tolerance versus sensitization for foods, the role of diagnostic testing for specific epitopes for food allergens, and the use of oral immunotherapy for IgE-mediated food allergy.

Index 835

FORTHCOMING ISSUES

Neuro-rhinology
Richard Harvey, MD, and
Carl Snyderman, MD,
Guest Editors

Vestibular Schwannoma
Fred Telischi, MD, and
Jacques Morcos, MD, *Guest Editors*

Cochlear Implants
J. Thomas Roland, MD, and
David Haynes, MD, *Guest Editors*

Telehealth in Otolaryngology
Michael Holtel, MD, and
Yehudah Roth, MD,
Guest Editors

Pediatric Otolaryngology Challenges in Multi-System Disease
Austin Rose, MD, *Guest Editor*

RECENT ISSUES

Dizziness and Vertigo across the Lifespan
Bradley W. Kesser, MD, and
A. Tucker Gleason, PhD, *Guest Editors*
April 2011

Oral Medicine
Vincent D. Eusterman, MD, DDS, and
Arlen Meyers, MD, MBA,
Guest Editors
February 2010

Head and Neck Ultrasound
Joseph Sniezek, MD, LTC, MC, USA,
and Robert Sofferman, MD,
Guest Editors
December 2010

RELATED INTEREST ARTICLE

In Immunology & Allergy Clinics, November 2010
Infectious Diseases in Asthma
Shyam Mohapatra, and Gary Hellermann, *Guest Editors*

Allergic Disorders Interface with Ear, Nose, and Throat Disorders

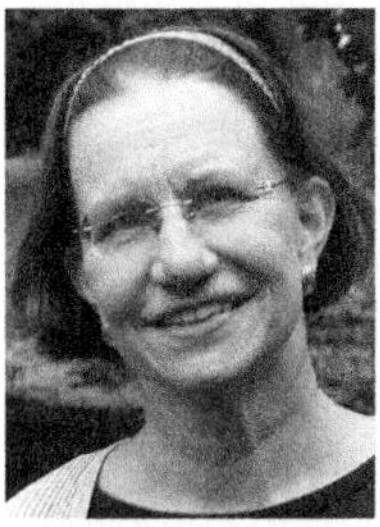
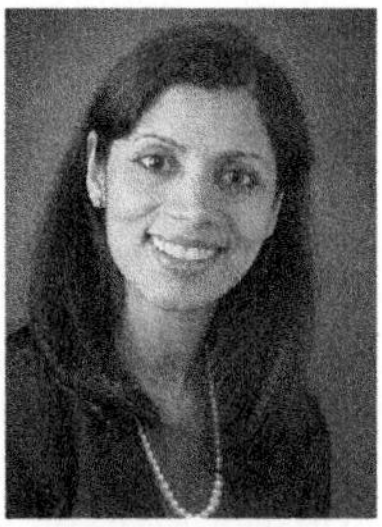

B.J. Ferguson, MD Suman Golla, MD
Guest Editors

Allergic rhinitis disproportionately affects the developed world and, although allergies are only rarely life threatening, they significantly impair quality of life.

For over half a century, the American Academy of Otolaryngic Allergy (AAOA), the oldest subspecialty organization under the umbrella of the specialty, Otolaryngology, has provided education and research opportunities to further our understanding of the interface of allergic disorders with ear nose and throat disorders.

In this 2011 *Otolaryngology Clinics of North America*, we have assembled distinguished and expert authors, all of whom are members of the AAOA. This *Clinics'* publication provides the most current opinion and evidence-based assessment of allergy as it relates to ear, nose, and throat disorders, as well as the lower airway—asthma, which is a frequent comorbidity of allergic rhinitis and patients with chronic rhinosinusitis, especially those with nasal polyps.

Currently, the most controversial aspect of allergy management in the United States is the role of sublingual immunotherapy (SLIT), which is not currently FDA approved, although quite commonly employed in Europe because of its excellent safety and efficacy profile. Brian Leatherman and Sandra Lin review the evidence for and against SLIT.

Even though allergy desensitization or more precisely, hyposensitization, is currently the only therapy that offers the potential for cure, and even though allergy desensitization is approaching its century anniversary, we still know little about the mechanisms of allergy desensitization. Karen Calhoun and Minka Schofield provide a quite readable article on our current understanding of allergic immunology and potential mechanisms of immunotherapy improvement.

The role of allergy in ear disorders is frequently overlooked and Jennifer Derebery and David Hurst provide articles that update our latest understanding of type I hypersensitivity in inner and middle ear disorders.

Finally, there are so many excellent contributions on diagnosis and management that to list them would be merely a relisting of the table of contents. We hope you enjoy

Otolaryngol Clin N Am 44 (2011) xv–xvi
doi:10.1016/j.otc.2011.04.002 oto.theclinics.com

and learn from this well-prepared, illustrated, and diagrammed volume as much as we have enjoyed working and learning from these experts.

B.J. Ferguson, MD
Division of Sino-Nasal Disorders and Allergy
Department of Otolaryngology
University of Pittsburgh School of Medicine
UPMC Mercy
Pittsburgh, PA, USA

Suman Golla, MD
University of Pittsburgh School of Medicine
UPMC Mercy
Pittsburgh, PA, USA

E-mail addresses:
fergusonbj@upmc.edu (B.J. Ferguson)
mishras@upmc.edu (S. Golla)

The Evolution of Understanding Inhalant Allergy

J. David Osguthorpe, MD*

KEYWORDS

• Inhalant allergy • Atopy • Immunotherapy • Skin testing
• Pharmacotherapy • Allergen • Immunoglobulin E

Key Points: Understanding Inhalant Allergy

- From the later half of the 1800s to the early 1900s, allergy, infectious disease, and immunology practitioners were one and the same, with the view that sensitivity to pollen toxin could be addressed in the same way vaccination or subcutaneous injection remedied susceptibility to bacterial diseases. It was not until 1955 that bacterial vaccines became uncommon in the treatment of intrinsic asthma or chronic rhinitis.
- In the first half of the twentieth century, the basis for much of what we currently practice, from skin testing to progressive dose escalation immunotherapy, was derived empirically from uncontrolled (single arm, unblinded) clinical studies with nonstandardized extracts. The efficacy of combining multiple allergens in a treatment regimen went largely unverified.
- In the 1920s, observations that house dust and climate allergens could cause rhinitis and exacerbate asthma failed to gain the attention of allergy practitioners. It was not until 1960s when dust mite was characterized that environmental modification joined the prior triad of treatment (counseling, pharmacotherapy, and immunotherapy).
- Oral immunotherapy was common in the United States until a multi-institutional trial in 1940, with the negative result now ascribed to the ineffective pill route of administration. Positive reports from European centers over the intervening period have caused a recent resurgence in interest.
- Beginning in the mid-1950s, clinical trials began to incorporate placebo controls and subject/doctor blinding, moving the practice of allergists from empiric- to evidence-based practices. Oral immunotherapy still trails injection therapy in corroborating data. Recently, organized allergy has promulgated practice parameters from patient testing to allergen standardization and administration and has agreed on standards for future studies.

Disclosure: The author has nothing to disclose.
Department of Otolaryngology-Head and Neck Surgery, Medical University of South Carolina, 135 Rutledge Avenue, Charleston, SC 29425, USA
* Surgical Service, 109 Bee Street, Ralph Johnson Veterans Administration Hospital, Charleston, SC 29401.
E-mail address: John.Osguthorpe@va.gov

Otolaryngol Clin N Am 44 (2011) 519–535
doi:10.1016/j.otc.2011.03.008
0030-6665/11/$ – see front matter. Published by Elsevier Inc.
oto.theclinics.com

EARLIEST HISTORY

The first inklings that one's native reaction to a toxic substance could be altered may have originated with Mithridates (131–63 BC), a king of Pontus in Asia Minor.[1,2] Because poison was a common way to dispatch rivals in those days, the king began ingesting small amounts of the potential poisons in gradually increasing doses until he developed resistance. Vague references to alterable capabilities of the immune system thereafter surfaced sporadically,[2] from Galen and others, but it was not until 1891 that Ehrlich[3] confirmed the ability to induce tolerance in mice fed ricin, a potent toxin, after a prolonged and gradual dose escalation. The distinction between resistance to toxin, or to infection, now known to be principally IgG and/or IgA mediated, and hypersensitivity diseases, principally IgE mediated or cell mediated, was indistinguishable to physicians until 1915 when verbiage related to a toxin (poison to infection) as the inciting factor for allergic rhinitis or asthma was abandoned in favor of the concept that such was a localized manifestation of anaphylaxis.[4] In 1923, an allergy interest group was formed, and subsequently the *Journal of Allergy*, within the members of the American Association of Immunologists, which itself did not have sufficient numbers to be self-sustaining until 1913.[2,5] Skepticism in the scientific community about both disciplines was characterized by an admonition to the society's first journal editor that "immunology is dead."[5]

EIGHTEENTH AND NINETEENTH CENTURY CONTRIBUTIONS

Many investigators in the eighteenth and early nineteenth centuries who empirically derived much of the basics of what is still practiced clinically, from skin testing to progressive allergen dose escalation, were themselves afflicted with allergic rhinitis, chronic rhinosinusitis, and/or asthma. Pharmacologic alternatives were sparse, and there was no agreement on the nature of inhalant sensitivities. An article by Bishop[6] in the first issue of *Laryngoscope* espoused a formula of morphine, atropine, and caffeine, laying the blame for seasonal rhinitis to an excess of uric acid in the blood. Adrenaline did not become commercially available until 1904, ephedrine until 1924, the first sedating antihistamine until 1936, and widespread release of steroid preparations until the mid-1950s.[1,7] Given this dearth of effective remedies, it is not surprising that many investigators devoted their professional careers sorting through the confusing, given few laboratory-based assays, morass of hypersensitivity disorders to identify effective treatments. The efforts of some prominent contributors in allergy and related immunology are detailed.

The concept of an epicutaneous or transcutaneous route for conferring resistance started in 1795 with Jenner,[8] who used a prick into a subject's skin to deliver material derived from a cowpox pustule, which over time afforded protection from the more virulent smallpox virus. Jenner named the process vaccination (Latin reference to cow). In 1879, Pasteur[9] demonstrated that a weak cholera strain given to chickens also provided protection from virulent strains and then replicated this procedure for anthrax in sheep. Pasteur chose a term just appearing in English literature, immunizes, for this phenomenon and, in 1884, successfully applied a series of graduated subcutaneous inoculations for rabies prevention. However, there were issues including significant reactions in some cases, now known to be from antineural autoantibodies. In the same time frame, Koch[10] reported delayed hypersensitivity responses in some samples in which he had given tuberculosis culture inoculations with the hope of conferring immunity. These untoward effects encouraged alternate approaches, and by 1891, von Behring and Kitasato[11] had successfully conferred passive immune protection to diphtheria in human patients injected with serum containing antitoxin from previously infected animals (usually horse).

However, reports of adverse reactions surfaced yet again, with the first fatality in 1896, soon joined by others, suppressing enthusiasm for passive immunization to other infectious diseases prevalent in that era. In an effort to identify what might be causing these issues and also to introduce some standardization to antisera preparations, Ehrlich[12] identified in the laboratory what is now known to be an antigen-antibody reaction as the culprit behind anaphylactic reactions to nonhuman sera.

The first description of the classic symptoms of hay fever and asthma were penned by Bostock[13] in 1819, describing his personal illness. It was not until 1872 that Wyman[14] tentatively identified pollen as a cause of autumn catarrh in the United States. The next year in England, Blackley[15] followed with the same observation and a critical concept, not fully accepted for hay fever until 1915 and asthma until the 1940s, that inhalant sensitivities were not the result of an infectious disease. Blackley was the first to try immunotherapy, a self-experimentation whereby he rubbed grass pollen into his abraded skin, following up in 1880 with observations on the cutaneous wheal, erythema, and pruritus response to what was essentially a scratch test and using such to detect and grossly quantitate patient sensitivity.[16]

EARLY TWENTIETH CENTURY CONTRIBUTIONS

The concepts of passive versus active immunity, anaphylaxis, and hypersensitivity were sorted out during the first 15 years of the twentieth century. von Pirquet[17]was able to distinguish a basic difference between systemic horse serum reactions and a local response to smallpox vaccination, stating that, "immunity and hypersensitivity can plus be closely related" and introducing the term allergy from *allos* (other or altered state) and *ergon* (work) for the former phenomenon.[18] von Pirquet proposed the term allergen for a substance that stimulates an organism to change its intrinsic response after prior exposure to that substance. Attempting to answer the question of why an immunized organism could be protected from or supersensitive to the same disease or substance, Pirquet tracked the progressively shortening interval to reactions to successive horse serum antitoxin injections in affected individuals, postulating a collision of antigen and antibody as per Ehrlich's concept. The investigator added the distinction that because of previous exposure, the body was changed by antibodies and hence the heightened response. How to minimize these adverse reactions consumed the efforts of many. In 1907, Besredka and Steinhardt[19] demonstrated in an animal model that injections of progressively larger but tolerable doses of antigen, like that of Ehrlich's mice fed ricin, eventually conferred protection from an adverse response. This observation reinvigorated clinical interest in injection therapy for hay fever and asthma, although there were still continuing issues (which continue today), with acute asthma attacks being incited in some.

Curtis[20] in the United States was an early proponent for injection therapy, albeit with very dilute pollen extracts. Although the details were sparse, Curtis reported some success with injection therapy as well as oral administration in the same dosages. In Germany, Dunbar[21] was still pursuing the antitoxin route then being practiced for diphtheria and tetanus, applying a horse and rabbit serum antipollen preparation variously into the conjunctiva, nose, or mouth or via aerosolized oral inhalation, inciting occasional life-threatening reactions, which convinced most investigators that passive immunization for hypersensitivity diseases was a dead end. However, the investigator did develop a method of testing, whereby pollen extracts were applied to a subject's conjunctiva to identify specific sensitivities. This diagnostic approach became widespread and was adopted by Noon[22] who was practicing at St Mary's Hospital in London, a major center for chest diseases.

Noon added a measure of quantification to the conjunctivally applied extracts, which he thought contained a plant toxin, setting that amount extracted from a thousandth part of a milligram (ie, a microgram) of a pollen sample as 1 "Noon unit." Noon subdivided patients into those who were very sensitive, reacting to 4 or fewer Noon units; those with intermediate sensitivity, reacting to a 70-unit threshold; and those who were nonallergic, reacting to no less than 20,000 units.[22,23] The investigator chose subcutaneous injections, still called inoculations, of the same extract as for testing preseasonally and/or coseasonally at 5- to 10-day intervals for 2 months (**Fig. 1**). Although Noon's approach varied considerably among patients, he seemed to use higher doses of the extract in lesser-sensitive patients. Noon eventually settled on an optimum interval between injections of 1 to 2 weeks and noted that local or systemic reactions increase if the injections were too frequent or excessive in extract dose. He documented diminished conjunctival reaction to allergen challenge after preseasonal therapy. Noon's personal issue with tuberculosis necessitated his withdrawal from practice (died 2 years later), and he transferred ongoing investigations to his partner and a hay fever sufferer, Freeman.[24] Freeman established that some symptom relief persisted for at least a year after discontinuing the injections and noted that some individuals were also less troubled by asthma.[23,24] The investigator introduced the concept of a placebo effect with immunotherapy, observing a "constant tendency to detect such improvements in adventitious fluctuations in health" and noting the potential for physician or patient bias or external circumstances such as a heavy or light pollen season. Freeman[25] marketed Noon's toxin solution via the Parke Davis pharmaceutical firm. By 1920, Freeman reported experience with more than 200 pollen-sensitive patients (no controls), had discarded the 2-per-day limitation of conjunctival testing in favor of batteries of scratch tests, and was experimenting with injections for food and animal sensitivities (**Fig. 2**). The investigator also suggested the option of rush immunotherapy over a day or two, an approach now used for vespid or in-hospital drug hyposensitization.[26]

EARLY ORGANIZATION OF ALLERGY TESTING AND TREATMENT

From 1914 to the 1950s, most published clinical allergy experience shifted from Europe to the United States, with Koessler[27] in Illinois and Goodale[28] in Massachusetts, the former investigator reporting positive results with 45 patients. Goodale had established

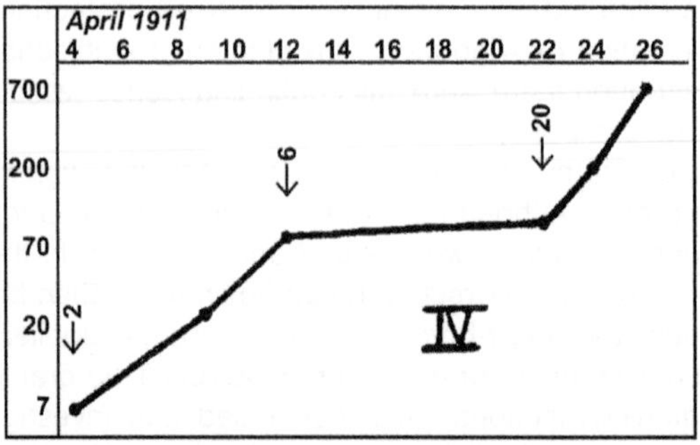

Fig. 1. The x-axis denotes the number of conjunctivally applied drops of timothy pollen extract in Noon units that were required to incite a response and the y-axis, when subcutaneous injections of such extracts were given during immunotherapy. The numbers adjacent to the arrows indicate the strength in Noon units of each injection. (*From* Noon L. Prophylactic inoculation against hay fever. Lancet 1911;177:153, figure 1; with permission.)

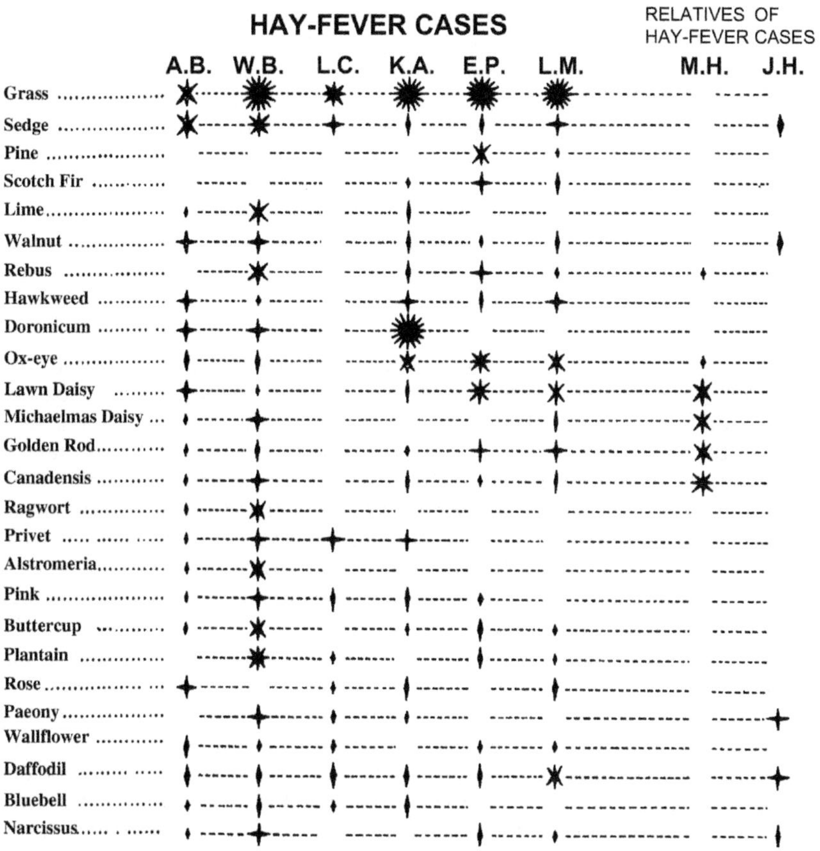

Fig. 2. Six-level classification of scratch test reactions to pollen extracts in 6 patients and 2 relatives of such. To some degree (details not fully clear), the starting dose for subcutaneous immunotherapy was determined by patient sensitivities (ie, lower starting dose if higher sensitivity). (*From* Freeman J. Toxic idiopathies: the relationship between hay and other pollen fevers, animal asthmas, food idiosyncrasies, bronchial and spasmodic asthmas. Proc R Soc Med 1920;13:137, diagram 7; with permission.)

the first university-based allergy clinic in the United States in the Department of Laryngology of the Massachusetts General Hospital, where he enjoyed a career-long collaboration with medicine colleagues Rackemann and Colmes[29] whose interest was asthma. A year later, Cooke established an allergy practice in the Department of Medicine at Cornell, where he also benefited from the presence of a learned colleague, Coca, who was running a fledgling immunology lab and later became the first editor of the *Journal of Immunology*.[5,29] Cooke, who in the 1920s was a founder of both the first US allergy society and the *Journal of Allergy*, was striving to understand a personal affliction.[30] He had had severe asthma during childhood, which vanished during sojourn in boarding school, and it became apparent that his major sensitivity was toward horses. During an obligatory 6-month internship rotation on a horse-drawn ambulance in New York City, Cooke observed that this would not have been possible save for his adrenaline kit, stating "I put as much adrenaline under my skin as any human being."[30] After assisting a tracheotomy in a patient with diphtheria, and hence obliged to a prophylactic injection of horse serum antitoxin, the investigator lapsed into unconsciousness for 10 hours, requiring intubation. In his 1915 publication,[4] choosing Goodale's preferred journal, *Laryngoscope*, Cooke eschewed pollen toxin as the source of hay fever in favor of the pollen inciting a sensitization that could manifest as either localized (rhinitis, asthma) or systemic anaphylaxis. The investigator postulated that immunity to infection likely resulted from induction of a widely circulating antibody, which for anaphylaxis was from a mostly tissue-fixed antibody. Observing that most sufferers had multiple sensitivities, Cooke preferred wide batteries of intracutaneous skin tests in a clinic session along with the scratch tests Freeman favored and prick tests that had been introduced in 1908 by Mantoux as he searched for the best method to apply a tuberculosis skin test. All 3 cutaneous testing methods remained in common use until 1987, when issues with reproducibility of scratch tests led the American Medical Association to recommend against routine use.[31–33] Cooke tested for a wide variety of pollens as well as foods, including lobster, although only treated for inhalants.[30] Extracts of varying strengths were used to classify patients into 4 levels of sensitivity, and to some degree, the initial injection dose was determined by such, ranging from 5 to 100 Noon units. Most treatment was preseasonal, although coseasonal was an option. The usual regimen was to start with a low dose and escalate weekly, beginning as Noon about 2 months before the relevant season. After a report on the aforementioned in 140 patients, Cooke teamed with VanderVeer (1916) to detail the medical histories, with emphasis on a possible inherited predilection to allergic diseases, of 621 patients.[34] The investigators noted a familial tendency for asthma, allergic rhinitis, angioneurotic edema, and immediate food sensitivities but had insufficient evidence to include eczema. However, by the 1920s, Coca was using atopy to describe the trio of hay fever, asthma, and eczema. The incidence of inhalant allergy in the New York area was estimated by Cooke at 10%, of whom 42% had multiple sensitivities.[34] Cooke noted that, "sensitized individuals transmit to their offspring not their own specific sensitization but an unusual capacity for developing bioplastic reactivities to any foreign protein." Although the conclusion was that hypersensitivity was transmitted as a dominant characteristic, it did not fit the simple mendelian pattern; so the question remained open.

Immunotherapy for asthma or rhinitis was confined to pollen sensitivities until 1921 when Kern[34] identified house dust as the causative agent in many cases. However, the major allergen, mite, was not isolated until 1959,[35] and extract preparations until then were as varied among practitioners and commercial sources as any in immunotherapy; not unexpectedly, reports on effectiveness varied. Cooke and others began adding dust and many other nonstandardized allergens into testing and treatment mixes, but there were few published reports, none major, establishing efficacy. It was not until 1954 that the first placebo-controlled trial of immunotherapy for basic pollen sensitivity was published.[36]

van Leeuwen and colleagues in 1924 observed the presence of climate allergens that could exacerbate asthma and rhinitis.[37] The first allergen-free hospital rooms were fitted, and the substantial relief produced in asthma patients brought to the attention of the medical community the potential effect of environmental modification beyond the simple advice to avoid outdoor activities during problematic pollen seasons. Without specifically identifying molds as the issue, the investigators established that damp sleeping quarters were bad for asthma patients, whereas dry mountain areas were favorable.[37–39] Curiously, recommendations for environmental measures for patient homes or places of employment did not gain traction in the allergy community until the 1980s when within a decade there was an explosion of publications distributed across the world's literature and the introduction of the hygiene hypothesis.[40,41]

EARLY USE OF BACTERIAL VACCINES FOR ALLERGY

Another common practice during the early years of immunotherapy was the use of bacterial vaccines for asthma and/or chronic rhinitis. This practice was first mentioned by Allen[42] who in 1908 applied an autologous nasopharyngeal vaccine for chronic rhinitis (infectious or allergic, it seems). Lowdermilk[43] advocated combining pollen and bacterial extracts in the same injection for the patient with both seasonal rhinitis and sinusitis issues. Bacterial vaccines were adopted for patients with sinusitis by Goodale and for selected asthma patients by his colleague, Rackemann,[29] who thought intrinsic asthma was possibly of bacterial origin, unlike the better-characterized extrinsic variety that was correctly ascribed to inhalant hypersensitivity.[1] Cooke[44] later became a proponent, correctly making the distinction that injections for allergies and those for bacterial issues caused different bodily responses, one being hyposensitization and the other immunity. This insight was confirmed by his colleague, Coca, who established in 1925 that a heat-labile reagin (now known to be IgE) was responsible for positive skin test results and hypersensitivity reactions and that a heat-stable antibody called blocking antibody (now known to be IgG) was induced by immunotherapy.[30,44–47] Enthusiasm for bacterial vaccines did not wane until the advent of antibiotic therapies in the 1940s allowed trials of such in asthma patients to no effect. As a final blow, in 1955, the first controlled study of bacterial vaccines was reported by Franklin, followed within a few years by other negative studies, removing mixed respiratory or autologous bacterial vaccines from the practices of most allergy practitioners (**Fig. 3**).[48]

POLLENS AND EARLY STANDARDIZATION ATTEMPTS

The distribution of various pollen types, and their seasonal variations in the United States (eg, earlier and shorter spring, summer, and fall seasons in northern

Results of Treatment

Score		H		F	
		Vaccine	Control	Vaccine	Control
−11	Worse ..	0	2	5	1
−7−10		1 } 6	1 } 5	3 } 12	1 } 10
−3−6		5	2	4	8
−2 +2	No change ..	13	13	11	12
+3+6	Improved ..	10	8	9	1
+7+10		16 } 31	9 } 21	15 } 27	14 } 23
+11		5	4	3	8
		50	39	50	45

Fig. 3. Experience of 2 investigators (H and F) with bacterial vaccine or saline placebo administered every 1 to 2 weeks for 1 year in 184 patients, divided into vaccine and placebo injection groups, with intrinsic asthma; vaccines were prepared per nasal swab results for each patient and variously included *Haemophilus influenzae*, *Streptococcus viridans*, *Moraxella catarrhalis*, and *Bacillus subtilis*. There were no symptom differences between the active and placebo arms at 1 year. (*From* Frankland A, Hughes W, Garrill R. Autogenous bacterial vaccines in the treatment of bronchial asthma. Br Med J 1955;2:943, table VII; with permission.)

locales), was ascertained by a nationwide survey of allergists by Durham in 1929.[49] Two years later, Thommen[50] cited 15 studies by different investigators, all but 1 of which detailed a positive experience with pollen extract therapy and also a few that included house dust. The investigator postulated guidelines for assessing the burgeoning number of potential allergens being added to immunotherapy regimens, with little to establish efficacy, by various allergy practitioners with internal medicine, pediatric, or otolaryngologic backgrounds, stating these allergens must be airborne and in sufficient quantities to incite a hypersensitivity response. It remains challenging (in fact impossible) to compare reports from the plethora of investigators in this era because most studies were small series with little standardization of skin testing or extract preparation beyond the basics described in 1911 by Noon. This lack of standardization was recognized by Coca[45] who developed an assay for the total nitrogen content in an extract, acknowledging that this and allergenic activity were not always identical. Then in 1933, Cooke and colleagues,[51] took another step toward allergen quantization with an assay of protein nitrogen units (PNUs), an alternative to the traditional weight per volume (W/V). Just as importantly, the investigators observed that the extract mixtures did not possess permanent potency but deteriorated depending on the passage of time, diluents selected, and other allergens in the mix. These laboratory-based advances encouraged the 2 precursor organizations of the American Academy of Allergy to meet in 1935 with the goal of standardizing practices.[52] The organizations were unable to reach a consensus but did concur that skin test results do not always correlate with patient manifestations and hence the clinical judgment of a trained practitioner was critical. There was no agreement on extract preparation/storage and also on an optimal testing method, with scratch, prick, and intradermal approaches common, and some preferred oral administration to injection administration of allergen. Black[53] had reported lower nasal responses to ragweed extract after oral immunotherapy, although 12 years later followed up with a wider yet less-favorable experience when comparing oral therapy with injection therapy.[54,55] Stier and Hollister (1937) reported a 3-year experience, achieving an improvement of 78% with oral drops of pollen allergen extracts in concentrations up to 1:100 W/V.[56] Bernstein and Feinberg[56] compared the amount of allergen that is required to produce equivalent relief if given orally versus subcutaneously and established that the oral route required the larger amount. Confusion was such that in 1940, Feinberg and colleagues[57] assembled a multiuniversity trial on 103 subjects who took oral immunotherapy or placebo and another 57 who took injections or placebo and found that although only 25% experienced relief with oral therapy, 56% did with shots (**Fig. 4**).[58] This diminished enthusiasm for oral therapy in the United States, although some investigators, such as Hansel, were still experimenting with sublingual drop administration in the 1970s.[57] This approach has since been demonstrated to be valid by the European allergy community, and hence, interest in this alternative among US practitioners has returned in the past decade.[59] It is notable that Feinberg and colleagues[57] chose to administer the oral extract in pill form, which is likely the reason that 12.5% of patients experienced major gastrointestinal symptoms, whereas current thinking specifies an interval of oral retention to allow uptake by Langerhans cells in the oral submucosa. The gastrointestinal reactions also limited enthusiasm for oral immunotherapy for contact dermatitis. Shelmire[60] had advocated a similar method for poison ivy after patch test verification of sensitivity, following a common remedy in the homeopathic, native American, and folk medicine communities in earlier decades.[1]

Summary of Study of Oral Pollen Therapy.
Rush Medical College, University of Chicago

Type of Cases	Oral Group*	Parenteral Group †
A. Total number of cases................	32	25
B. In 1938, hay fever only.............	18	10
C. In 1938, hay fever and asthma....	14 (44% of A)	15 (60% of A)
Treatment in 1939 Season		
D. Average number of doses...........	40	14.4
Variation............................	(23–62)	(7–21)
E. Average maximum daily dose......	116,000	2,452
Variation............................	(60,000–120,000)	(700–4,500)
F. Average total course dose...........	3,237,000	16,817
Variation............................	(675,000–5,113,000)	(1,930–41,320)
Results of Treatment		
G. In 1939, hay fever only.............	10	10
H. In 1939, hay fever and asthma....	22 (69% of A)	15 (60% of A)
I. In 1939, asthma for first time....	9 (50% of B)	2 (20% of B)
Comparison with 1938 Senson		
J. Symptoms same	3 (10%)	7 (28%)
K. Symptoms better	8 (25%)	14 (56%)
L. Symptoms worse	21 (65%)	4 (16%)

* Received oral pollen and saline injections.
† Received pollen extract injections and placebo capsules.

Fig. 4. Oral pollen immunotherapy, in pill form, was compared with subcutaneous immunotherapy for grass pollen delivered coseasonally. Allergen doses (nonstandardized extracts) were much higher in the oral than in the subcutaneous preparations, and gastrointestinal side effects in the former group were severe in 12.5% and minor in another 12.5%. No anaphylactic reactions were encountered. (*From* Feinberg S, Foran F, Lichtenstein M. Oral pollen therapy for ragweed pollinosis. J Am Med Assoc 1940;115:27, table 2; with permission.)

Hansel, called the "father of otolaryngic allergy" after the publication of his textbook on allergy and rhinology in 1936, had also served as a president of the American College of Allergy.[61,62] The investigator advocated intradermal testing for quantification of sensitivity, selecting a 1:10 serial dilution technique, which became a common tool in basic clinical investigations, including that by Voorhorst and colleagues[63] in 1964 when establishing dust mite as a major allergen and the current regimen for vespid sensitivity testing.[32,62,64,65] Rinkel,[65] a brief understudy of Hansel's, in 1949 introduced a 1:5 variation that became the standard within the otolaryngologic community.[66,67] By whatever scheme, the serial dilution approach not only identified the degree of patient sensitivity to a particular allergen but also served as a rough guideline to the extract concentration at which immunotherapy could be safely initiated.[32,66,68] Serial dilution was also adopted by the US Food and Drug Administration (FDA), a 1:3 approach described by Turkeltaub and colleagues[68] in 1986 to quantify in subjects of known sensitivity the potencies of extracts submitted for commercial distribution.

BEGINNING OF PLACEBO-CONTROLLED TRIALS IN IMMUNOTHERAPY

The 1950s ushered in the first large evidence-based studies of skin testing and immunotherapy protocols and the following decade, the first useful laboratory assays beyond the crude measures for reagin and blocking antibody and passive transferability with the Prausnitz-Kustner technique. The aforementioned said, it was remarkable what the allergy practitioners and immunologists previously detailed had accomplished with limited investigations with nonstandardized extracts in modest patient populations. The downside was that there remained a wide variety of practices, some now known to be suboptimal to ineffective, that warranted scrutiny via an evidence-based approach. Feinberg and colleagues[57] in their placebo-controlled study of oral immunotherapy in 1940, selected an ineffective route for administration. It was not until 1954 that Franklin and Augustin,[36] in the same London hospital in which Noon had practiced, reported a placebo-controlled trial of injection immunotherapy on 200 subjects. The investigators compared crude pollen extract (little changed from Noon's) with a purified pollen protein (PNU, as Cooke advocated) and phenolized saline. There was a response greater than 75% to the pollen extracts, and 33% for the saline group, establishing what was first described by Freeman[25] as the placebo response (25%–35%) intrinsic to allergen therapies. As mentioned previously, Frankland and colleagues[48] had reported a controlled, and negative, study of bacterial vaccines that same year. In 1965, Lowell and Franklin[69] published a double-blind placebo-controlled (DBPC) study using ragweed symptom and patient medication scores as outcomes measures, setting a new baseline for the minimum measures for randomization and outcomes measures expected for allergy-related studies. The investigators suggested that serial measurement of neutralizing or blocking antibody might in the future be suitable to quantitate response to immunotherapy independent of cumbersome clinical trials, a goal still not met. In 1968, Norman and colleagues[70] adopted the DBPC approach to a 4-year comparison of whole ragweed extract with the newly identified major allergen in ragweed, antigen E, the latter better tolerated both systemically and locally. To ensure that the placebo group is not detected by subjects or practitioners, the investigators added histamine to the placebo injections. Antigen E in micrograms was 200 times more active than the W/V extract and 20 times more active than the PNU preparations. The investigators verified Cooke's[51] observation (1933) that the potency of extract solutions varied with the diluent and time and recommended a 50% glycerol solution for the storage of concentrates. Immunotherapy was proposed, rather than the commonly used desensitization, as the most accurate reflection of the changes that take place, observing that although reagin levels did not change much over the course of therapy, blocking antibody levels increased more than 100 times.[71]

Studies from the 1980s to the present reflect the improving pharmacologic alternatives to immunotherapy, with cromolyn commercially available in the late 1970s, second-generation (nonsedating) antihistamines in the early 1980s, and topical steroids without major mucosal or hypothalamic/pituitary suppression in the later 1980s.[7] Hence, immunotherapy for just single-season pollen sensitivities came into question, and allergy organizations adopted verbiage that reflected environmental modification, if feasible, and initiation of pharmacotherapy before resorting to injection therapy. By the time of the study by Durham and colleagues[71] in 1999 on immunotherapy for timothy sensitivity, control subjects were allowed effective pharmacotherapy (with minimal side effects) as a real-world assessment of any added benefits from immunotherapy. This study, a landmark as those mentioned in the prior paragraph, established that after 3 years of immunotherapy, there was

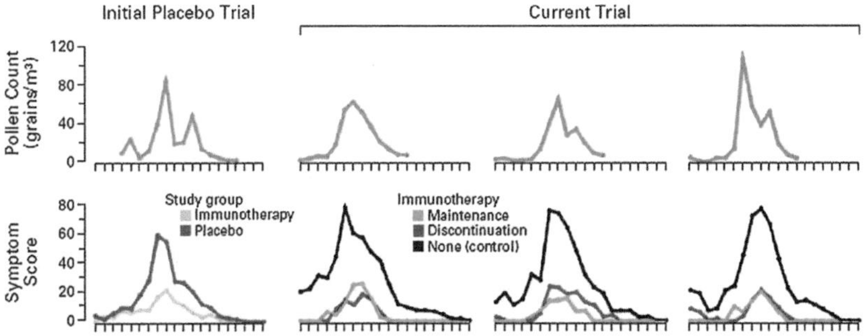

Fig. 5. Graphs depicting grass pollen counts over the course of a year (peak counts in summer) in which the placebo group was given subcutaneous saline/histamine and the active group immunotherapy ("initial placebo trial"). Then, after 3 years of immunotherapy, the study extended 3 further years ("current trial") during which those initially given immunotherapy were split into 2 groups, 1 receiving placebo shots and 1 completing 3 more years of immunotherapy (for a total of 6 years). There were no detectable differences between those receiving 3 versus 6 years of immunotherapy, and both groups experienced significantly fewer in-season symptoms than those on medication alone (all groups were permitted rescue medication in season). (*From* Durham S, Walker S, Varga E, et al. Long term clinical efficacy of grass pollen immunotherapy. N Engl J Med 1999;341:471, figure 1; with permission.)

no difference in the symptoms or medication requirements of those whose shots continued for 3 further years versus those who received 3 years of histamine-spiked placebo injections and that both groups did better than control subjects (**Fig. 5**). This study established that 3 years of immunotherapy with adequate levels of major allergen provided long-term benefits (5 years at least, per continuing follow-up of participants) and patients with moderate to severe symptoms from a particular allergen, even if seasonal, could achieve benefit beyond that afforded by pharmacotherapy alone.

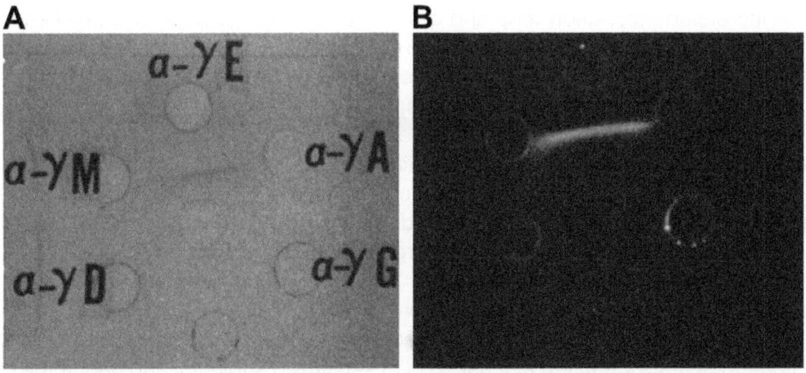

Fig. 6. Radioimmunodiffusion analysis of reagin-rich serum from a ragweed-sensitive patient. The serum is in the center well, and around such are arrayed solutions of antibodies specific to each immunoglobulin, including the newly isolated IgE, which had paralleled the concentration of reagin in the patient's serum. Ergo, IgE = reagin, first identified as a marker of inhalant allergies by Coca[46] in 1925. (*From* Ishizaka K, Ishizaka T. Identification of gamma E antibodies as the carrier of reaginic activity. J Immunol 1967;99:1194, figure 5; with permission.)

ANTIGEN STANDARDIZATION

Durham colleagues' study benefited from progress in allergen standardization, a widely held goal since promulgation of PNU by Cooke and colleagues.[51] Progress had begun in 1959 with the isolation of the key allergenic fraction of house dust by Vannier and Campbell[35] and 3 years later with the identification of antigen E as the major ragweed allergen by King and Norman.[72] In 1967, Voorhorst and colleagues[63] established mite as Vannier's allergen, important in both perennial allergic rhinitis and asthma.[62] Ishizaka and Ishizaka[73] that same year documented reagin to be IgE (**Fig. 6**) and set others on a track, which by 1975 led to the first commercial availability of an allergen-specific IgE immunoassay, although such was not endorsed by the American Medical Association as an alternative to skin testing and a guide to the initial starting dose until 1986.[74] There followed a quest to identify the major allergens of common inhalant sensitizers, thereby allowing extract standardization sufficient for consideration by the US FDA (www.fda.gov). After acceptance of amb 1 as the major allergen in short ragweed in 1975, the major allergen for vespid was endorsed in 1981, cat in 1983, house dust mite in 1990, and many grasses in 1998.[75] At present, 19 allergens are certified for commercial use; however, there are none for molds, cockroach, or many tree or weed pollens or for oral administration (by mid-2009, 4 allergens for oral administration were authorized in Germany but only 1 throughout the European Union).[59] On parallel course, there were dose-ranging studies that have established for standardized allergens the cumulative injected dose that afforded relief in most patients, replacing prior empiric-based strategies with the vaguely characterized end points of a maximum tolerated dose, optimum dose, or symptom-relieving dose.[76–78]

IN VITRO ALLERGY SCORING AND ALLERGY SCREENS

Practitioners initially struggled to correlate the degree of patient sensitivity as evidenced by skin testing to that of the radioactive counts reported in the early radioallergosorbent assays (now largely replaced by enzyme linked immunosorbent assays, which eschew the handling and storage issues of radioactive tracers). Several scoring systems were proposed. In 1977 Fadel and Nalebuff, modifying the technique with an increased incubation time and other changes, constructed a 6-level scoring system that roughly correlated with a 1:5 intradermal skin titration technique.[79–81] The progressively increasing number of commercially available allergens both for skin (more than 200, most nonstandardized)[59,76] and in vitro testing led to the concept of allergy screens to identify those in a patient suspected of significant inhalant sensitivities, and on which it would be cost-justifiable to proceed with a full battery of tests, usually 20 to 30 allergens deemed likely culprits based on patient history. In 1982 King,[81] and later Nalebuff,[82] documented that a geographically adjusted in vitro screen of 8 to 10 carefully selected allergens was sufficiently efficient to identify more than 90% of those who would have 1 or more major sensitivities detected by a full battery of tests. This cost-effective approach was confirmed by a 2009 Pan-European study (more than 3000 subjects) that confirmed that an 8 to 10 allergen battery of prick tests identified at least 95% of sensitized subjects, and hence the cost to the nationalized health insurance systems of a full test battery could be justified.[83]

RECENT REVIEWS AND GUIDELINES

The aforementioned advances in extract standardization, specification of effective doses, and the like were supported by increasingly sophisticated laboratory assays. Although Cooke, courtesy of Coca, had a crude assay for reagin in 1925,[44] by 1999,

Durham had sufficient technology to establish per skin biopsy T-cell and interleukin 4 infiltrations at allergen injection sites.[72] Recent investigators have access to a wide gamut of specific T-cell identifiers with their associated cytokines and even some of the genetic switches relevant to allergy and asthma. The reader is referred to recent summaries of this fascinating area, which have allowed clinicians to tie patient responses to serum parameters, adding a further layer of objectivity to many recent trials.[77,84–86] With the earlier-mentioned allergen and laboratory advances, organized allergy again sought to standardize evaluation and treatment methods. Meta-analyses, including a Cochrane Review in 2007, had confirmed that appropriately administered injection immunotherapy (1) improved patient quality of life, (2) diminished medication use and the development of new sensitivities or asthma, and (3) ameliorated nasal, conjunctival, and, to a lesser degree, bronchospastic issues.[78,87–89] A similar review in a 2009 World Allergy Organization position paper on oral immunotherapy reflected much the same, although not as clearly because of a wide heterogeneity of studies, a paucity of standardized allergen preparations for sublingual use, and continuing uncertainties about allergen dosing, administration schedule, and treatment duration.[59,90,91] Recent guidelines by organizations in the United States (2008, injection therapy)[88,89] and Europe (2009, injection and sublingual therapies)[59,90,91] for future clinical trials specify allergens of known potency for which handling and administration must be detailed. Both subjects and practitioners must be blinded as to randomly assigned treatment versus placebo arms, and the investigation must encompass sufficient subjects to power statistically valid conclusions.[92,93] A related initiative is the CREATE project, funded by an agency of the European Union, to construct via recombinant technology the major allergens of common inhalant offenders, the ultimate in allergen standardization and well beyond the current FDA-approved standardized extracts, which although achieving extract purity much better than W/V or PNU, allow for up to a 4 times variation among commercial preparations.[94] Not ready for commercial release, progress has been made with replication of the major allergens of birch and of timothy pollens.

SUMMARY

This article summarizes the developments that led to the current approach to immunotherapy. These developments were characterized in the early years by empirically derived successive approximations to arrive at effective injection regimens, in the middle years by a sorting through of the wide variations in practice with placebo-controlled clinical trials, and more recently by a closer association of clinical and laboratory measures to better define evidence-based practices. The pace of investigation along with the scientific quality continues to increase. As per a PubMed (www.pubmed.gov) search, there were more than 1000 articles on inhalant allergy in 2009. Two entities deserve recognition for the encouragement of, frequently with funding, current pursuits in clinical and bench research that will determine the next article on the understanding of the treatment of inhalant sensitivities. These are the National Institute of Allergy and Infectious Diseases (www.niaid.gov) within the National Institutes of Health of the United States and the Global Allergy and Asthma Network (www.ga2len.net) supported by the European Union's Framework Program for Research.

REFERENCES

1. Cohen S, Evans R. Allergen immunotherapy in historical perspective. Clin Allergy Immunol 2008;21:1–19.

2. Silverstein A, Bialasiewicz A. History of immunology. Cell Immunol 1980;51:151–67.
3. Ehrlich P. Experimentelle intersuchungen uber immunitat. Dsch Med Wochenschr uber ricin 1891;17:976 [in German].
4. Cooke R. The treatment of hay fever by active immunization. Laryngoscope 1915;25:108–12.
5. Saunders J, Cruse J, Cohen S, et al. The AAI, 1913–1988, in the first century of immunology. J Immunol 1988;141:S37–54.
6. Bishop S. Hay fever and its successful treatment. Laryngoscope 1896;1:21–8.
7. Simons F, Akdis C. Histamine and H1-antihistamines. In: Adkinson N, Bochner B, Busse W, et al, editors. Middleton's allergy. 7th edition. Philadelphia: Mosby Elsevier; 2009. p. 1518–47.
8. Jenner E. An inquiry into the causes and effects of the variolae. London: Sampson Low, Soho; 1798.
9. Pasteur L. Method pour prevenir la rage après morsure. C R Acad Sci (Paris) 1885;101:765 [in French].
10. Koch R. Forsetzung der Muttheilungen uber ein hermittel gegen tuberculose. Dtsch Med Wochenschr 1891;9:101–3 [in German].
11. Behring von E, Kitasato S. Ueber das zustandekommen der diphtheria-immunitat und der tetanus-immunitat bei thieren. Dtsch Med Wochenschr 1890;16:1113 [in German].
12. Ehrlich P. Die wertbestimmunung des diphtherieheislserums. Klin Jb 1897;6:299 [in German].
13. Bostock J. Case of periodical affection of the eyes and chest. Med Chir Trans 1819;10:161.
14. Wyman M. Autumnal catarrh. Cambridge (MA): Hurd and Houghton; 1872.
15. Blackley C. Experimental researches on the causes and nature of catarrhus aestivus. London: Balliere, Tindall, Cox; 1873.
16. Blackley C. Hay fever. London: Balliere, Tindall, Cox; 1880.
17. von Pirquet C. Allergie. Munchen Med Wchnschr 1906;53:1457 [in German].
18. Dworetzky M, Cohen S. Pioneers and milestones. J Allergy Clin Immunol 2002;109:722–6.
19. Besredka A, Steinhardt E. De l'anaphylaxie et de l'antianaphylaxie vis-à-vis due serum de cheval. Ann Inst Pasteur 1907;21:117 [in French].
20. Curtis H. The immunizing cure of hay fever. N Y Med News 1900;37:16.
21. Dunbar W. The present state of our knowledge of hay-fever. J Hyg 1902;13:105.
22. Noon L. Prophylactic inoculation against hay fever. Lancet 1911;177:1572–3.
23. Dworetzky M. Noon and Freeman. J Allergy Clin Immunol 2003;111:1148–50.
24. Freeman J. Further observations on the treatment of hay fever by hypodermic inoculations of pollen vaccine. Lancet 1911;178:814–7.
25. Freeman J. Toxic idiopathies: the relationship between hay and other pollen fevers, animal asthmas, food idiosyncrasies, bronchial and spasmodic asthmas. Proc R Soc Med 1920;13:129–48.
26. Reisman R, Rose N, Witebsky E, et al. Penicillin allergy and desensitization. J Allergy 1962;33:178–87.
27. Koessler K. The specific treatment of hay-fever by active immunization. Ill Med J 1914;24:120.
28. Goodale J. Pollen therapy in hay fever. Boston Med Surg J 1915;173:42.
29. Rackemann F, Colmes A. Studies in asthma: the clinical characteristics of hypersensitiveness. J Allergy 1929;1:2–11.

30. Dworetzky M, Cohen S. Pioneers and milestones. J Allergy Clin Immunol 2002; 110:674–80.
31. American Medical Associations Council on Scientific Affairs. In vivo diagnostic testing and immunotherapy for allergy. Report 1. JAMA 1987;258:1361–7.
32. Gordon B. Allergy skin tests for inhalants and foods. Otolaryngol Clin North Am 1998;31:35–53.
33. Cooke R, VanderVeer A. Human sensitization. J Immunol 1916;1:201–305.
34. Kern R. Dust sensitization in bronchial asthma. Med Clin North Am 1921;5:751.
35. Vannier W, Campbell D. The isolation and purification of purified house dust allergen fraction. J Allergy 1959;30:198.
36. Frankland A, Augustin R. Prophylaxis of summer hay-fever and asthma: a controlled trial comparing crude grass pollen extracts with the isolated main protein component. Lancet 1954;263:1055–7.
37. Spieksma F, Dieges P. The history of the finding of the house dust mite. J Allergy Clin Immunol 2004;113:573–6.
38. van Leeuwen WS. Asthma and tuberculosis in relation to "climate allergens". BMJ 1927;2:344–7.
39. van Leeuwen WS. Ueber die bedeutung allergenfreier kammern fur diagnose und therapie allergischer krankheiten. Dtsch Med Wochenschr 1928;23: 703–7 [in German].
40. Platts-Mills T, Vaughm J, Carter M. The role in intervention in established allergy avoidance of indoor allergens in the treatment of chronic allergic disease. J Allergy Clin Immunol 2000;106:787–804.
41. Liccardi A, Custovic G, Cassoli M. Avoidance of allergen and air pollutants in respiratory allergy. Allergy 2001;56:705–22.
42. Allen R. The common cold: its pathology and treatment with especial reference to vaccine therapy. Lancet 1908;172:1659–65.
43. Lowdermilk R. Hay-fever. J Am Med Assoc 1914;63:141–2.
44. Cooke R. Studies in the specific hypersensitiveness. New etiologic factors in bronchial asthma. J Immunol 1922;7:147.
45. Coca A. Studies in specific hypersensitiveness XV. The preparation of fluid extracts and solutions for use in the diagnosis and treatment of allergies. J Immunol 1922;7:163.
46. Coca A, Grove E. Studies in hypersensitiveness XIII. A study of the atopic reagins. J Immunol 1925;10:445.
47. Levine P, Coca A. Studies in hypersensitiveness XXI. J Immunol 1926;11:435–48.
48. Frankland A, Hughes W, Garrill R. Autogenous bacterial vaccines in the treatment of bronchial asthma. Br Med J 1955;2:941–4.
49. Durham O. Cooperative studies in ragweed pollen incidence. J Allergy 1929;1: 12–21.
50. Thommen A. In: Coca A, Walzer M, Thommen A, editors. Asthma and hay fever in theory and practice. London: Balliere, Tindall, Cox; 1931. p. 511–5, p. 757–84.
51. Stull A, Cooke R, Tenant J. The allergen content of protein extracts. J Allergy 1933;4:455.
52. American Academy of Allergy. Report of Joint Committee on Standards. J Allergy 1935;6:408.
53. Black J. The oral administration of pollen. J Lab Clin Med 1927;12:1156.
54. Black J. The oral administration of ragweed pollen. J Allergy 1939;10:156.
55. Stier R, Hollister G. Desensitization by oral administration of pollen extracts. Northwest Med 1937;36:166.

56. Bernstein T, Feinberg S. Oral ragweed therapy. Clinical results and experiments in gastrointestinal absorption. Arch Intern Med 1938;2:297–304.
57. Feinberg S, Foran F, Lichtenstein M. Oral pollen therapy for ragweed pollinosis. J Am Med Assoc 1940;115:23–9.
58. Hansel F. Sublingual testing and therapy. Trans Am Soc Opth Otolaryngology Allergy 1970;11:93–103.
59. Bousquet J, Casale T, Lockey R, et al. Sublingual immunotherapy: World Allergy Organization position paper 2009. Allergy 2009;64:S1–59.
60. Shelmire B. Contact dermatitis from vegetation: patch testing and treatment with plant oleoresins. South Med J 1940;38:337.
61. Hansel F. Allergies of the nose and paranasal sinuses. St Louis (MO): CV Mosby; 1936.
62. Osguthorpe J. The evolution of otolaryngic allergy. Otolaryngol Head Neck Surg 1996;114:515–24.
63. Voorhorst R, Spieksma-Boezeman M, Spieksma F. Is a mite the producer of the housedust allergen. Allerg Asthma (Leipz) 1964;10:329–34.
64. Voorhorst R, Spieksma F, Varekamp H, et al. The house dust mite (Dermatophagoides pteronyssinus) and the allergens it produces. J Allergy 1967;39:325–39.
65. Rinkel H. The whealing response of the skin to serial testing. Ann Allergy 1949;7:120–6.
66. Mabry R. Skin endpoint titration technique. Washington, DC: American Academy of Otolaryngic Allergy; 1989.
67. Osguthorpe J. Evolution to current otolaryngic allergy techniques. Otolaryngol Clin North Am 1998;31:1–10.
68. Turkeltaub P, Rastogi S, Baer H. Quantitative intradermal test procedure to determine relative potency of allergenic extracts using parallel line bioassay. In, Methods of the laboratory of allergenic products DBP, OBRR, CDB, FDA. Washington, DC: US Government Printing Office; 1986.
69. Lowell F, Franklin W. A double blind study of the effectiveness and specificity of injection therapy in ragweed hay fever. N Engl J Med 1965;273:675–9.
70. Norman P, Winkenwerder W, Lichtenstein L. Immunotherapy of hay fever with ragweed antigen E. J Allergy 1968;42:93–108.
71. Durham S, Walker S, Varga E, et al. Long term clinical efficacy of grass pollen immunotherapy. N Engl J Med 1999;341:468–75.
72. King T, Norman P. Isolation studies of allergens from ragweed pollen. Biochemistry 1962;1:709–20.
73. Ishizaka K, Ishizaka T. Identification of gamma E antibodies as the carrier of reaginic activity. J Immunol 1967;99:1187–98.
74. American Medical Associations Council on Scientific Affairs. In vitro tests for allergy. Report II. JAMA 1987;258:1639–43.
75. Nelson H. Preparing and mixing allergen vaccines for subcutaneous immunotherapy. Clin Allergy Immunol 2008;21:303–20.
76. Osguthorpe J. Immunotherapy. Curr Opin Otolaryngol Head Neck Surg 2010;18:206–12.
77. Calderon M, Alves B, Jacobson M, et al. Allergen injection immunotherapy for seasonal allergic rhinitis. The Cochrane Library 2008;4:1–86. Available at: www.cochranelibrary.com. Accessed March 15, 2011.
78. Emanuel I. In vitro testing for allergy diagnosis. Otolaryngol Clin North Am 2003;36:879–93.

79. Nalebuff D. In vitro testing methodologies: evolution and current status. Otolaryngol Clin North Am 1992;25:27–42.
80. Sogg A. Comparative skin and RAST test results. Laryngoscope 1985;95:1213–5.
81. King W. Efficacy of a screening radioallergosorbent test. Arch Otolaryngol Head Neck Surg 1982;108:91–5.
82. Nalebuff D. Use of RAST screening in clinical allergy. Ear Nose Throat J 1985;64:107–10.
83. Bousquet P, Burbach G, Heinzerling L, et al. GA2LEN skin test study III. Allergy 2009;11:1656–62.
84. James L, Durham S. Update on the mechanisms of allergen injection immunotherapy. Clin Exp Allergy 2008;38:1074–89.
85. Akdis C, Akdis M. Mechanisms and treatment of allergic disease in the big picture of regulatory T cells. J Allergy Clin Immunol 2009;123:735–46.
86. Miossec P, Korn T, Kuchroo V. Interleukin-17 and type 17 helper T-cells. N Engl J Med 2009;361:888–98.
87. Passalacqua G, Durham S. Allergic rhinitis and its impact on asthma update. J Allergy Clin Immunol 2007;119:881–91.
88. Wallace D, Dykewicz M, Bernstein D, et al. The diagnosis and management of rhinitis: an updated practice parameter. J Allergy Clin Immunol 2008;122:S1–84.
89. Brozek J, Bousquet J, Baena-Cagnani C, et al. Allergic rhinitis and its impact on asthma (ARIA) guidelines. J Allergy Clin Immunol 2010;126:466–76.
90. Bousquet P, Calderon M, Demoly P, et al. The Consolidated Standards of Reporting Trials (CONSORT) Statement applied to allergen-specific immunotherapy with inhalant allergens: a Global Allergy and Asthma European Network (GA2LEN) article. J Allergy Clin Immunol 2011;127(1):49–56.
91. Nieto A, Mazon A, Pamies R, et al. Sublingual immunotherapy for allergic respiratory diseases. J Allergy Clin Immunol 2009;124:157–61.
92. Brozek J, Aki E, Alonso-Coello P, et al. Grading quality of evidence and strength of recommendations in clinical practice guidelines. Allergy 2009;64:669–77.
93. Bousquet P, Brozek J, Bachert C, et al. The CONSORT statement checklist in allergen-specific immunotherapy. Allergy 2009;64:1737–45.
94. Van Ree M, Chapman M, Ferreira F, et al. The CREATE project. Allergy 2008;63:310–26.

Epidemiology of Allergy

Charles S. Ebert Jr, MD, MPH[a,*], Harold C. Pillsbury III, MD[b]

KEYWORDS

• Allergy • Epidemiology • Asthma • Atopy • Food allergy

Key Points: Epidemiology of Allergy

- The prevalence of atopic disease has reportedly been on the rise in the United States, where an estimated 50 million Americans (1 in 5) have allergic disease.[1] When combined with comorbid conditions, atopic disease is considered the most common chronic disease in the United States.[2]
- Clear evidence supports the united airway concept where upper and lower airways influence each other in response to allergy via a complex interaction of neurologic, immunologic, and allergic responses involved in inflammation.
- Due to the high prevalence of aeroallergic disease, there is a significant economic burden of these disease processes on the health care system and society as a whole—in 1996, the cost of allergic rhinitis, in terms of direct medical expenditures, exceeded $3 billion and more than $6 billion was spent on prescription medications for the treatment of allergic rhinitis (AR) in 2000. Indirect costs associated with AR were reported to include 3.5 million lost workdays and 2 million missed school days each year.[3]
- In the United States, aeroallergic disease is found in all geographic regions. The prevalence of AR tends to be higher in the Southeastern portion of the country, however, followed by the Central Northeast, Pacific, and Middle Atlantic regions.[3]
- The estimated rates of clinical food allergy in the United States range from 3.5% to 6%.[4,5] Patients with other atopic diseases, such as asthma, allergic rhinitis, and eczema, have a higher prevalence of food allergy[4] whereas those with asthma and food allergy are at increased risk for episodes of life-threatening asthma exacerbations.[6]

This work has no funding support.
[a] Division of Rhinology, Allergy, and Sinus Surgery, Department of Otolaryngology/Head and Neck Surgery, University of North Carolina School of Medicine at Chapel Hill, CB# 7070, Chapel Hill, NC 27599-7070, USA
[b] Department of Otolaryngology/Head and Neck Surgery, University of North Carolina School of Medicine at Chapel Hill, CB# 7070, Chapel Hill, NC 27599-7070, USA
* Corresponding author.
E-mail address: cebert@med.unc.edu

Otolaryngol Clin N Am 44 (2011) 537–548
doi:10.1016/j.otc.2011.03.001 oto.theclinics.com
0030-6665/11/$ – see front matter

Arthur Coca and Robert Cooke introduced the concept of atopy (Greek *a* [without] and *topy* [place]) in an article read at the annual meeting of the American Association of Immunologists in 1922.[7] Atopy referred to a collection of disease processes in patients who had any form of allergic disease, where "the individuals as a group possess a peculiar capacity to become sensitive to certain proteins in which their environment and habits of life expose them."[7] Since this early account, atopy now commonly refers to hypersensitivity to antigens mediated by IgE and represents a wide spectrum of disorders.[8]

Atopic disease afflicts an estimated 50 million Americans (1 in 5).[1] Allergic disease is the fifth leading chronic disease in the United States among all ages and the third most common chronic disease among children under 18.[9] When combined with comorbid conditions (**Fig. 1**), atopic disease is considered the most common chronic disease in the United States.[2]

Evidence supports that the upper and lower airways influence each other in response to allergy.[10–12] This complex interaction of neurologic, immunologic, and allergic responses involved in inflammation is the foundation of concept of the united airway, which holds that allergic stimulation in one part of the airway can have an adverse effect on other aspects of the airway.[10–13] Marple[10] showed a concordance of allergic disease, specifically AR with asthma, otitis media, nasal polyposis, and chronic rhinosinusitis. Furthermore, a longitudinal, population-based study found that patients with AR had an increased risk for development of asthma, nearly 4-fold.[10,14]

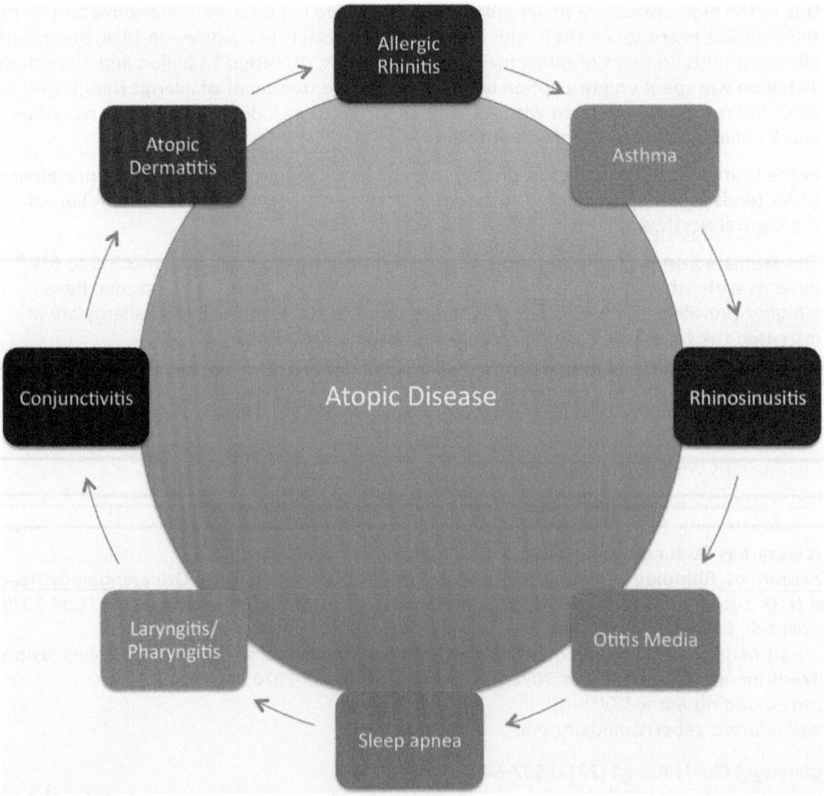

Fig. 1. Atopic diseases and associated conditions.

The sequelae of inhalant and food allergies may present in many organ systems but patients frequently report symptoms affecting the eyes, nose, ears, and oral cavity as well as the upper and lower airways.[15] Because otolaryngologists have expertise in examination of the end organs of allergic disease, they are in a unique position to diagnose and care for those with allergic disease and to appreciate the interrelationships of the united airway. It is important for clinicians to understand the epidemiology of atopic disease to determine its causes as well as to be aware of the natural history to develop effective treatment and prevention strategies. This article focuses on the epidemiology of inhalant allergies causing AR and asthma as well as IgE-mediated food allergies.

Prevalence of Aeroallergic Disease

Asthma and other IgE-mediated diseases represent significant health problems throughout the world. The World Health Organization estimates that nearly 300 million people worldwide have asthma.[16] In the United States, the prevalence of asthma is approximately 7% of the population.[17] A reliable estimate of the prevalence of AR is difficult to obtain due to frequent misclassification bias and varied research study design.[3,18] AR is more prevalent than asthma, however, with estimates of prevalence ranging from 10% to 20% (500 million) worldwide[19] and in the United States ranging from 10% to 40%.[15,20–22] A national survey of 35,757 households in the United States identified 500 children who were diagnosed with AR by a health care provider found the prevalence of AR to be 13% in children.[23] Another comprehensive national survey that included 2500 adults diagnosed with AR and 400 health care practitioners who treat AR found the prevalence in adults to be 14%.[24] Asthma and respiratory allergies often coexist in the same patients (the united airway) with approximately 19% to 38% of those with AR having asthma.[17,25] Of those with asthma, between 50% and 85% of patient have some form of rhinitis.[20]

The prevalence of atopic disease has reportedly been on the rise in the United States and around the world, although rates may have plateaued recently, according to the International Study of Asthma and Allergies in Childhood, which reported that the lifetime prevalence rates of atopic disease stabilized at 20%.[13,26–28] This plateau is a mixture of a substantial increase in prevalence of atopic disease in Mexico, Chile, Kenya, Algeria, and Southeast Asia, with decreases in New Zealand and the United Kingdom, which previously had high rates.[13,27,28]

Asthma and AR have also begun to demonstrate changes in prevalence patterns, with lower rates in many English-language and Western European countries and with concomitant higher rates in the developing world—Africa, Latin America, and parts of Asia.[28,29] The cause of these variations is not fully understood. Increased urbanization, however, in parts of the developing world may contribute to these trends due to the higher prevalence of aeroallergic disease in urban settings compared with rural environments.[30]

The hygiene hypothesis is often used to explain these disparities. This hypothesis holds that modifications in the environment by industrialization/urbanization have led to reduced microbial exposure in early life in contrast to farming/rural societies.[30] It is thought that increasing urbanization is associated with improved hygiene, a reduced exposure to infectious agents (biasing the immune system away from a helper T cell type 1 immune-mediated response), and thus higher prevalence of allergy.[31]

The hygiene hypothesis, however, does not fully explain the observed increase in allergic disease in certain areas. For example, in the inner cities of the United States, children have high rates of allergy and a very high prevalence of asthma (39.8%—nearly

6 times the national rate for children).[32] Similarly, African children who move to large cities with supposed improved hygiene have experienced increases in infections, wheezing, and diagnosed asthma.[30]

The increased severity of asthma in North American cities could be explained by several factors, including prolonged time indoors; high exposure to dust mite, cockroach, or rodent allergens; and extreme sedentary lifestyle/obesity.[30] Other factors, such as exposure to elevated concentrations of fossil fuel–generated air pollution, increasing dust mite populations, and decreased home/workplace ventilation as well as the development of sensitization to a variety of novel cross-reacting exotic food and pet allergens, may result in a lower tolerance to pollens: a reverse case of immunotherapy.[26,33,34]

Climate change/global warming may also contribute to prevalence changes in aeroallergic disease. A recent review of climate change and allergic disease by Shea and colleagues[16] reported that climate change measurably affects "the timing, distribution, quantity, and quality of aeroallergens," thereby altering the distribution and severity of allergic disease. It was anticipated that worsening pollution and altered locoregional pollen production would lead to worsening of aeroallergic disease with more symptomatic days and reduced quality of life if trends of climate change continue.[16]

Burden of Aeroallergic Disease

Secondary to the high prevalence of aeroallergic disease, there is a significant economic burden of these disease processes on health care systems and society as a whole. In 1994, the total cost for the care of asthma in the United States was $10.7 billion.[35] Direct medical costs of asthma care (which included hospitalizations, doctors' visits, and medications) comprised $6 billion and indirect costs (workdays lost, time lost from school, and costs attributed to asthma deaths) were $4.64 billion.[35] In 1996, the cost of allergic rhinitis, in terms of direct medical expenditures, exceeded $3 billion and an additional $4 billion was ascribed to exacerbations of concomitant conditions, such as asthma and otitis media.[3] In addition, more than $6 billion was spent on prescription medications for the treatment of AR in 2000. Indirect costs associated with AR were reported to include 3.5 million lost workdays and 2 million missed school days each year.[3] Nathan and colleagues[3] also noted that traumatic injuries in the workplace were connected with the use of sedating antihistamines for self-treatment of AR symptoms.

Druss and colleagues[36] reported that health care costs of persons with asthma in the United States were more than $27 billion (1996 dollars), whereas total societal costs (including work loss) of persons with asthma exceeded $31.2 billion. It also seems that lower socioeconomic groups may have a higher prevalence and incidence of asthma than other groups, which places further strain on the health care system.[37]

The enormous economic burden is not limited to the United States. The Global Initiative for Asthma reviewed cost-of-illness studies on asthma and found that asthma costs in developed countries averaged an annual societal burden ranging from $326 to $1315 (1991 US dollars) per afflicted person.[38] Furthermore, approximately 40% to 50% of the total asthma costs were attributed to direct medical expenditures.[38] These cost studies of aeroallergic disease demonstrate the enormous economic burden in both the United States and around the world.[38]

In addition, allergic disease exerts significant indirect costs on society. For example, Bousquet and colleagues[39] reported that increased severity of AR had adverse affects on quality of life—sleep, activities of daily living, and professional performance. Camelo-Nunes and Sole reported that the symptoms of nasal obstruction that occur with AR result in poor sleep quality, which ultimately results in poor cognition, daytime somnolence, reduction in professional performance, and risk for work-related accidents.[40] In a survey involving individuals with AR, 68% of those with perennial AR and 48% of those with seasonal AR reported that the disease interfered with their sleep.[41] The impact of allergic disease would dramatically increase when the disruptions of daily life caused by associated conditions, such as asthma, sinusitis, laryngitis, otitis media, are included in the equation (see **Fig. 1**).

Gender and Age Distribution of Aeroallergic Disease

Although men and women share identical mechanisms that activate the immune system, there is a clinical preponderance of women affected with atopic disease.[42] In the National Health Interview Survey, Pleis and colleagues[43] found that women were more likely to have been told they had asthma, hay fever, sinusitis, or chronic bronchitis than were men. In addition, the survey of the burden of allergic disease in the United States found that the prevalence of physician-diagnosed allergic disease was more common in women (34.3%) compared with men (27%).[3] In another large cohort of patients with difficult-to-treat asthma, women had more asthma control problems and lower asthma-related quality of life compared with men ($P<.0001$).[44] Asthma triggers, allergic rhinitis, and atopic dermatitis were also more frequently found in female subjects.[44] These gender-related differences have several explanations. One explanation includes the estradiol-receptor–dependent mast-cell activation. Perimenopausal and postmenopausal women have been reported to increasing rates of asthma, wheeze, and AR.[42] This association may indicate that women ultimately become hypersensitive to their own sex hormones.[42,45] Other explanations include misclassification bias and female preponderance to self-reporting disease.[42]

In contrast to adults, male children seem more frequently affected with asthma or atopic disease than female children. The male-to-female ratio of children who have atopic disease is approximately 1.8:1.[8] In the National Health Interview Survey, boys (17%) were more likely than girls (11%) to have ever been diagnosed with asthma.[46]

It also seems that respiratory allergic disease varies with age, with symptoms peaking in childhood and adolescence with the mean age of onset between the years 8 and 11.[3,26] A nested case-control study from Tucson, Arizona, found annual incidence of asthma was 1.4% for boys and 0.9% for girls in the 0-year to 4-year age group, 1.0% for boys and 0.7% for girls in the 5-year to 9-year age group, and 0.2% for boys and 0.3% for girls in the 10-year to 14-year age group.[47] Although the incidence of asthma in this study declined with age, the prevalence rates were comparatively constant.[47] The prevalence of AR tends to be lower in children than adults and lower after 65 years of age than in younger adults.[48]

An early age at onset of symptoms may ultimately result in a gradual progression of atopic disease. This phenomenon is referred to as the atopic march. The presumed method of sensitization is via the skin where possible defects in the epidermal barrier lead to later sensitization in the airways.[28] This march is characterized by the development of atopic dermatitis followed by a sequence of food allergy, rhinitis, and/or asthma, where symptoms may develop, subsequently fade away, or persist for several years.[28,49]

There is some conflicting evidence as to whether or not race plays a significant role in allergic disease. In a study of children without personal or family history of allergic disease and a low socioeconomic class who underwent skin testing, the investigators reported an increased risk among African American children for sensitization to any allergen (odds ratio [OR] 2.17; 95% CI, 1.23–3.84) and sensitization to outdoor allergens (OR 2.96; 95% CI, 1.52–5.74]).[50] In another study, white children were found more likely to have had hay fever (10%) than African American children (8%).[46] In a population-based cohort study, Yang and colleagues[51] concluded that the disparity in allergic sensitization by race could be due to environmental factors rather than genetic differences. Overall, the influence of racial and/or genetic factors is complex and difficult to separate from environmental influences and changes due to emigration.

Despite the impact of environmental influences, there are some genetic links to allergic diseases. Chromosome 5 has been thought to be involved in the regulation of total IgE concentration, whereas chromosome 11q has been associated with the high total IgE concentration or specific IgE.[52] In addition, chromosome 14 has been linked to eczema and specific HLA haplotypes are linked to the development of IgE.[52] Despite the evidence for genetic propensity to allergic disease, it is unlikely that geographic disparities in disease prevalence between those of similar genetic background or the increase in allergic disease over the previous decades can be explained by solely a genetic cause.[52]

Geographic Distribution of Aeroallergic Disease

Atopic disease generally decreases from north to south in the Northern Hemisphere and from south to north in the Southern Hemisphere.[52–55] A survey of representative samples of 20- to 44-year-old men and women mainly in Europe, North Africa, India, North America, Australia, and New Zealand revealed the median prevalence of AR was 22%, with a substantial variation across regions. AR decreased with geographic latitude, however.[55] Latitude is typically considered a proxy for ultraviolet solar exposure (ie, radiation that reaches the earth's surface is inversely related to latitude). Therefore, the variations in prevalence of atopic disease reflect climatic differences responsible for different pollen seasons and population lifestyle as well as different building construction. Furthermore, a higher number of less developed countries are found in the lower latitudes/tropical regions, which correlates with fewer medical resources so that allergic diseases go underdiagnosed.[54] Other explanations may be related to socioeconomic status. There is a reported lower frequency of immunologic diseases in populations with a low socioeconomic status. For example, there is a positive correlation between the incidence of asthma in 12 European countries and the gross national product.[54]

In the United States, it seems that aeroallergic disease is found in all geographic regions. The prevalence of AR tends to be higher, however, in the Southeastern portion of the country followed by the Central Northeast, Pacific, and Middle Atlantic regions.[3] A related comorbid condition may also have some regional distribution characteristics. Pleis and colleagues[43] noted that the percentage of adults with sinusitis was higher in the South than in any other region of the United States.

Risk Factors for Allergic Disease

Atopic diseases are multifactorial processes and linked by a complex combination of hereditary and environmental factors. The strongest risk factor for development of AR is a family history of primary relative with atopy.[15,22,48] When each parent is atopic, there is a 50% chance that the offspring will develop atopic disease.[8] This risk increases to nearly 72% when both parents have an identical type of allergy (asthma or atopic dermatitis). When neither of the parents has atopy, however, there is only a chance of 13% that their children will develop atopic disease. When one parent or sibling is atopic, the risk of atopy in another child is nearly 30%.[8] The concordance for AR is higher in inmonozygotic (identical) twins compared with dizygotic (fraternal), approximately 0.45 and 0.25, respectively.[48] Genetics factors cannot fully explain the concordance of atopy, however, in identical twins.[48]

There are additional risk factors for atopic disease. The season of birth may play a role in the development of allergic disease.[55] In Japan, investigators have found a significantly higher proportion of the children with AR born between August and October than during the rest of the year.[56] Another study found atopic disease was higher in children born in the autumn and winter (September to February) compared with the spring and summer months.[57] Male gender during childhood may also be a risk factor (female gender as an adult has not been clearly identified as a risk factor).[26]

Increases in pollution (eg, nitrogen and diesel particles) as well as tobacco smoke exposure may increase the risk for atopic disease.[26,58] Many studies in various parts of the world have shown a substantial and constant association between elevated levels of particulate pollutants and an increase in allergic conditions.[58] Exposure to tobacco smoke has been shown to increase the risk of developing wheezing, and infants exposed to secondhand smoke have nearly a 4-fold increase in airway hyper-responsiveness to histamine challenge.[8] In addition, smoking exposure has been shown to increase the number of emergency department visits made by children who have asthma to 3.1 visits annually compared with 1.8 visits annually in children who are not exposed to secondhand smoke.[8]

Dietary changes, such as increased use of food colorings/preservatives, increased sodium intake, and decreased fruit, vegetable, and fish consumption, have been linked to the increased prevalence of atopic disorders.[26] Furthermore, increased caloric intake combined with lack of exercise (childhood obesity) has been suggested as a risk factor for asthma.[58] Population studies have shown that those patients who have a family history of atopy and obesity have a higher incidence of asthma than other subgroups.[8,26,58] African American race is a risk factor for asthma, which is 2.5 times more prevalent among African Americans than among whites.[8] Elevated serum IgE levels in childhood (before age 6) and increased allergens in the environment are other potential risk factors.[21,59,60]

Higher socioeconomic status and education may also play a role in development of atopic disease. Children with a parent who has more than a high school diploma are more likely to have respiratory asthma or AR than children with parents who have less education.[46]

In contrast, several factors may offer protection from developing allergic rhinitis. These factors include possible exposure to environments associated with increased childhood infections, such as a large families and day care, and antibiotic restraint for childhood infections.[15,21,60]

IgE-Mediated Food Allergies

Food allergy is the term used to describe an immunologic response to food.[61] Because diets in developed countries have been modified over the past 30 years, sensitivity to foods, specifically milk, eggs, and fish, is relatively common in childhood.[52,61,62] For adults, the picture is more complicated due to frequent reports of intolerance to foods not typically seen on food challenge testing or by specific assessment of IgE.[52] Bias in study populations and poor diagnostic methodologies make it difficult to accurately assess current prevalence and patterns of food allergy.[61]

Nevertheless, the estimated rates of clinical food allergy in the United States range from 3.5% to 6%.[4,5] In a study of 8203 participants with IgE-measured food allergy in the National Health and Nutrition Examination Survey, the estimated prevalence of clinical food allergy was 2.5%, with the highest rates seen in children(4.2% ages 1–5 years and 3.8% in those ages 6–19 years).[4] According to a recent report from the Centers for Disease Control and Prevention, childhood food allergies have increased 18% from 1997 to 2007, with an nearly 3.9% of children having a food allergy.[62]

Although an allergic response may be caused by practically any food, nearly 90% of all food allergic reactions are due to milk, soy, eggs, wheat, peanuts, tree nuts, fish, and shellfish.[9,61] Current estimated rates of specific food allergies in infants/children and adults are in **Table 1**.

Food allergies In the United States account for approximately 125,000 emergency department visits[63] and 53,700 episodes of anaphylaxis[64] each year. Deaths related to food allergy typically are reported form anaphylactic reactions to peanuts and tree nuts. These deaths are usually related to delayed treatment with epinephrine and occur more often in teens and young adults with asthma and a previously diagnosed food allergy.[61,65]

It has been commonly thought that food allergies in children resolve by 3 years of age. Recent studies report, however, that only approximately 11% of children with egg allergy and 19% with milk allergy resolved by 4 years of age.[66,67] Yet, nearly 80% of children resolved these allergies by age 16.[66,67] Peanut allergy, considered a persistent allergy, may resolve in approximately 20% of children by school age, although recurrence of peanut allergy has also been described.[61]

Patients with other atopic diseases, such as asthma, allergic rhinitis, and eczema, have a higher prevalence of food allergy.[4] In a study using serologic data from children and adults, Liu and colleagues[4] reported that the odds of patients with food allergy and asthma experiencing severe exacerbations were 6.9 times higher than those without food allergy. In addition, those with hay fever (AR) and asthma are at an increased risk for food allergy or food sensitization (**Table 2**).[4] Roberts and colleagues[6] found 54% of children with asthma requiring intubation due to a severe asthma exacerbation had a food sensitization, and regression analysis revealed that food allergy (5.89; 1.06–32.61) was independently associated with life-threatening asthma.

Young age (1–19), male gender, and non-Hispanic African American race/ethnicity also have been identified as significant risk factors for food allergy. The odds of African American males having food allergy were 4.4 times higher than others in the general population.[4] With regard to food-specific allergy, Sicherer and colleagues[68] found distinct racial differences in the self-reporting of shellfish allergy, where African American reported it more frequently than white subjects. In another study, Branum and

Table 1
Estimated prevalence of food allergy to specific foods in North America

Prevalence	Children (%)	Adults (%)
Milk	2.5	0.3
Egg	1.5	0.2
Peanut	1	0.6
Tree nuts	0.5	0.6
Fish	0.1	0.4
Shellfish	0.1	2.0
Wheat, soy	0.4	0.3

Data from Sicherer SH, Sampson HA. Food allergy. J Allergy Clin Immunol 2010;125(2 Suppl 2): S116–25.

Table 2
Prevalence and risk of food allergy/sensitization in diagnosed asthma and hay fever (allergic rhinitis)

	Asthma		Hay Fever	
Food Sensitization/allergy	**Prevalence (%)**	**OR**	**Prevalence (%)**	**OR**
Milk	9.1	2.0	6.8	1.9
Egg	8.2	2.9	6.9	2.6
Peanut	13.3	2.3	15.0	3.4
Shrimp	9.1	1.9	7.3	1.7

Data from Liu AH, Jaramillo R, Sicherer SH, et al. National prevalence and risk factors for food allergy and relationship to asthma: results from the National Health and Nutrition Examination Survey 2005–2006. J Allergy Clin Immunol 2010;126(4):798–806, e713; and Sicherer SH, Sampson HA. Food allergy. J Allergy Clin Immunol 2010;125(2 Suppl 2):S116–25.

Lukacs[69] found higher rates of sensitization to shrimp, milk, and peanuts among non-Hispanic African American children than other children.

SUMMARY

Atopic disease represents a wide spectrum of disorders characterized by hypersensitivity mediated by IgE.[8] The sequelae of inhalant and food allergies may present in many organ systems and frequently involves the eye, ear, nose, throat, and the upper and lower airways. The prevalence of atopic disease is increasing and currently affects an estimated 50 million Americans (1 in 5).[1] The prevalence of AR ranges from 10% to 20% (500 million) worldwide[19] and from 10% to 40% in the United States.[15,20–22]

Evidence supports that the upper and lower airways influence each other in response to allergy via a complex interaction of neurologic, immunologic, and allergic responses involved in inflammation.[10–12] This concept of the united airway holds that allergic stimulation in one part of the airway can have an adverse effect on other aspects of the airway.[10–13] For example, a patient with AR may also have with asthma, otitis media, nasal polyposis, and/or chronic rhinosinusitis.[10] Furthermore, patients with asthma and AR have a higher prevalence of food sensitization and food allergy.[4] Estimated rates of clinical food allergy in the United States range from 3.5% to 6%.[4,5]

Because otolaryngologists have expertise in examination of the end organs of allergic disease, they are in a unique position to diagnose and care for those with allergic disease and to appreciate the interrelationships of the united airway.

REFERENCES

1. Airborne allergens: something in the air. NIH Publication No. 03–7045; National institute of allergy and infectious diseases. U.S. Department of Health and Human Services; 2003. Available at: http://www.niaid.nih.gov/topics/allergicdiseases/documents/airborne_allergens.pdf. Accessed March 23, 2011.
2. Prevalence of selected chronic conditions. Hyattsville (MD): National Center for Health Statistics; 1994.
3. Nathan RA, Meltzer EO, Derebery J, et al. The prevalence of nasal symptoms attributed to allergies in the United States: findings from the burden of rhinitis in an America survey. Allergy Asthma Proc 2008;29(6):600–8.
4. Liu AH, Jaramillo R, Sicherer SH, et al. National prevalence and risk factors for food allergy and relationship to asthma: results from the National Health and

Nutrition Examination Survey 2005–2006. J Allergy Clin Immunol 2010;126(4): 798, e713–806.
5. Bock SA. Prospective appraisal of complaints of adverse reactions to foods in children during the first 3 years of life. Pediatrics 1987;79(5):683–8.
6. Roberts G, Patel N, Levi-Schaffer F, et al. Food allergy as a risk factor for life-threatening asthma in childhood: a case-controlled study. J Allergy Clin Immunol 2003;112(1):168–74.
7. Lieberman PL, Kaliner MA, Lockey RF, et al. The allergy archives: pioneers and milestones. J Allergy Clin Immunol 2006;117(2):478–82.
8. Nimmagadda SR, Evans R 3rd. Allergy: etiology and epidemiology. Pediatr Rev 1999;20(4):111–5 [quiz: 116].
9. Asthma and allegy foundation of America. Allergy facts and figures. Available at: http://www.aafa.org/display.cfm?id=9&sub=30#_ftnref2. Accessed November 25, 2010.
10. Marple BF. Allergic rhinitis and inflammatory airway disease: interactions within the unified airspace. Am J Rhinol Allergy 2010;24(4):249–54.
11. Lundblad L. Allergic rhinitis and allergic asthma: a uniform airway disease? Allergy 2002;57(11):969–71.
12. Compalati E, Ridolo E, Passalacqua G, et al. The link between allergic rhinitis and asthma: the united airways disease. Expert Rev Clin Immunol 2010;6(3):413–23.
13. Shaaban R, Zureik M, Soussan D, et al. Allergic rhinitis and onset of bronchial hyperresponsiveness: a population-based study. Am J Respir Crit Care Med 2007;176(7):659–66.
14. Thomas M. Allergic rhinitis: evidence for impact on asthma. BMC Pulm Med 2006; 6(Suppl 1):S4.
15. Franzese CB, Burkhalter NW. The patient with allergies. Med Clin North Am 2010; 94(5):891–902.
16. Shea KM, Truckner RT, Weber RW, et al. Climate change and allergic disease. J Allergy Clin Immunol 2008;122(3):443–53 [quiz: 454–5].
17. Meltzer EO, Hadley J, Blaiss M, et al. Development of questionnaires to measure patient preferences for intranasal corticosteroids in patients with allergic rhinitis. Otolaryngol Head Neck Surg 2005;132(2):197–207.
18. Settipane RA, Charnock DR. Epidemiology of rhinitis: allergic and nonallergic. Clin Allergy Immunol 2007;19:23–34.
19. Brozek JL, Bousquet J, Baena-Cagnani CE, et al. Allergic Rhinitis and its Impact on Asthma (ARIA) guidelines: 2010 revision. J Allergy Clin Immunol 2010;126(3):466–76.
20. Ryan MW. Asthma and rhinitis: comorbidities. Otolaryngol Clin North Am 2008; 41(2):283–95, vi.
21. Skoner DP. Allergic rhinitis: definition, epidemiology, pathophysiology, detection, and diagnosis. J Allergy Clin Immunol 2001;108(1 Suppl):S2–8.
22. Sibbald B. Epidemiology of allergic rhinitis. Monogr Allergy 1993;31:61–79.
23. Meltzer EO, Blaiss MS, Derebery MJ, et al. Burden of allergic rhinitis: results from the Pediatric Allergies in America survey. J Allergy Clin Immunol 2009;124(3 Suppl): S43–70.
24. Meltzer EO. Allergic rhinitis: the impact of discordant perspectives of patient and physician on treatment decisions. Clin Ther 2007;29(7):1428–40.
25. Bousquet J, Khaltaev N, Cruz AA, et al. Allergic Rhinitis and its Impact on Asthma (ARIA) 2008 update (in collaboration with the World Health Organization, GA(2) LEN and AllerGen). Allergy 2008;63(Suppl 86):8–160.
26. Schoenwetter WF. Allergic rhinitis: epidemiology and natural history. Allergy Asthma Proc 2000;21(1):1–6.

27. Williams H, Stewart A, von Mutius E, et al. Is eczema really on the increase worldwide? J Allergy Clin Immunol 2008;121(4):947, e915–954.
28. Spergel JM. Epidemiology of atopic dermatitis and atopic march in children. Immunol Allergy Clin North Am 2010;30(3):269–80.
29. Pearce N, Ait-Khaled N, Beasley R, et al. Worldwide trends in the prevalence of asthma symptoms: phase III of the International Study of Asthma and Allergies in Childhood (ISAAC). Thorax 2007;62(9):758–66.
30. Platts-Mills TA, Erwin E, Heymann P, et al. Is the hygiene hypothesis still a viable explanation for the increased prevalence of asthma? Allergy 2005;60(Suppl 79): 25–31.
31. Nicolaou N, Siddique N, Custovic A. Allergic disease in urban and rural populations: increasing prevalence with increasing urbanization. Allergy 2005;60(11): 1357–60.
32. McLean DE, Bowen S, Drezner K, et al. Asthma among homeless children: undercounting and undertreating the underserved. Arch Pediatr Adolesc Med 2004; 158(3):244–9.
33. Linneberg A. Hypothesis: urbanization and the allergy epidemic–a reverse case of immunotherapy? Allergy 2005;60(4):538–9.
34. Mosges R, Klimek L. Today's allergic rhinitis patients are different: new factors that may play a role. Allergy 2007;62(9):969–75.
35. Weiss KB, Sullivan SD, Lyttle CS. Trends in the cost of illness for asthma in the United States, 1985–994. J Allergy Clin Immunol 2000;106(3):493–9.
36. Druss BG, Marcus SC, Olfson M, et al. Comparing the national economic burden of five chronic conditions. Health Aff (Millwood) 2001;20(6):233–41.
37. Ellison-Loschmann L, Sunyer J, Plana E, et al. Socioeconomic status, asthma and chronic bronchitis in a large community-based study. Eur Respir J 2007;29(5): 897–905.
38. Weiss KB, Sullivan SD. The health economics of asthma and rhinitis. I. Assessing the economic impact. J Allergy Clin Immunol 2001;107(1):3–8.
39. Bousquet J, Neukirch F, Bousquet PJ, et al. Severity and impairment of allergic rhinitis in patients consulting in primary care. J Allergy Clin Immunol 2006; 117(1):158–62.
40. Camelo-Nunes IC, Sole D. Allergic rhinitis: indicators of quality of life. J Bras Pneumol 2010;36(1):124–33.
41. Blaiss Mr T, Philpot E. A study to determine the impact of rhinitis on sufferers sleep and daily routine. J Allergy Clin Immunol 2005;115(2 Suppl):S197.
42. Jensen-Jarolim E, Untersmayr E. Gender-medicine aspects in allergology. Allergy 2008;63(5):610–5.
43. Pleis JR, Ward B, Lucas JW, et al. Summary Health Statistics for U.S. Adults: National Health Interview Survey, 2009. Data From the National Health Interview Survey No. Hyattsville, Maryland. Vital Health Stat 10 2010;249:1–86.
44. Lee JH, Haselkorn T, Chipps BE, et al. Gender differences in IgE-mediated allergic asthma in the epidemiology and natural history of asthma: Outcomes and Treatment Regimens (TENOR) study. J Asthma 2006;43(3):179–84.
45. Roby RR, Richardson RH, Vojdani A. Hormone allergy. Am J Reprod Immunol 2006;55(4):307–13.
46. Bloom BC, Freeman G. Summary Health Statistics for U.S. Children: National Health Interview Survey, 2009. Hyattsville, Maryland. Vital Health Stat 10 2010; 247:1–37.
47. Guerra S, Sherrill DL, Martinez FD, et al. Rhinitis as an independent risk factor for adult-onset asthma. J Allergy Clin Immunol 2002;109(3):419–25.

48. Sly RM. Epidemiology of allergic rhinitis. Clin Rev Allergy Immunol 2002;22(1):67–103.
49. Shaaban R, Zureik M, Soussan D, et al. Rhinitis and onset of asthma: a longitudinal population-based study. Lancet 2008;372(9643):1049–57.
50. Stevenson MD, Sellins S, Grube E, et al. Aeroallergen sensitization in healthy children: racial and socioeconomic correlates. J Pediatr 2007;151(2):187–91.
51. Yang JJ, Burchard EG, Choudhry S, et al. Differences in allergic sensitization by self-reported race and genetic ancestry. J Allergy Clin Immunol 2008;122(4):820, e829–827.
52. Jarvis D, Burney P. ABC of allergies. The epidemiology of allergic disease. BMJ 1998;316(7131):607–10.
53. Worldwide variation in prevalence of symptoms of asthma, allergy, rhinoconjuctivitis, and atopic eczema: ISAAC. The International Study of Asthma and Allergies in Childhood (ISAAC) Steering Committee. Lancet 1998;351(9111):1225–32.
54. Bach JF. The effect of infections on susceptibility to autoimmune and allergic diseases. N Engl J Med 2002;347(12):911–20.
55. Wjst M, Dharmage S, Andre E, et al. Latitude, birth date, and allergy. PLoS Med 2005;2(10):e294.
56. Saitoh Y, Dake Y, Shimazu S, et al. Month of birth, atopic disease, and atopic sensitization. J Investig Allergol Clin Immunol 2001;11(3):183–7.
57. Nilsson L, Kjellman NI. Atopy and season of birth. Allergy 1996;51(2):138–9.
58. Kaiser HB. Risk factors in allergy/asthma. Allergy Asthma Proc 2004;25(1):7–10.
59. Weeke ER. Epidemiology of allergic diseases in children. Rhinol Suppl 1992;13:5–12.
60. Ceuppens J. Western lifestyle, local defenses and the rising incidence of allergic rhinitis. Acta Otorhinolaryngol Belg 2000;54(3):391–5.
61. Sicherer SH, Sampson HA. Food allergy. J Allergy Clin Immunol 2010;125(2 Suppl 2):S116–25.
62. Branum AM, Lukacs SL. Food allergy among U.S. children: trends in prevalence and hospitalizations. NCHS Data Brief 2008;(10):1–8.
63. Ross MP, Ferguson M, Street D, et al. Analysis of food-allergic and anaphylactic events in the National Electronic Injury Surveillance System. J Allergy Clin Immunol 2008;121(1):166–71.
64. Decker WW, Campbell RL, Manivannan V, et al. The etiology and incidence of anaphylaxis in Rochester, Minnesota: a report from the Rochester Epidemiology Project. J Allergy Clin Immunol 2008;122(6):1161–5.
65. Bock SA, Munoz-Furlong A, Sampson HA. Further fatalities caused by anaphylactic reactions to food, 2001–2006. J Allergy Clin Immunol 2007;119(4):1016–8.
66. Savage JH, Matsui EC, Skripak JM, et al. The natural history of egg allergy. J Allergy Clin Immunol 2007;120(6):1413–7.
67. Skripak JM, Matsui EC, Mudd K, et al. The natural history of IgE-mediated cow's milk allergy. J Allergy Clin Immunol 2007;120(5):1172–7.
68. Sicherer SH, Munoz-Furlong A, Sampson HA. Prevalence of seafood allergy in the United States determined by a random telephone survey. J Allergy Clin Immunol 2004;114(1):159–65.
69. Branum AM, Lukacs SL. Food allergy among children in the United States. Pediatrics 2009;124(6):1549–55.

Types of Rhinitis

Kevin F. Wilson, MD[a,*], Matthew E. Spector, MD[b], Richard R. Orlandi, MD[a]

KEYWORDS

• Rhinitis • Allergic • Nonallergic • Occupational • Vasomotor • Irritant • Atrophic

Key Points: Types of Rhinitis

- Chronic rhinitis can be broadly classified into allergic, infectious, or nonallergic or noninfectious.
- Because of overlapping symptoms, the types of rhinitis are distinguished mainly by a careful history and, when indicated, allergy testing.
- The pathophysiology of nonallergic rhinitis likely involves a combination of inflammatory and neurogenic mechanisms that are poorly understood.
- The differential diagnosis is broad, and causes may include both local and systemic factors.
- Treatment involves having the patient avoid the offending agent, when possible, and use appropriate medications to control the predominant symptoms.

Rhinitis is a familiar disorder well known to primary care and specialty clinics alike. It affects up to 20% of the general population[1] and is one of the most common reasons for presentation to an otolaryngologist's office.[2]

Rhinitis is defined as inflammation of the nasal mucosa. This inflammation may be caused by a variety of factors, including infectious agents, allergies, irritants, medications, and hormones, among others. Associated symptoms may include excessive mucus production, nasal congestion, pain, pressure, sneezing, and pruritus. Acute rhinitis is often caused by infectious agents, such as viruses or bacteria, and is commonly associated with sinus inflammation as part of acute rhinosinusitis. More commonly, rhinitis presents as ongoing persistent symptoms, termed chronic rhinitis.

Chronic rhinitis can be broadly classified into allergic, infectious, or nonallergic-noninfectious. Allergic rhinitis (AR) is defined as IgE-mediated inflammation of the

No funding support.
Disclosure: Dr Orlandi is a consultant for Entellus.

[a] Division of Otolaryngology—Head and Neck Surgery, University of Utah, 50 North Medical Drive, SOM 3C120, Salt Lake City, UT 84132, USA
[b] Department of Otolaryngology, University of Michigan, 1500 East Medical Center Drive, TC 1904, Ann Arbor, MI 48109, USA
* Corresponding author.
E-mail address: kevin.wilson@hsc.utah.edu

Otolaryngol Clin N Am 44 (2011) 549–559
doi:10.1016/j.otc.2011.03.016
0030-6665/11/$ – see front matter. Published by Elsevier Inc.
oto.theclinics.com

nasal mucosa after allergen exposure. It is definitively diagnosed through allergy testing, with either skin testing or serum-specific IgE antibody testing. Nonallergic rhinitis (NAR) is diagnosed when the history and physical examination are consistent and proper allergy testing is negative. Of patients seen with chronic rhinitis, approximately 50% of them will have allergic rhinitis as demonstrated on allergy testing.[3] The remainder are given the diagnosis of nonallergic rhinitis. The latter is a broad category that includes a myriad of causes, some known, and some unknown.

Nasal symptoms characteristic of NAR are often indistinguishable from those that occur in AR. A careful history is important in establishing a diagnosis and distinguishing the two entities. Within the category of nonallergic rhinitis are various described entities relating to the causative factor. These include irritant, medication-induced, hormonal, atrophic, nonallergic rhinitis with eosinophilia syndrome (NARES), and smoking. When no causative agent is found, the patient is given the diagnosis of idiopathic rhinitis.

PATHOPHYSIOLOGY

The mechanisms that cause symptoms of rhinitis are complex and are likely multifactorial. Proposed contributions include chronic inflammatory and neurogenic sources.

Chronic Inflammation

It is well established that in allergic rhinitis, there is an influx of inflammatory cells and mediators into the nasal mucosa as they respond to the offending antigen. These mediators result in venous engorgement, increased nasal secretions and tissue edema, causing the classic symptoms of nasal congestion, sneezing, rhinorrhea, and pruritus.[4,5] There are likely similarities in nonallergic rhinitis patients as well, though the relation is not as clear-cut.

Powe and colleagues[6] examined inferior turbinectomy specimens from allergic, nonallergic, and normal patients. They found significantly more nasal mucosa mast cells and eosinophils in the rhinitic patients compared with the normal individuals. They concluded that idiopathic and allergic rhinitic mucosa show similarities in their inflammatory infiltrate suggesting that both groups share a similar cellular immunopathology.

In contrast, a study by van Rijswijk and colleagues[7] found no difference in nasal mucosal lymphocytes, antigen-presenting cells, eosinophils, macrophages, monocytes, mast cells, and other IgE-positive cells between idiopathic rhinitis patients and controls.

Neurogenic Mechanisms

The sensory nerves of the nose arise from the olfactory nerves as well as from the ophthalmic (through the ethmoidal nerve) and maxillary (through the nasopalatine nerve) branches of the trigeminal nerve. In the neurogenic model of rhinitis, exaggerated responses to environmental or endogenous stimuli occur because neural activity is upregulated as a result of a pathologic process, primarily of an inflammatory nature. In this case, a stimulus of average intensity generates exaggerated symptoms. This phenomenon is known as neural hyperresponsiveness and is believed to play an important role in the clinical presentation of nasal disease.

The neural regulation of the upper airways is complex and consists of a number of interacting nervous systems. Sensory, parasympathetic, and sympathetic nerves regulate epithelial, vascular, and glandular processes in the nasal mucosa. The sensory, parasympathetic, and sympathetic neural systems contain heterogeneous populations of nerve fibers with unique combinations of neurotransmitters and neuropeptides.

In 1959, Malcomson[8] stated that idiopathic rhinitis was caused by an autonomic imbalance. Normally, increased sympathetic tone in nasal blood vessels leads to vasoconstriction.[9] Underactivity of the sympathetic nervous system leads to nasal obstruction. Overactivity of the parasympathetic system also leads to rhinorrhea.[10]

In addition, perivascular and intraepithelial nonadrenergic, noncholinergic, sensory nerve fibers contain neuropeptides. These neuropeptides are locally released from peptidergic neurons (unmyelinated C-fibers or "pain fibers") in the nasal mucosa after activation by nonspecific stimuli, and can be responsible for the symptoms of idiopathic rhinitis.[11,12,13]

Progression to Allergic Rhinitis

Patients diagnosed with NAR typically have persistent symptoms, yet they are generally not followed up with further allergy management. Rondon and colleagues[14] studied patients diagnosed with nonallergic rhinitis on the basis of rhinitis symptoms and negative skin prick testing and negative serum specific IgE on initial testing. They were reevaluated 3 to7 years later with clinical questionnaires, spirometry, skin prick testing, and measurement of serum-specific IgE to common aeroallergens. They found that patients with NAR generally experienced worsening disease (52%), with an increase in the persistence (12%), severity of nasal symptoms (9%), and new comorbidities (24%) over time. The most frequent comorbidities at reevaluation were asthma (increasing from 32% to 55%) and conjunctivitis (from 28% to 43%), followed by chronic rhinosinusitis. Sensitization to aeroallergens not present at the initial evaluation was detected by means of skin prick testing, serum-specific IgE measurement, or both in 24% of the patients. They concluded that NAR may progress to AR over time and recommended that these patients be periodically reevaluated for allergy.

CLASSIFICATION

The classification of rhinitis is broad and, as previously mentioned, the most important diagnostic tool is the history. After excluding allergic rhinitis through history and appropriate allergy testing as indicated, a diagnosis of nonallergic rhinitis can be made. Often the term "vasomotor rhinitis" is used after ruling out allergy as the underlying cause: this term should only used for cases that are idiopathic and after other causes of nonallergic rhinitis are excluded. Rhinitis can be classified based on multiple criteria and associated factors. The most common and clinically important forms are presented in **Box 1**. Although this is not exhaustive, it will give the reader a firm basis of understanding of these disorders.

Allergic Rhinitis

Allergic rhinitis is the most common type of rhinitis. It can be categorized into three basic subgroups: seasonal, perennial, and occupational. IgE mediates immunologic responses to different allergens. Tree, grass, and weed pollens generally cause seasonal symptoms. Mold spores may cause seasonal and perennial symptoms. Indoor allergens such as dust mites, pet dander, and molds usually cause perennial symptoms. Occupational rhinitis is triggered by exposure to allergens or irritants in the workplace.

Allergic rhinitis symptoms include early and late responses. Seasonal or intermittent allergy exposures yield classic "acute phase" symptoms such as pruritus, sneezing,

Box 1
Classification of rhinitis

- Allergic rhinitis
  - Perennial rhinitis
    - Seasonal rhinitis
- Nonallergic rhinitis
  - Atrophic rhinitis
    - Surgery
    - Cocaine abuse
    - Aging
  - Emotional rhinitis
  - Exercise-induced rhinitis
  - Gustatory rhinitis
  - Hormone-related rhinitis
    - Hypothyroidism
    - Pregnancy
    - Menstrual cycle
    - Oral contraceptives
  - Idiopathic (vasomotor) rhinitis
  - Infectious rhinitis
    - Acute (usually viral)
    - Chronic (rhinosinusitis)
  - Irritant- or chemical-induced rhinitis
    - Temperature
    - Humidity
    - Perfumes
    - Cleaning agents
    - Cosmetics
    - Air pollution
    - Tobacco smoke
  - Medication-related rhinitis
    - Rhinitis medicamentosa
    - Other drugs
  - Nonallergic rhinitis with eosinophilia syndrome (NARES)
  - Systemic diseases
    - Autoimmune disorders
    - Vasculitides
    - Hormone disturbances

watery rhinorrhea, and acute conjunctivitis. On the other hand, perennial antigens such as cat dander or dust mite antigen can yield a more subtle presentation, with year-round "late-phase" symptoms such as congestion and rhinorrhea. Seasonal and perennial allergic rhinitis can be associated with systemic symptoms, including malaise, weakness, and fatigue. Patients with seasonal and perennial allergic rhinitis also may have asthma and eczema. Inasmuch as classic acute phase allergic symptoms may be blunted with constant antigen exposure, allergy testing may be beneficial in cases with only the more subtle late phase symptoms.

Hormone-related Rhinitis

Hormone-related rhinitis has been described in multiple disease processes as well as physiologic states. A neurogenic mechanism is proposed but is unclear. Disturbances in thyroid hormone (mainly hypothyroidism) and growth hormone (acromegaly) may have prominent nasal congestion and rhinorrhea. Estrogen and progesterone assert at least part of their effects on vascular smooth muscle, and hormonal rhinitis can develop during the menstrual cycle, puberty, or more commonly pregnancy. Pregnancy-induced rhinitis is probably the most common and well-known form of hormone-related rhinitis. It is diagnosed in a pregnant patient with rhinitis lasting 6 or more weeks without other causative agents, which disappears after delivery.[15] Estrogen levels are correlated with the severity of rhinitis symptoms and are the most severe in the second trimester.[16]

Medication-related Rhinitis

Medication-induced rhinitis is related to the neurogenic mechanism or local inflammatory effects of the offending agent and can be difficult to diagnose given the broad range of drugs available to patients.[17] Broad categories of medications include the antihypertensives, antidepressants, psychotropics, phosphodiesterase type 5 inhibitors (eg, sildenafil, vardenafil), and antiinflammatories. Many of these medications act at receptors that are ubiquitous throughout the body, including the nasal mucosa. The antiinflammatories exert a local effect and have a well-known mechanism of increased leukotriene production, leading to asthma and reactive airway disease in susceptible patients. This is termed aspirin-exacerbated respiratory disease (AERD).[17]

Intranasal decongestants such as oxymetazoline deserve specific mentioning. Extended use of topical α-adrenergic medications may result in rebound nasal congestion, termed "rhinitis medicamentosa." These patients also have characteristic-appearing erythematous nasal mucosa, which may be prone to bleed, as opposed to other drug-induced rhinitis.[18] Cocaine can act in a similar mechanism, resulting in rebound congestion. As mentioned previously, exogenous estrogen or progesterone agents can lead to rhinitis, which is reversible with discontinuation of medications.

Irritant-related Rhinitis

Irritant-related rhinitis involves an occupational or environmental exposure that causes symptoms. In this case, the agent causes an irritation rather than an allergic response. A spatial and temporal relationship of the exposure and associated symptoms is usually necessary to make the diagnosis, although sometimes it can be a difficult part of the history to assess. Some of the more common culprits are industrial chemicals, wood dust, tobacco smoke, paint fumes, hairspray, perfumes, and other fragrances. The diagnosis can be further strengthened by concurrent lower respiratory symptoms. Confirmation can be performed with a nasal provocation test under a controlled setting in clinic.[19] Environmental exposures, including weather or pressure changes, air pollution, cleaning agents, exercise, or even emotional situations, have been described. Ingestion of foods causing rhinitis characterized primarily by profuse, clear anterior rhinorrhea is termed gustatory rhinitis and is more common with spicy foods.[20]

Atrophic Rhinitis

Atrophic rhinitis is characterized by atrophy of the nasal mucosa, including mucus glands and nerves. It can be primary or secondary and is due to the replacement of the normal ciliated columnar epithelium of the nasal mucosa by stratified squamous epithelium. Primary atrophic rhinitis can occur as the result of aging, heredity, infection, or even nutritional deficiencies.[21] In Western civilization, the most common risk factor for primary atrophic rhinitis is age, with the majority of patients being diagnosed after 40.[22] Secondary atrophic rhinitis can be due to surgery (excessive removal of turbinates), radiation, longstanding cocaine abuse, or infections (eg, leprosy, syphilis, rhinoscleroma). These factors may cause destruction of nasal structures leading to atrophic changes. With chronic changes in airflow patterns and mucous secretion, there is decreased stimulation to the olfactory mucosa as well as the trigeminal afferents leading to a sense of congestion.[22] In addition to rhinitis, patients may present with foul smelling crusts or nasal obstruction with sensations of pain and pressure.

Systemic Diseases

Numerous systemic diseases can affect the nose, resulting in rhinitis. Granulomatous diseases (Wegener granulomatosis, sarcoidosis, Churg-Strauss syndrome), autoimmune diseases (lupus, Sjögren syndrome, pemphigoid), cystic fibrosis, tuberculosis, and ciliary dyskinesia all can have nasal manifestations of rhinitis.[23] When a patient's symptoms are not controlled with maximal medical management or the nasal mucosa demonstrates unusual features such as scarring (pemphigoid), excessive bleeding, and crusting (Wegener), or submucosal cobblestoning (sarcoidosis), other systemic causes must be considered.

Signs of granulomatous disease include persistent inflammation and crusting (Wegener), ulceration, nasal masses, submucosal nodules or cobblestoning (sarcoid), extranasal manifestations, and systemic symptoms. Autoimmune diseases can involve the complex process of antigen-antibody interaction in the nose and may result in mucosal ulceration (pemphigoid, lupus), dryness and crusting (Sjögren), and recurrent infections.[24] Sinonasal involvement in cystic fibrosis varies with the mutation status of the patient. Nasal polyps are present in most patients with the most common mutation ΔF508 and is frequently associated with the presence of bacterial biofilm infections, usually *Staph aureus* or *Pseudomonas*. Tuberculosis commonly affects the nasopharynx and can result in nasal inflammation and rhinorrhea.[25] Primary ciliary dyskinesia results in nasal symptoms as the patient cannot clear the mucus produced. It should be suspected in patients with stagnant clear secretions on the floor of the nose. The diagnosis can be confirmed with a mucociliary transport saccharine test.

NARES

NARES exhibits symptomatology similar to allergic rhinitis (nasal congestion, sneezing, rhinorrhea, nasal and ocular pruritus), but allergy testing is negative.[26,27] A distinguishing feature of NARES is the presence of eosinophils, usually 10% to 20% on nasal smears.[28] Although the overactivation of mast cells in the setting of chronic inflammation plays a role in the development of NARES, there is a lack of understanding of the exact pathophysiology. NARES patients can develop nasal polyposis and aspirin sensitivity, but this is not always the case.[28] NARES has also been associated with the severity of obstructive sleep apnea.[29] The diagnosis is made by history, physical examination, and negative serologic or skin testing, and is confirmed by the presence of prominent eosinophilia within the nasal mucosa on cytology. On physical examination, the turbinates of NARES patients often appear pale and boggy. These patients are more responsive to treatment with nasal corticosteroids compared with other patients with nonallergic rhinitis. The differentiation is important to aid in adequate symptom relief.[30]

Idiopathic Rhinitis

Idiopathic rhinitis (aka vasomotor rhinitis) should be a diagnosis of exclusion after an exhaustive history and physical examination. The pathogenesis of this condition is unclear. Increased sensitivity to environmental factors (eg, climate change, pollution, strong odors, perfumes) may trigger symptoms. This is the most common diagnosis within the subtypes of nonallergic rhinitis. On examination of nasal cytology, there is typically an absence of eosinophils, plasma cells, and mast cells compared with allergic rhinitis.[31] Without typical causative factors, vasomotor rhinitis is thought to be due to an imbalance of the neurogenic mechanisms described previously.[9,31]

DIAGNOSIS

Differentiating AR from NAR is important, but can be challenging, given the similarity in presentation and overlapping symptoms. However, a comprehensive history usually suggests the correct diagnosis. History-taking should focus on symptom onset, duration, chronicity, and severity. Rhinitis that appears later in life is more likely to be nonallergic.[3] Environmental and occupational triggers should be sought. Seasonal variation, environmental influences, and exposures should be elucidated. Medical history, comorbidities, and family history are all important and help to differentiate NAR from AR. Previous treatments and their efficacy are also important to elicit.

The differential diagnosis for acute symptoms lasting only a few days is relatively small and often suggests a viral origin. An acute exposure to an irritant or allergen can also give these acute symptoms, as can a nasal foreign body (especially if unilateral in children). The differential diagnosis of chronic rhinitis, however, is much broader.

An environmental trigger, whether allergic or irritant, should be sought. Seasonal variations in symptoms suggest allergic rhinitis. Age can help to differentiate AR from NAR (80% of allergic rhinitis patients have the onset before age 20).[3] Family history is important because allergic rhinitis and asthma both run in families. Comorbidities, especially those relating to atopy (asthma and eczema), can help steer the diagnosis. Finally, the success of past and current treatments may help identify the cause and direct future treatment.

A focused physical examination should follow the history. Acute viral rhinitis will tend to cause more generalized symptoms, including fevers, muscle aches, and fatigue. Patients with chronic allergic symptoms may have allergic shiners (ie, blue-gray or purple discoloration under the lower eyelids) or they may breathe preferentially through their mouths. Conjunctivitis can be a component of allergic rhinitis or acute viral upper respiratory infection (URI). A careful examination of the nose is important to identify structural abnormalities, polyps, mucosal swelling, foreign bodies, and discharge. Nasal endoscopy can enhance visualization and allow examination for signs of nasal polyps or sinusitis, but it is not always necessary. Examining the pharynx for enlarged tonsils or postnasal drip also can help identify viral causes or chronic drainage from chronic rhinitis. Lymphadenopathy with associated symptoms may suggest a viral or bacterial cause of rhinitis. Wheezing or eczema suggests an allergic cause.

Allergy Testing

There is debate as to when allergy testing is indicated in the rhinitic patient. Gendo and Larson[32] performed an extensive systematic review of the evidence on allergy testing and recommended that in general, physicians should select tests that will change outcomes or treatment plans; that empiric treatment is appropriate in patients with classic symptoms; that diagnostic tests may be appropriate if severe symptoms or an unclear diagnosis is present, or if the patient is a potential candidate for allergen avoidance treatment or immunotherapy; and that observation may be appropriate for patients with mild symptoms or an unclear history.

Allergy testing is useful to identify IgE-mediated disease, as this can have an effect on management. It usually involves one or more of the following methods: skin prick testing, intradermal testing, and allergen-specific IgE antibody testing. There are advantages and disadvantages to each, and the ultimate decision on which method to use often depends on the familiarity and preference of the physician and patient. The diagnosis of nonallergic rhinitis is made after eliminating allergic or IgE-mediated causes, often through allergy testing.

TREATMENT

As there are a myriad of causes of rhinitis, so there are a myriad of treatments. The treatment chosen for the specific patient is dictated by the underlying cause. Because the cause is not always apparent, as in idiopathic rhinitis, the treatment should be tailored toward the most troublesome symptoms of the patient.

If a cause is identified, such as an offending trigger, patient education regarding environmental modification and avoidance, if possible, should be employed. For temporary conditions, such as rhinitis of pregnancy, reassurance and counseling may be all that is needed. For those who desire pharmacologic treatment, several classes of drugs can be used.

Intranasal corticosteroids (INS) are FDA-approved for the treatment of rhinitis. The mechanism of action, presumably, relates to its antiinflammatory effects on the nasal mucosa. Fluticasone was shown to decrease the number of CD3+ cells, the amount of major basic protein, and the number of tryptase-positive cells in subjects with nonallergic rhinitis. It also lowered mRNA expression for interleukin (IL)-4 and IL-5.[33] In randomized clinical trials, INS have been shown to be effective in reducing symptoms, though it can take several weeks to reach maximal treatment effect.[34,35] This treatment is especially effective for NARES patients. However, for many NAR patients, INS alone is not as effective as in AR.

Oral antihistamines have not been shown to be effective in treating NAR. However, the intranasal antihistamine azelastine is FDA-approved for both AR and NAR.[36] In clinical trials, azelastine has been shown to reduce symptoms of rhinitis, including postnasal drainage, sneezing, rhinorrhea, and congestion.[37] These multicentered, placebo-controlled trials studied azelastine for the treatment of nonallergic vasomotor rhinitis. Over 200 patients were evaluated. The response rate of between 82% and 85% was significantly higher than the placebo response of 73%. The high placebo response is expected because saline nasal spray also has been shown to have a beneficial effect in this disorder.

Given that NAR is a non–IgE-mediated condition, the mode of action of azelastine in NAR is not clear, partially because the pathophysiology of this condition itself is uncertain. However, there are several possible mechanisms. including a decrease in neurokinin,[38] the prevention of mast cell degranulation,[39] a reduction in eosinophil accumulation associated with a decrease in expression of adhesion molecules,[40] and a decrease in the synthesis of inflammatory cytokines and nitric oxide via an effect on transcription mediated through NF-kB.[41]

Patients with predominantly secretory or rhinorrhea symptoms, especially vasomotor rhinitis, may benefit from an anticholinergic agent such as ipratropium nasal spray, 80 mcg up to four times a day.[42] Intranasal cromolyn has not been shown to be effective in treating this disorder. For those patients with congestion, a slow-release oral decongestant may provide relief, though significant side effects may result.[43] Even a simple intranasal saline spray may be all that is required for symptomatic improvement.

Patients with rhinitis medicamentosa attributable to over-use of topical α-adrenergic agonist medications should be weaned off these agents over 7 to 10 days while using an intranasal steroid. The patient may also require a short course of oral prednisone tapering over 7 to 10 days. Nonallergic rhinitis with eosinophilia syndrome is best treated with intranasal steroids. Treatment of rhinitis associated with a systemic disease should be directed at the underlying disease process. Management of atrophic rhinitis may include nasal saline irrigation and antibiotics. If an anatomic abnormality exists such as a deviated septum or nasal valve collapse, surgical intervention may be indicated.

REFERENCES

1. Bousquet J, Van Cauwenberge P, Khaltaev N. Allergic rhinitis and its impact on asthma (ARIA). J Allergy Clin Immunol 2001;108:S147–334.
2. Woodwell DA. Office visits to otolaryngologists 1989–90, national ambulatory medical care survey. Vital and Health Statistics of the CENTERS FOR DISEASE CONTROL AND PREVENTION/National Center for Health Statistics. Adv Data 1992;222:1–12.
3. Dykewicz MS, Fineman S, Skoner DP, et al. Diagnosis and management of rhinitis: complete guidelines of the Joint Task Force on Practice Parameter in Allergy, Asthma and Immunology. American Academy of Allergy, Asthma, and Immunology. Ann Allergy Asthma Immunol 1998;81:478–518.
4. Bentley AM, Jacobson MR, Cumberworth V, et al. Immunohistology of the nasal mucosa in seasonal allergic rhinitis: increases in activated eosinophils and epithelial mast cells. J Allergy Clin Immunol 1992;89:877–83.
5. Braunstahl GJ, Overbeek SE, Fokkens WJ, et al. Segmental bronchoprovocation in allergic rhinitis patients affects mast cell and basophil numbers in nasal and bronchial mucosa. Am J Respir Crit Care Med 2001;164:858–65.
6. Powe DG, Huskisson RS, Carney AS, et al. Evidence for an inflammatory pathophysiology in idiopathic rhinitis. Clin Exp Allergy 2001;31:864–72.
7. van Rijswijk JB, Blom HM, KleinJan A, et al. Inflammatory cells seem not to be involved in idiopathic rhinitis. Rhinology 2003;41:25–30.
8. Malcomson KG. The vasomotor activities of the nasal mucous membrane. J Laryngol Otol 1959;73:73–5.
9. Kimmelman CP, Ali GH. Vasomotor rhinitis. Otolaryngol Clin North Am 1986;19: 65–71.

10. Jones AS, Lancer JM. Vasomotor rhinitis [editorial]. Br Med J (Clin Res Ed) 1987; 294:1505–6.
11. Baraniuk JN, Kaliner MA. Neuropeptides and nasal secretion. J Allergy Clin Immunol 1990;86:620–7.
12. Fang SY, Shen CL. Neuropeptide innervation and neuroendocrine cells in allergic rhinitis and chronic hypertrophic rhinitis. Clin Exp Allergy 1998;28:228–32.
13. Lacroix JS, Kurt AM, Pochon N, et al. Neutral endopeptidase activity and concentration of sensory neuropeptide in the human nasal mucosa. Eur Arch Otorhinolaryngol 1995;252:465–8.
14. Rondon C, Dona I, Torres MJ, et al. Evolution of patients with nonallergic rhinitis supports conversion to allergic rhinitis. J Allergy Clin Immunol 2009;123: 1098–102.
15. Ellegård EK. Clinical and pathogenetic characteristics of pregnancy rhinitis. Clin Rev Allergy Immunol 2004;26:149–59.
16. Fokkens WJ. Thoughts on the pathophysiology of nonallergic rhinitis. Curr Allergy Asthma Rep 2002;2:203.
17. Varghese M, Glaum MC, Lockey RF. Drug-induced rhinitis. Clin Exp Allergy 2010; 40:381–4.
18. Ramey JT, Bailen E, Lockey RF. Rhinitis medicamentosa. J Investig Allergol Clin Immunol 2006;16:148–55.
19. Airaksinen L, Tuomi T, Vanhanen M, et al. Use of nasal provocation test in the diagnostics of occupational rhinitis. Rhinology 2007;45:40–6.
20. Raphael G, Raphael MH, Kaliner M. Gustatory rhinitis: a syndrome of food-induced rhinorrhea. J Allergy Clin Immunol 1989;83:110.
21. Sanico A, Togias A. Noninfectious, nonallergic rhinitis (NINAR): considerations on possible mechanisms. Am J Rhinol 1998;12:65–72.
22. Moore GF, Freeman TJ, Ogren FP, et al. Extended follow-up of total inferior turbinate resection for relief of chronic nasal obstruction. Laryngoscope 1985;95: 1095.
23. Tami TA. Granulomatous diseases and chronic rhinosinusitis. Otolaryngol Clin North Am 2005;38:1267–78.
24. Robson AK, Burge SM, Millard PR. Nasal mucosal involvement in lupus erythematosus. Clin Otolaryngol 1992;17:341–3.
25. Alobid I, Guilemany JM, Mullol J. Nasal manifestations of systemic illnesses. Curr Allergy Asthma Rep 2004;4:208–16.
26. Jacobs RL, Freedman PM, Boswell RN. Nonallergic rhinitis with eosinophilia (NARES syndrome): clinical and immunologic presentation. J Allergy Clin Immunol 1981;67:253.
27. Dykewicz MS, Hamilos DL. Rhinitis and sinusitis. J Allergy Clin Immunol 2010; 125:S103–15.
28. Ellis AK, Keith PK. Nonallergic rhinitis with eosinophilia syndrome. Curr Allergy Asthma Rep 2006;6:215–20.
29. Kramer MF, de la Chaux R, Fintelmann R, et al. NARES: a risk factor for obstructive sleep apnea? Am J Otolaryngol 2004;25:173–7.
30. Mullarkey MF, Hill JS, Webb DR. Allergic and nonallergic rhinitis: their characterization with attention to the meaning of nasal eosinophilia. J Allergy Clin Immunol 1980;65:122–6.
31. Smith TL. Vasomotor rhinitis is not a wastebasket diagnosis. Arch Otolaryngol Head Neck Surg 2003;129:584.
32. Gendo K, Larson EB. Evidence-based diagnostic strategies for evaluating allergic rhinitis. Ann Intern Med 2004;140:278–89.

33. Condo H, Nachtigal D, Frenkiel S, et al. Effect of steroids on nasal inflammatory cells and cytokine profile. Laryngoscope 1999;109:91–7.
34. Lieberman P. Treatment update: non-allergic rhinitis. Allergy Asthma Proc 2001; 22:199–202.
35. Scadding GK, Lund VJ, Jacques LA, et al. A placebo-controlled study of fluticasone propionate aqueous nasal spray and beclomethasone dipropionate in perennial rhinitis: efficacy in allergic and non-allergic perennial rhinitis. Clin Exp Allergy 1995;25:737–43.
36. Bosquet J, van Cauwenberge P, Khaltaev N, et al. Allergic rhinitis and its impact on asthma (ARIA). In collaboration with the World Health Organization. Executive Summary of the Workshop Report. Allergy 2002;57:841–55.
37. Banov CH, Lieberman P. Efficacy of azelastine nasal spray in the treatment of vasomotor (perennial nonallergic) rhinitis. Ann Allergy Asthma Immunol 2001; 86:28–35.
38. Shinoda M, Watanabe N, Suko T, et al. Effects of substance P (SP) and vasoactive intestinal peptide (VIP) in nasal secretions. Am J Rhinol 1997;11:237–41.
39. Takao A, Shimoda T, Matsuse H, et al. Inhibitory effects of azelastine hydrochloride in alcohol-induced asthma. Ann Allergy Asthma Immunol 1999;82:390–4.
40. Ciprandi G, Prozanto C, Passlacqua G, et al. Topical azelastine reduces eosinophilic activation and intracellular adhesion molecule-1 expression on nasal epithelial cells: an anti-allergic activity. J Allergy Clin Immunol 1996;981:1088–96.
41. Yoneda K, Yamamoto T, Ueta E, et al. Suppression by azelastine hydrochloride of NF-kappa B activation involved in generation of cytokines and nitric oxide. Jpn J Pharmacol 1997;73:145–53.
42. Bronsky EA, Druce H, Findlay SR, et al. A clinical trial of ipratropium bromide nasal spray in patients with perennial nonallergic rhinitis. J Allergy Clin Immunol 1995;95:1117–22.
43. Kaliner M. Progressive management strategies in the treatment of rhinitis. Allergy Asthma Proc 2003;24:163–9.

Differential Diagnosis in Allergy

Robert J. Stachler, MD*, Samer Al-khudari, MD

KEYWORDS

- Allergy differential diagnosis • Otologic diseases
- Otitis media with effusion • Eustachian tube dysfunction
- Ménière's disease • Nonallergic rhinitis
- Laryngopharyngeal reflux • Eosinophilic esophagitis

Key Points: Differential Diagnosis in Allergy

- A thorough history and physical examination of the head and neck is paramount to an appropriate diagnosis of allergic and nonallergic diseases
- Otologic disease can be mediated by allergic and nonallergic mechanisms
- Structural anatomic problems—tonsillar and adenoid hypertrophy, septal deviation, nasal masses, laryngeal, and pharyngeal masses—should be readily diagnosed and managed to give the patient the best outcome
- Laryngopharyngeal reflux and eosinophilic esophagitis commonly mimic each other, with the latter often mediated by food hypersensitivities.

OVERVIEW: DIFFERENTIAL DIAGNOSIS OF ALLERGY

An otolaryngic allergist addresses a vast myriad of complaints. Many conditions need to be ruled out before the diagnosis of allergy can be made. This article discusses the differential diagnoses that need to be considered during the allergic evaluation. Using a local-regional discussion, the initial step in creating a differential diagnosis is a thorough history and physical examination of the head and neck. The physical examination should include a complete ear, nose, and throat evaluation with a microscopic ear examination and/or endoscopic nasal endoscopy, if indicated. The larynx and supraglottic area can be visualized with a mirror, a straight rod (using a 30°–70° scope), or a flexible fiberoptic scope, if the anatomy or gag reflex precludes the aforementioned techniques. Cincik and Ferguson[1] noted patients preferred examinations

The authors have nothing to disclose.
Department of Otolaryngology Head and Neck Surgery, Henry Ford Health Systems, 2799 West Grand Boulevard K8, Detroit, MI, USA
* Corresponding author.
E-mail address: rstachl1@hfhs.org

Otolaryngol Clin N Am 44 (2011) 561–590
doi:10.1016/j.otc.2011.03.017
oto.theclinics.com

with a 30° rigid scope. This technique afforded superior visualization of the nose and larynx. Videostroboscopy of the larynx is reserved for specific voice complaints or vocal dysfunction. Swallowing and laryngopharyngeal reflux complaints may require transnasal esophagoscopy. **Table 1** lists a few of the common conditions that may be confused with allergy, which are outlined in the following sections.

OTOLOGIC CONDITIONS

There are many otologic conditions that may have a similar presentation to allergy. Otitis media (OM) refers to an inflammatory condition of the middle ear and does not refer to etiology or pathogenesis. OM has been subdivided into various subcategories: otitis media with effusion (OME), acute otitis media (AOM), recurrent acute otitis media (RAOM), and chronic otitis media with effusion (COM) Middle ear effusion is defined by the type of fluid noted behind the tympanic membrane. The fluid may be thick and viscous (mucoid), thin and watery (serous), or purulent (filled with pus). The duration of the disease is also used to classify the process: acute (0–3 weeks), subacute (3–12 weeks), and chronic (longer than 12 weeks).

Otitis Media with Effusion

OME is defined as a middle ear space with fluid in the absence of an acute ear infection. OM and OME represent greater than 2.2 million episodes diagnosed per year in the United States.[1–3] OME is most prevalent in early childhood. Screening surveys have reported a point prevalence of middle ear effusion from infancy to age 5 years to range between 15% and 40%. The peak incidence is in the winter months.[3–8] Allergy has been believed to play a major role in OME and is detailed in the article by Hurst elsewhere in this issue.[9] On otoscopy, fluid is present without evidence of infection (**Fig. 1**). Many investigators have established a link between IgE-related diseases and OME.[9–12]

Acute Otitis Media

AOM is a viral or bacterial infection associated with fever, ear pain, irritability, and may be associated with a concurrent upper respiratory tract infection. AOM is the most common childhood infection for which antibiotics are prescribed in the United States.[13–15] The diagnosis is most closely associated with otoscopic findings of tympanic membrane bulging or redness. Coker and colleagues[16,17] determined that otoscopic findings were critical in detecting the disease relative to subjective findings or complaints. The diagnosis of RAOM is made when recurrent ear infections are noted. The exact underlying mechanism is poorly understood and multifactorial. Risk factors associated with developing RAOM include male gender, sibling history of recurrent OM, early occurrence of infection, day-care attendance, parental

Table 1
Common conditions confused with allergy

Otologic Conditions	Nasal Conditions	Laryngeal Conditions
Otitis media	Septal deviation	Laryngeal masses or tumors
Eustachian tube dysfunction	Nasal tumors	Laryngopharyngeal reflux
Otitis externa	Nasal irritants	Dysphagia
Ménière's disease	Chronic sinusitis	Eosinophilic esophagitis
	Medication rhinitis	Globus (foreign body sensation)
	Nonallergic rhinitis	—

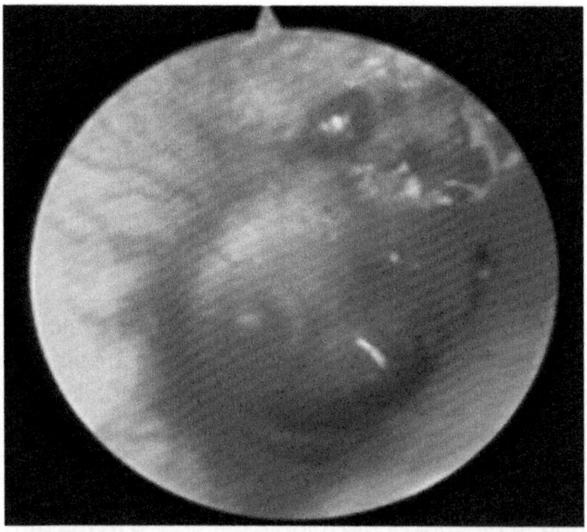

Fig. 1. Serous otitis media. Air fluid levels and "air bubbles" are present.

smoking, absence of breastfeeding, and second-hand smoke.[7] A meta-analysis by Uhari and colleagues[18] found that sibling history, day-care attendance, parental smoking, breastfeeding less than 3 months, and pacifier use are significant risk factors for AOM. COM has also be linked to underlying allergy (see Hurst and Venge[9]).

EUSTACHIAN TUBE DYSFUNCTION

The eustachian tube connects the middle ear with the pharynx. It is a key component of the middle ear cleft, which consists of the middle ear, the mastoid, and the eustachian tube. The tube extends from the anterior inferior portion of the middle ear to the nasopharynx. In adults the tube is 15 mm below the tympanic ostium at an angle 45°

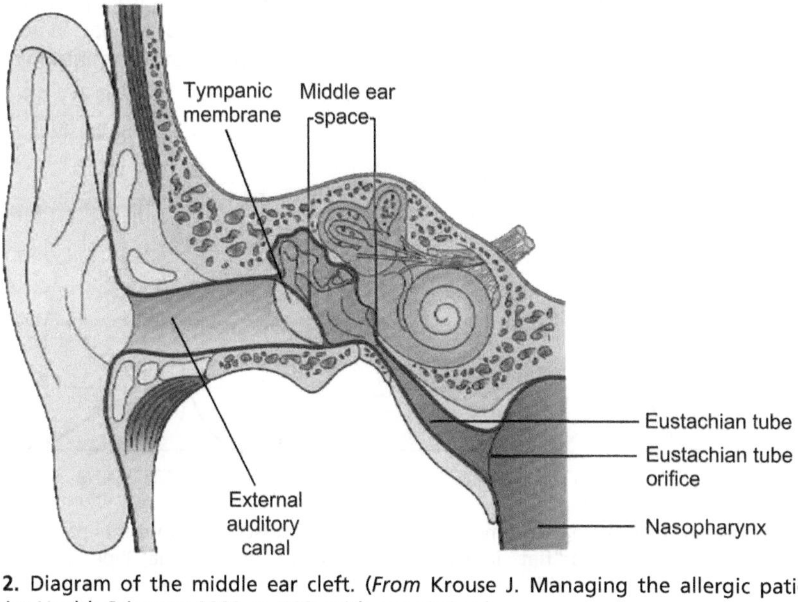

Fig. 2. Diagram of the middle ear cleft. (*From* Krouse J. Managing the allergic patient. Elsevier Health Sciences; 2008. p. 183; with permission.)

from the horizontal plane (**Fig. 2**).[19,20] In children the tube is significantly shorter, and is at an angle 10° from the horizontal plane.[19] This anatomic difference makes the middle ear cleft more vulnerable to inoculation with bacteria from nasopharyngeal secretions. The act of swallowing causes the tensor veli palatinae muscle to open and close the tube in order to ventilate the middle ear with atmospheric pressure.[19,21] The eustachian tube appropriately allows secretions to drain from the middle ear into the nasopharynx, and also offers protection from the nasopharyngeal secretions.[22–24]

Mechanisms of Eustachian Tube Dysfunction

Three main theories exist to explain why OM or OME develop. Some researchers believe that local inflammation at the nasal side causes retrograde edematous spread up the tube to cause obstruction. Others believe in a mucociliary dysfunction mechanism that results in physical stasis of secretions, resulting in mechanical blockage of the tube.[22,25] The last theory proposed describes the direct inflammatory changes within the tube itself that result in edema, vascular engorgement, and hypersecretion of the lining of the tube. A closure of the middle ear space to the atmosphere occurs.[26] Once the middle ear space is closed off, the air diffuses into the bloodstream (nitrogen first, then oxygen). The loss of air causes a negative pressure relative to the surrounding tissues. This negative pressure causes retraction of the tympanic membrane. The negative pressure developed results in a transudate to develop in the middle ear space.[26,27] Patients may complain of fullness or a pressure sensation in the ear. The tympanogram may be a B or C type, depicting fluid or a negative pressure, respectively (**Fig. 3**). The clinician must determine a cause for the tubal dysfunction and must carefully evaluate the ear and the nasopharynx for abnormalities.

Contact Dermatitis or Dermatophytid of the Ear

Contact dermatitis (A Gel and Combs type 4 hypersensitivity reaction, T-cell medicated) can occur as a result of using certain shampoos, perfumes, creams, or lotions. The metal in an ear ring (chromium or nickel) may cause a localized reaction (scaling, edema, erythema of the ear lobe). Ear drops or ear molds (made from plastic) from hearing aids may cause similar reactions in the canal or concha of the ear. In addition to contact hypersensitivities, the external ear is a common site of a dermatophytid or

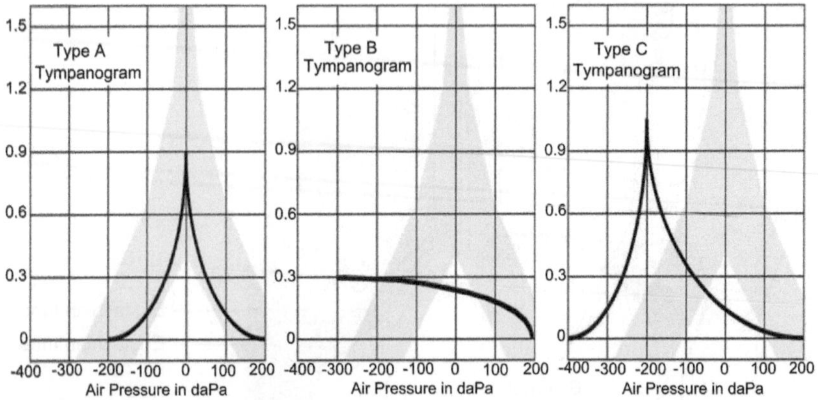

Fig. 3. Representative tympanograms: Type A, "normal pressure" in a normal patient; Type B, commonly referred to as "flat" in a patient with serous otitis media; Type C, "negative pressure" seen in patients with eustachian tube dysfunction. (*Courtesy of* Dr Brad Stach, Detroit, MI.)

ID reaction, characterized by preauricular or postauricular fissures and skin eruptions around the ear. This condition is a result of hematogenous spread of fungi or their allergic products (antigens) from the primary site of the fungal infection, usually the feet, to an alternative site on the body. Classic sites of the primary fungal infection are toe or fingernails, the skin, or vagina. *Tricophyton, Oidiomycetes* (Candida), and *Epidermophyton* are collectively referred to as TOE fungi, and are the most common fungi responsible for this reaction.[28–30] On identification of a possible ID reaction, the otolaryngic allergist should investigate fungal infections in other areas of the body so to not overlook these abnormalities.

Ménière's Disease and its Mimics

There has been growing evidence that Ménière's disease is partly related to allergic disease; this is comprehensively reviewed in the article elsewhere in this issue on Ménière's disease. Ménière's disease is characterized by aural fullness, fluctuating hearing loss, tinnitus, and vertigo. Patients with Ménière's disease may be disproportionately afflicted by benign positional vertigo (BPV). Aural fullness can be simulated by eustachian tube dysfunction and Ménière's disease. Tinnitus is frequently associated with sensorineural hearing loss; however, when this hearing loss is in the low frequencies, the likelihood that Ménière's disease is the cause is greater than for the more common high-frequency hearing loss associated with presbycusis and loud noise exposure.

NASAL CONDITIONS

The differential diagnosis for nonallergic nasal congestion is large. Nasal congestion may occur as a result of the normal ebb and flow of the autonomic nervous system (the nasal cycle), or may occur with changes in the environment or inflammation locally at the mucosal level due to antigens. Nasal congestion may be the result of mucosal edema from an infection or hormonal changes. Physiologic nasal congestion appears to have the greatest effect on the turbinates. Usually this is not a problem unless a significant septal deviation or turbinate hypertrophy exists. Anterior rhinoscopy will miss significant pathology, especially when there is a septal deviation or when the turbinates obstruct and limit the examination. The most anterior source of nasal obstruction, often missed on examination with a nasal speculum or nasal endoscopy, is obstruction at the nasal valve. The nasal valve is located at the caudal end of the upper lateral cartilage, bound by the septum and the anterior border of the inferior turbinate. This valve provides 50% of the total airway resistance.[31] Turbinate hypertrophy and nasal valve collapse are common findings, both of which give the sensation of obstruction to the patient.[32] It is important to determine whether the turbinate will respond to topical decongestion. Unresponsive turbinates suggest autonomic dysregulation and may need to be addressed surgically. Blue, boggy turbinates (**Fig. 4**) suggest nasal allergy or nonallergic rhinitis with eosinophilia, and require further workup.

Choanal atresia/stenosis is a cause of nasal obstruction, but is usually diagnosed at birth if bilateral; however, unilateral atresia may escape diagnosis for many years. Cleft palate may present with excessive secretions in the nose resulting from the palatal defect. Clefts are also associated with significant feeding issues in early infancy.

Nasal Masses

Nasal masses or enlarged adenoids cause nasal obstruction. Enlarged adenoids may need to be removed if they are obstructing the posterior nasopharynx. A differential diagnosis for tumors in the nasal cavity includes chordoma, chemodectoma,

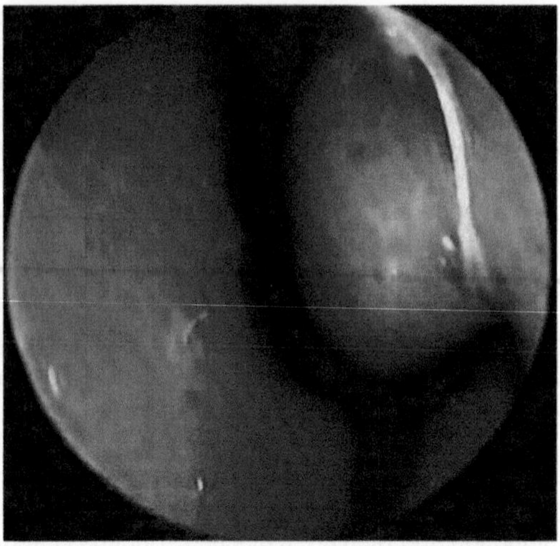

Fig. 4. Pale and boggy inferior turbinates in a patient with allergic rhinitis.

neurofibroma, angiofibroma, inverting papilloma, squamous cell carcinoma, sarcoma, encephalocele, or meningocele.

Nasal Irritants

There are several substances that may cause nasal irritation resulting in mucosal edema and erythema. Chemical exposures may result in type 1 (immediate) or type 4 (delayed) Gel and Coombs reactions. Repeated exposures are usually necessary to develop allergic reactions to various chemicals.[33,34] There are more than 3800 different chemical compounds in cigarette smoke that cause increased sensitivity of the airways to allergens. Passive smoking in children has been shown to lead to higher rates of childhood infections, higher middle ear effusion rates, decreases in pulmonary function tests, increased childhood asthma rates, and sudden infant death syndrome.[35,36]

"Sensory irritation" is acute and reversible eye, nose, and throat irritation that occurs after exposure to coarse particulate matter or water-soluble gases or vapors.[37] Nonallergic, noninfectious building-related illness or "sick building syndrome" is predominantly related to sensory irritation.[38] Indoor irritations include extremes of temperature or humidity, combustion products (poorly functioning combustion appliances, cigarette smoke, improper exhaust ventilation), volatile organic compounds (from furnishings) or reactive chemicals, such as cleaning products (ammonia, chlorine).[39] Environmental control with subsequent reduction of exposure to the noxious substance is recommended, if possible, to reduce nasal exposure.

Nonallergic Rhinitis

Nonallergic rhinitis (NAR) is defined as any nonimmune-related rhinitis, and consists of a cluster of syndromes that cause rhinitis. In 1998 Dykewicz and colleagues[40] noted, in a guideline of the Joint Task Force on Practice Parameters in Allergy, Asthma, and Immunology, that 50% of the patients who presented for allergic rhinitis actually had some other form of rhinitis. NAR may be triggered by endogenous or exogenous stimuli. The nose responds similarly in inflammation and irritation: sneezing, congestion, rhinorrhea, and itching. This response leads to similar presentation for allergy and NAR. NAR is considered a "diagnosis of exclusion" by many allergists. After allergy testing is negative, it is the clinician's responsibility to determine which diagnostic category best describes the patient's complaints.

Settipane and Lieberman[41] divided nonallergic rhinitis into 12 categories (**Box 1**). The different types are described briefly here. A complete description by Wilson and colleagues is available elsewhere in this issue and is beyond the scope of this article.

Vasomotor Rhinitis (Idiopathic Rhinitis)

In the article by Settipane and Klein,[42] vasomotor rhinitis (VMR) was the most common diagnosis in 61%, nonallergic rhinitis with eosinophilia syndrome (NARES) in 33%, sinusitis in 16%, BENARS (blood eosinophilia nonallergic rhinitis syndrome) in 4%, elevated IgE in 12%, and hypothyroid state in 2% of patients. VMR implies idiopathic, perennial, nonallergic rhinitis with a negative skin test, normal IgE levels, and with no inflammatory changes on nasal cytology. VMR symptoms are more obstructive/congested as compared with sneezing, rhinorrhea, and itching. Itching, sneezing, and eye irritation are more commonly seen in allergic rhinitis. At present, this disorder is thought to be related to excessive parasympathetic activity or reduced sympathetic activity of the nasal mucosa. There are other theories that have been proposed but lack definitive evidence.[43]

NARES

This disorder was first described by Mullarkey and colleagues[44] in 1980. Patients with NARES typically have more intense nasal symptoms of watery rhinorrhea, pruritus, sneezing paroxysms, hypoanosmia, and have negative skin or in vitro tests for allergy. Nasal smears are characterized by diffuse eosinophilia. Fifteen percent to 33% of the adults with NAR are found to have this condition.[42,44] NARES may be associated with Samter's triad (asthma [non-IgE mediated], aspirin sensitivity, and nasal polyposis) or may be a variant of this disease. BENARS is felt to be a subset of NARES, and is defined by elevated numbers of eosinophils in the peripheral blood.

Box 1
Types of nonallergic rhinitis

Vasomotor rhinitis (unknown etiology)

NARES (nonallergic rhinitis with eosinophilia syndrome)

Basophilic/metachromatic nasal disease

Conditions associated with sinusitis

Nasal polyp rhinitis

Metabolic conditions

Vaculitities/autoimmune and granulomatous diseases

Drug-induced rhinitis

Structurally related rhinitis

Atrophic rhinitis

Physical/irritative rhinitis

Occupational rhinitis

Data from Settipane RA, Lieberman P. Update on nonallergic rhinitis. Ann Allergy Asthma Immunol 2002;86:494–508.

Basophilic/Metachromatic Nasal Disease

Basophilic/metachromatic nasal disease, also known as nasal mastocytosis, is very similar to NARES, as both require histologic diagnoses.[45,46] The hallmark of this disease is mast cell infiltration of the tissue (>2000 per mm^3) with eosinophilia. Patients typically complain of nasal blockage, congestion, and rhinorrhea in comparison with the sneezing and pruritus seen in NARES. Pale boggy and bluish turbinates may be seen on examination. In contrast to NARES, nasal basophilic/metachromatic disease is not associated with nasal polyps, aspirin sensitivity, or asthma. Its etiology is currently unknown.

Conditions Associated with Sinusitis and Nasal Polyps

Chronic rhinitis does have a propensity to be associated with sinusitis, and is very common in our patient population.[47] These conditions are covered in other articles in this issue.

METABOLIC CONDITIONS

There are numerous metabolic conditions that can be a cause of NAR. Pregnancy, hypothyroidism, oral contraceptives, and estrogen replacement have all been associated with rhinitis. Rhinitis of pregnancy is characterized by obstruction and nasal congestion. There are a few theories regarding the physiologic cause of rhinitis of pregnancy. One is that the circulating blood volume is elevated, which may lead to venous pooling and nasal congestion. The second theory is nasal congestion arising from progesterone-induced smooth muscle relaxation. The third theory is nasal congestion due to the direct effects of estrogen on the nasal mucosa. Direct stimulation of the mucosa by estrogen causes nasal mucosal gland hyperactivity,[48–50] which results in excessive, thick secretions leaving the patient congested. It is imperative that these patients be treated conservatively.

Vasculitities/Autoimmune and Granulomatous Diseases

There are several systemic diseases that may cause rhinitis. Churg-Strauss vasculitis,[51] systemic lupus erythematosus,[52] relapsing polychondritis,[53] and Sjögren syndrome[54] are autoimmume-related diseases associated with nasal complaints. Granulomatous diseases, such as sarcoidosis[55] and Wegener granulomatosis,[56] have been noted to cause common nasal symptoms and should be considered in the differential of systemic diseases that may cause rhinitis.

Drug-Induced Rhinitis

There are several drugs that cause nasal side effects (**Box 2**). Aspirin and nonsteroidal anti-inflammatory medications are associated with upper airway reactions including nasal polyposis and asthma. Psychotropic agents (ie, thioridazine, amitriptyline, perphenazine) and antihypertensive medications (ie, α-blockers, β-blockers, angiotensin-converting enzyme [ACE] inhibitors, vasodilators) may cause nasal congestion or other nasal symptoms. Oral contraceptives and/or hormonal replacement are well-known causes of rhinitis.[57,58] With the increased use of phosphodiesterase type 5 inhibitors in men with erectile dysfunction, rhinitic complaints should trigger a discussion on medication use. Cocaine and topical decongestants/vasoconstrictors (ie, oxymetazoline, xylometazoline, phenylephrine, ephedrine) have been associated with rhinitis medicamentosa, and cause rebound nasal congestion and rhinitis. Decongestant use should be addressed when these types of complaints are mentioned during a patient encounter.

Box 2
Drugs with nasal side effects

Aspirin

Nonsteroidal anti-inflammatory medications

Psychotropic medications

Antihypertensive medications

- α-blockers and β-blockers
- ACE inhibitors
- Vasodilators

Exogenous hormones

Topical decongestants

Structurally Related Rhinitis

Anatomic defects account for 5% to 10% of the complaints in nonallergic rhinitis. The structural abnormalities that may cause rhinitis include nasal septal deviation, turbinate hypertrophy, adenoid hypertrophy, nasal valve collapse, or masses. These conditions are described in detail in previous sections of this article.

Atrophic Rhinitis

Atrophic rhinitis is typically encountered in too aggressive turbinate reduction, granulomatous diseases, trauma, radiation damage, and chronic cocaine use. In undeveloped countries, bacterial infestation secondary to *Klebsiella pneumoniae* subspecies *ozaenae* causes nasal cavity crusting, bleeding, fetor, and mucosal atrophy, also leading to atrophic rhinitis. The nasal mucosa changes from a functional ciliated columnar respiratory epithelium to a nonciliated squamous metaplasia type that is nonfunctional. Mucociliary clearance and neurologic regulation no longer occur. The patient complains of nasal congestion and obstruction due to the loss of the normal laminar flow of the nasal cavity. These patients' nasal cavities are usually widely patent on examination despite subjective obstruction.[59]

Physical/Irritant Rhinitis

This category includes physical changes in the environment including temperature, barometric pressure, inhaled substances, and ingested foods. Cold temperature changes have been reported to result in profuse rhinorrhea.[60,61] Facial pressure, headaches, and rhinorrhea are common nasal complaints in patients who are exposed to extreme changes in barometric pressures (ie, aviation workers and mountain climbers). Mast cell degranulation and stimulation of irritated nerve endings are felt to be the offending mechanism's pathophysiology.[61,62] Gustatory rhinitis occurs when a patient ingests a certain food, usually hot or spicy: mucoid or watery rhinorrhea ensues.[41,63,64] This reaction occurs acutely and lasts as long as the person is ingesting the inciting substance. Raphael and colleagues[65] have theorized that the afferent sensory nerves are stimulated. This stimulation activates the parasympathetic nerves that supply the nasal mucosal glands, which causes the rhinorrhea and associated sweating and epiphora that may accompany the symptom complex. However, skin testing with abstracts of the suspected foods is commonly negative.

Air pollution can occur indoors or outdoors. Known substances to cause nasal irritation include dust, sulfur dioxide, formaldehyde, wood smoke, cigarette smoke, ozone, and volatile chemicals.[66] Patients complain of dryness, sneezing, congestion, and rhinorrhea. The exact mechanism is unknown but has been theorized in the section on nasal irritants in this article.[33,34] Ozone and volatile chemicals have been shown to induce a neutrophilic influx in the mucosa.[67]

Occupational Rhinitis

The incidence of occupational rhinitis is estimated to be 5% to 15%.[68] A complete medical and workplace history is important because these patients have multiple complaints, including sensory abnormalities with altered sensations of smell. Patients may also have nosebleeds, crusting, impaired mucociliary transport, and nasal hyperactivity. Immunologic hyperreactivity is discussed in previous sections. Allergens may include animal proteins, wheat, latex, pyrethrum in insecticides or other garden products, acid anhydrides in adhesives, and toluene in body spray paints.[69,70] Annoyance reactions occur in patients with heightened olfactory awareness. These patients complain about perfumes, exhaust fumes, room deodorizer, cleaning agents, floral fragrances, and cosmetics. Irritant reactions occur when a specific respiratory irritant is inhaled beyond a threshold level. Air pollution and ozone are examples of irritants in large cities that are discussed regularly in the news. Tobacco smoke, toluene, paint fumes, nitrogen oxide, and formaldehyde are other examples of nasal irritant.[71] Chronic exposure to formaldehyde, wood, leather, dust, nickel, or chlorophenol is associated with hypertrophic mucosa, metaplasia, and carcinoma in some cases.[68] A corrosive reaction results after exposure to high concentrations of soluble chemical gases causing inflammation to nose, mouth, ocular mucosa, and skin. Mucosal and skin burns as well as ulcerations may occur. Chemicals known to cause corrosive reactions include ammonium chloride, vinyl chloride, hydrochloric acid, organophosphates, and acrylamide. Irritants cause neurogenic inflammation, which is believed to be the predominant pathway model for chemical sensitivity.[72] Irritant receptors on sensory nerves (ie, C fibers) induce neuropeptide release. Vasodilation and edema ensue, which results in a nonimmune-mediated inflammation.

ORAL CAVITY CONDITIONS

There are not many oropharyngeal mimics of allergy. Otolaryngic allergists should be comfortable diagnosing cobblestoning and/or redness on the mucosa of the posterior pharyngeal wall, when it exists, from chronic postnasal drainage and discharge. Tonsillitis, both exudative and nonexudative, should be straightforward. It is important that tonsillar and adenoid hypertrophy be recognized and removed when appropriate. In early childhood, "failure to thrive" and obstructive sleep apnea are common manifestations of children with clinically significant adenotonsillar hypertrophy. Prompt recognition and removal is most effective in these cases.[73]

Otolaryngologists are often called to see patients with lip or tongue swelling caused by angioedema in the emergency room (**Fig. 5**). A significant percentage of the patients are found to have angioedema from ACE inhibitors.[74] This response is felt to be non-IgE mediated and is related to the kinin metabolic pathway. One-third of patients with angioedema are admitted to hospital, while one-tenth require intensive care[75] dependent on the etiology and severity. Patients may complain of cough while on ACE inhibitors. This response tends to occur in females more readily than in males, and seems to occur early in therapy.[76,77] The cough is restricted to patients on ACE inhibitors and is not found in those on ACE blockers. Rarely, C-1 esterase inhibitor

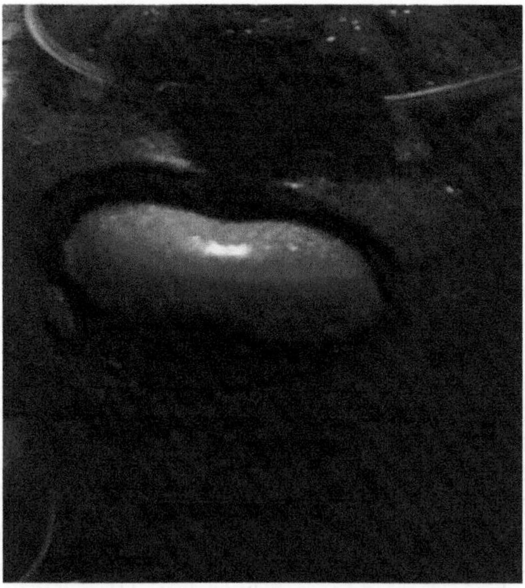

Fig. 5. Tongue and lip swelling in a patient with angiotensin-converting enzyme inhibitor–related angioedema.

levels need to be checked to rule out hereditary angioedema. Angioedema may also occur in severe anaphylaxis. Other signs and physical findings are usually present in these patients.

LARYNGEAL CONDITIONS

There are numerous laryngeal conditions that need to be ruled out before an allergic laryngeal diagnosis may be considered. Many conditions are diagnosed with a complete history and physical examination, including a laryngeal mirror examination or a flexible fiberoptic examination. Benign and malignant laryngeal lesions are considered in the differential diagnosis. Acute laryngitis needs to be differentiated from chronic laryngitis. Acute laryngitis may occur as a result of an acute infectious cause (bacterial or viral) or may occur in the setting of acute anaphylaxis or supraglottitis with vocal changes, but is almost always self-resolving within several months. Chronic laryngitis may be the result of vocal misuse, allergic changes, or laryngopharyngeal reflux (LPR). LPR is one of the most commonly encountered diagnoses associated with the symptom of postnasal drainage or vocal complaints. Often patients may exhibit both signs and symptoms of allergic laryngitis and LPR.

Laryngopharyngeal Reflux

Gastroesophageal reflux (GER) is the retrograde movement of stomach contents into the esophagus in the absence of belching or vomiting.[78–80] Gastroesophageal reflux disease (GERD) occurs when GER is associated with other signs, symptoms, or complications. LPR is retrograde flow of reflux material into the esophagus and larynx.

It is estimated that 30% of Americans suffer from GERD, while 7% to 10% experience daily heartburn and 25% to 30% have weekly symptoms.[78,81–83] Between 25 and 75 million Americans are affected by GERD.[83] Thirteen percent of all Americans use antacids 2 or more times a week.[83] The estimate of GERD in patients presenting to the otolaryngology clinic is been estimated to be 4% to 10%.[84] Fifty percent of the patients who were evaluated for speech and voice disorders in the clinics of Koufman and colleagues[85] had LPR.

Laryngeal inflammation is responsible for the signs and symptoms of LPR. These symptoms include a globus sensation, throat clearing, vocal fatigue, voice breaks, sore throat, neck pain, excessive throat mucus, chronic or nighttime cough, dysphagia, odynophagia, postnasal drip, halitosis, ear pain, laryngospasm, asthma exacerbation, diminished singing range, heartburn or regurgitation, and hoarseness. In addition, LPR can occur in a subpopulation of patients who do not have classic GERD. These patients present with laryngeal findings without the classic heartburn and substernal pain seen in GERD patients.[86] Belafsky and colleagues[87] developed a Reflux Symptom Index (RSI), which includes a self-administered survey of 9 questions used to assess patients with LPR. The instrument has proved to be reproducible and valid.[88] Each question has a rating from 0 (no problem) to 5 (severe problem). A score of 10 or greater is associated with a high likelihood of a positive dual-channel pH probe.[89] In another study, these investigators demonstrated that improvements in the RSI were noted before changes in physical findings occurred.[90]

Diagnosis is made using direct visualization of the vocal folds with a mirror examination, an endoscope, or a videostrobe. Physical findings seen in patients with reflux include laryngeal edema, loss of clear epithelial markings, hypervascularity of the posterior commissure and arytenoids, hyperkeratosis of the posterior commissure (pachydermia), increased mucous production, laryngeal ulceration, granuloma formation, subglottic stenosis, and pseudosulcus formation. This thickening of the undersurface of the vocal fold extends from the anterior portion of the vocal fold to the posterior commissure (**Figs. 6** and **7**). By contrast, true sulcus vocalis involves the free edge of the vocal fold and extends to the vocal process. The presence of pseudosulcus is sensitive and specific for reflux 70% and 77% of the time, respectively.[89] Other studies found the positive predictive value of pseudosulcus in detecting LPR to be 90%.[91]

A Reflux Finding Score has also been developed by Belafsky and colleagues.[88] This scale evaluates 8 findings associated with reflux. Seven of these findings involve edematous changes to the larynx and associated structures. Only one finding is associated with redness or erythema of these structures. Scores may range from 0 to 26. A score of 7 or higher is associated with a positive pH probe with a 95% certainty.

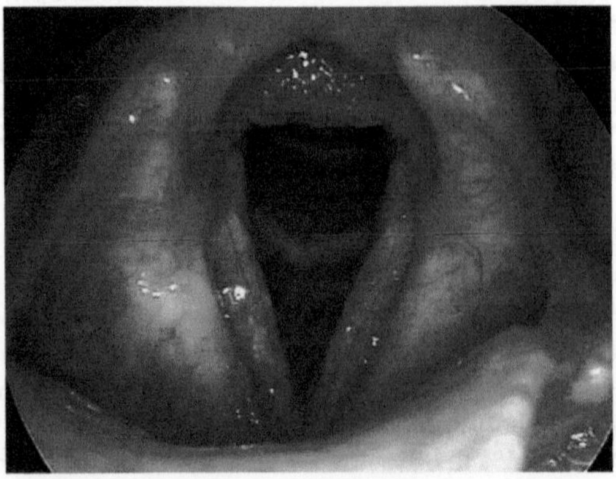

Fig. 6. Severe laryngeal pachydermia in a patient with laryngopharyngeal reflux. (*Courtesy of* Dr Glendon Gardner, Detroit, MI.)

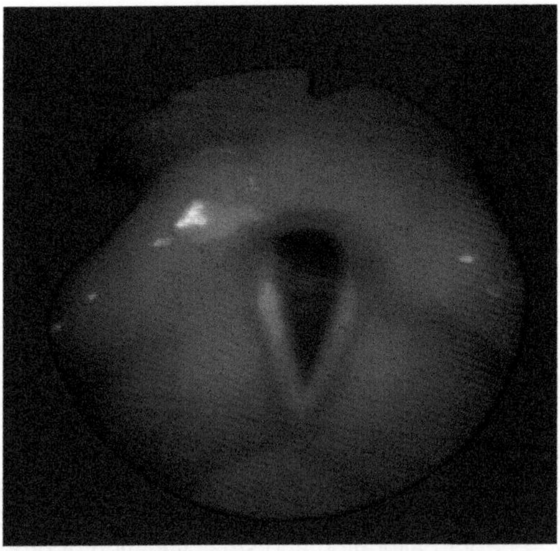

Fig. 7. Posterior glottic edema and erythema in a patient with laryngopharyngeal reflux.

Overall, this suggests that among all the aforementioned reflux findings, the clinical hallmark of extraesophageal reflux (EER) is edema as a result of reflux-induced trauma to the larynx.[89,92–94] EER is synonymous with the term LPR for the purposes of this article.

Diagnostic Testing for LPR

Diagnostic tests used to assess for reflux include an esophagogram, sensory testing with endoscopy, pH testing, monometry, impedance testing, and direct biopsy using transnasal endoscopy. A barium esophagogram may be useful to assess the esophagus for any type of structural or functional abnormality. An esophagogram is usually ordered together with a dynamic swallowing study to evaluate the whole swallowing mechanism at one time. The dynamic swallow is often performed with a speech and language pathologist. Findings that may be seen with this test include strictures, rings, webs, hiatal hernia, erosive esophagitis, candida esophagitis, cricopharyngeal bars, extrinsic compression, motility disturbances, aspiration, residuals in the pharynx, diverticula, and underlying neoplastic processes. Unfortunately, the sensitivity of the esophagogram in detecting EER is low (20%–60%) and its specificity is 64% to 90%, with an accuracy of 69%.[95]

Laryngeal Sensory Testing

Laryngeal sensory testing has been shown to be helpful in identifying EER.[94,96] The posterior laryngeal edema that results from reflux may be quantified with sensory testing. A pressure-generated pulse of air is delivered to the vocal fold, and the laryngeal adductory reflex is initiated to contract the vocal fold. As the edema progresses on the vocal fold, the puff of air required to elicit a response becomes much greater (5 mm or more). This test was found to be as sensitive and specific for reflux as the pH probe (50% and 83%, respectively). As patients improved with treatment, the pulse of air required to elicit a response decreased as the "neuropathy due to edema" improved.[96] Unfortunately, this method functions most as a research tool, as many otolaryngologists do not use a sensory testing device.

pH Probe Testing

The dual pH probe is considered the gold-standard test to assess for reflux. There is considerable controversy regarding the technique and what is considered a "normative" value. In addition, patient tolerance for the procedure is often poor. Merati and colleagues[97] performed a meta-analysis on 16 studies in the literature and found that laryngeal probe acid exposure time was reliable in differentiating patients with LPR from normal subjects. Some of the patients in this study who were considered to have LPR actually would have normal pH probes by gastroenterology criteria. These patients may have been suffering from other conditions such as nonacid reflux, sinusitis, allergies, and postnasal drip.[86] Dual pH probes are the accepted devices to identify EER. Postma[98] demonstrated that 59% of the patients he studied would have been inappropriately diagnosed as having a negative pH probe based on only one esophageal probe. The pharyngeal sensor was needed to make the diagnosis.[98,99] Fourteen percent of Koufman's patients[85] had a positive upper probe result despite a normal esophageal pH acid exposure time. Although the pH probe is the gold standard, the test is invasive, has a sensitivity of only 75% to 80%, and the false-negative rate may approach 50%.[100] Poor calibration and small variation of probe placement may affect the results.[98] Close monitoring of patient activities during the test is essential. Patient positioning, diet, reflux symptoms, and smoking habits should be carefully monitored.

While there is general agreement for normative values from the distal esophageal probe in determining whether reflux is present, controversy exists regarding the normative values of the proximal pH probe. Most researchers have agreed that a pH drop to 4 or less is considered pathognomonic for EER.[98,101] Others have documented that a small percentage of their normal subjects had proximal pH probe drops to 4 or less.[102–104] Still others such as Hanson and colleagues,[100] Contencin and Narcy,[105] and Koufman[106] believe these criteria to be too rigorous and note that pepsin, the main cause of tissue inflammation and damage, is active at pH levels of 5 or greater. In addition, reflux-related damage has been noted for days after the inciting event. In the larynx, defenses against reflux are virtually nonexistent on a mucosal level. Therefore, negative probe results need to be interpreted carefully. There are also vagally mediated reflux reflexes eloquently described by Shaker,[107] such as the glottic closure reflex and the cricopharyngeal/upper esophageal sphincter contraction reflexes, which may cause globus and laryngospasm in the face of distal esophageal exposure to acid.[107,108]

Wireless pH probe technology has been explored as an alternative to traditional pH probes. These probes consist of a transnasally or transpharyngeally placed capsule that may be attached to the mucosa of the esophagus; the sensor then detaches from the wall in about 3 days. A remote monitor on the waist records the data. These devices are capable of a longer recording time, providing more data for analysis. Their major limitation is that the proximal probe often cannot be placed close to the upper esophageal sphincter because of sensation at this area.[109–112]

Mechanisms of Acidic and Nonacidic Refluxate Damage to the Mucosa

Recent work by Johnston colleagues[113] has shown that pepsin exists in the laryngeal epithelium in reflux patients. When pepsin is incorporated into the cell via endocytosis, cellular cytotoxic events can occur. Pepsin does not require the presence of acid to remain active. Some investigators have suggested that pepsin may cause the depleted levels of carbonic anhydrase noted in the esophageal mucosa of LPR patients.[114–116] Carbonic anhydrase (CA) and its related isoenzymes CA-I through

CA-IV are present in esophageal mucosa where they can convert carbon dioxide into bicarbonate, which can move into the extracellular space and neutralize the acid. Decreased levels of the isoenzyme CA-III were found in the vocal fold epithelium of LPR patients.

Bile salts and acids in nonacidic refluxate may also cause damage to the laryngeal mucosa. Sasaki and colleagues[117] demonstrated that the bile salts taurocholic acid and chenodeoxycholic acid in an acidic and basic pH, respectively, produced laryngeal inflammation comparable to hydrochloric acid at a pH of 1.2. Localized inflammation clearly is the hallmark of this disease process, and needs to be reversed in order for healing to take place.

Monometry

Monometry is useful to assess for esophageal dysmotility and for weakness of the upper and lower esophageal sphincter contraction. Dysmotility is common in EER and can include ineffective motility, hypertensive lower esophageal sphincter, nutcracker esophagus (esophageal spasm), and achalasia.[118] Monometry has not been considered a useful a tool for diagnosing EER because of the short duration of testing, which may not accurately assess the transient relaxations of the lower esophagus that are thought to be important in the pathogenesis of EER.[95]

Impedance Testing

The multichannel intraluminal impedance device uses a pH sensor to detect nonacidic gastroesophageal reflux. Using electrical conductivity of the bolus in the esophagus, the device is able to distinguish between solid or liquid as well as direction of flow, antegrade or retrograde. Using the pH sensor, acid events are delineated from nonacid events.[119–123] Because persistent symptoms even after adequate acid-suppressive therapy have been attributed to nonacidic reflux events, impedance testing is likely to play a larger role in the diagnosis of this disease process in the future.

Transnasal Esophagoscopy

Further diagnostic testing may include transnasal esophagoscopy (TNE) with biopsy, which may show inflammatory changes to the esophageal mucosa. A diagnosis is made from looking at the amount of eosinophils per high-power field (HPF) that are present (in 5 or more fields). These histologic changes are felt to represent pathologic changes in the lining of the esophagus, even when the esophagus appears "normal." TNE has been found to be more than adequate to evaluate the esophagus. Dickman and colleagues[119] have demonstrated that the esophageal assessment is sufficient to diagnose reflux-related disease in patients with traditional esophageal reflux symptoms such as heartburn, regurgitation, and dysphagia, but who do not have gastric or duodenal symptoms such as abdominal pain, nausea, or a history of gastric or duodenal ulcer. Complete assessment of the stomach and duodenum is not necessary. TNE can be used to evaluate the esophagus in patients with suspected reflux disease to rule out Barrett esophagitis as well as adenocarcinoma. The presence of acid-induced reflux causes changes in the stratified squamous epithelium converting it to columnar epithelium normally present in the stomach mucosa. This condition is called Barrett esophagitis. Barrett esophagitis has been linked to adenocarcinoma.[124–127] Because the incidence of adenocarcinoma has risen significantly in the United States and western Europe (in some studies: 175%), early diagnosis of Barrett esophagitis may prevent patients from progressing on to adenocarcinoma. Similarly, early adenocarcinoma lesions may be identified before they are far advanced and cause dysphagia. Five-year survival rates of early esophageal cancer are 80% to 90%; but 5-year survival for symptomatic esophageal cancer is less than 10%.[127] Because cough and hoarseness are better predictors for esophageal adenocarcinoma than heartburn or regurgitation, patients with persistent laryngopharyngeal symptoms despite antireflux treatment should have an esophageal endoscopy.[128] TNE is safer than a traditional endoscopy, and avoids the cardiac and pulmonary complications associated with this procedure.[129,130]

ALLERGIC LARYNGITIS

Among voice specialists, it is well known that allergies play a significant role in patients with vocal complaints. Unfortunately, there have been few human or animal investigations that substantiate the current clinical findings. Chadwick[131] suggested that both upper and lower airway allergic inflammation can cause primary and secondary biomolecular and biomechanical laryngeal disturbance. Corey and colleagues[132] noted 2 types of allergic laryngitis: (1) acute, IgE-mediated (anaphylactic), (2) chronic, delayed, cyclic, non-IgE mediated. Research suggests that there are acute IgE-medicated laryngeal responses elicited by patients who were allergic to dust mites. Using antigen challenges, these patients were noted to have throat clearing, shortness of breath, bronchospasm, wheezing, coughing, and reduced FEV_1 (forced expiratory volume in 1 second) values.[133] The study was terminated prematurely, due to acute asthma exacerbation in 1 of 3 subjects studied and moderate side effects of wheezing and coughing in another of the 3. Chronic, non-IgE mediated reactions tended to be nonspecific and were difficult to differentiate from rhinitis, vocal abuse, lower airway reactions, and LPR.

The signs and symptoms that suggest allergic laryngitis are very similar to those seen in LPR: odynophagia, hoarseness, throat clearing, vocal cord edema, and coughing.[134,135] The otolaryngologist needs to carefully attempt to differentiate between the two when possible. Naito and colleagues[136] studied 30 patients with chronic laryngeal allergy who tested positive on skin testing for inhalant allergies and had laryngeal examinations. A characteristic finding for laryngeal allergy in this study was pale, glistening, and edematous arytenoid mucosa. Corey[137] evaluated more than 200 videostroboscopic images in patients who complained of nasal allergies and dysphonia. Her patients noted limitations in pitch range, frequent throat clearing, postnasal drip, chronic cough, and globus sensation. Findings consistent with laryngeal allergy included mild vocal fold edema, sticky-thick endolaryngeal secretions bridging the larynx, mildly edematous arytenoids, and hyperactive laryngeal reflexes. The viscous, thick mucous secretions seemed to be the most noteworthy finding of laryngeal allergy. In another study in the voice laboratory at Wayne State University, investigators examined two groups of patients: control (nonallergic) and dust mite–allergic individuals with allergic symptoms.[138] In an attempt to eliminate bias from reflux findings, all patients with reflux histories (GERD or EER) were eliminated from the study. Results from 15 different comparative phonation and respiration subsystem analyses showed no significant differences between the two groups of subjects. It is clear that future research is needed to help delineate specific laryngeal allergic findings from other complex and closely related clinical conditions.

EOSINOPHILIC ESOPHAGITIS

Eosinophilic esophagitis (EE) is a "new" disease identified in patients with esophageal eosinophilia unresponsive to the medical or surgical treatments of GERD. Confusion surrounding the diagnosis and management of these patients made it imperative that a precise definition and consensus statement be drafted. A multidisciplinary task force developed a systemic review and consensus recommendation for diagnosis and treatment of EE.[139] This panel described EE as a clinicopathologic disease characterized by (1) symptoms including, but not restricted to, food impaction and dysphagia in adults, feeding intolerance and GERD symptoms in children; (2) greater than or equal to 15 eosinophils per HPF; (3) exclusion of other disorders associated with similar clinical, histologic, or endoscopic features (especially GERD). The other conditions associated with eosinophageal eosinophilia are eosinophilic gastroenteritis, Crohn's disease, connective tissue disease, hypereosinophilic syndrome, infection, and drug hypersensitivity response.[140]

There has been a fourfold increase of disease prevalence in children with EE in the Midwest United States occurring from 2000 to 2003,[141] with an incidence of 1:10,000 children per year. This number remained constant over a 4-year period in Cincinnati. The prevalence of EE in Switzerland is 1:4000 patients.[142] EE occurs in 6% of the patients with esophagitis and in 6.5% of all adult patients undergoing endoscopy.[139,143] EE is common in young males with atopy.[139] It is frequently found in younger patients, but may be found in patients older than 90 years.[144] EE is a chronic disease without spontaneous remission.[145] Seasonal variations are seen in the disease and in inhalant allergens.[146] It has been identified in all continents except Africa.

Signs and Symptoms, and Presentation of Eosinophilic Esophagitis

EE's variable disease presentation initially made the disease difficult to define and diagnose. EE may present differently in various age groups. Children may present with failure to thrive, emesis, abdominal pain, dysphagia, GERD-like symptoms (heartburn and regurgitation), and food intolerance.[141,146–149] Adults tend to present with recurrent dysphagia and food impactions. These symptoms are usually refractory to antireflux treatment. The dysphagia is felt to be the result of impaired circular and longitudinal muscle function that occurs directly as a result of eosinophilic infiltration of the muscle. It improves once the condition has been adequately treated.[149–151]

Diagnosis and Histopathology of Eosinophilic Esophagitis

As stated previously, there is no diagnostic test for EE. EE is a clinicopathologic diagnosis based on the amount of eosinophils per high power field (eos/HPF) noted in a biopsy specimen in patients with clinical signs and symptoms of the disease. The threshold for diagnosis is 15 eos/HPF. A lower level of eos/HPF (>6) indicates GERD, whereas higher levels, 20–24 eos/HPF, tend to indicate EE, especially when patients are on anti-GERD therapy.[152,153] The number and location of the biopsies obtained is critical in making the diagnosis. At least 3 biopsies from the mid or distal esophagus are recommended, as the sensitivity for detecting EE is 97% when 3 or more biopsies are obtained.[139,154] EE appears to affect the entire esophagus, whereas in GERD eosinophils may be localized in the distal esophagus. EE may also be associated with mucosal changes, such as: basal cell hyperplasia and papillary thickening, not seen in GERD.[155,156] The diagnosis of EE is straightforward when endoscopic and radiographic findings of strictures, mucosal rings, ulcerations, whitish papules, and polyps are encountered (**Fig. 8**).[148,157] Thirty percent of the patients with EE have a normal endoscopy,[158] which make biopsies essential in making the appropriate diagnosis.

Pathogenesis of Eosinophilic Esophagitis

EE is significantly associated with atopy based on multiple co-occurrence studies, experimental animal studies, and the known success of avoidance-diets (allergen avoidance). Most patients are allergic to both food and aeroallergens, as determined

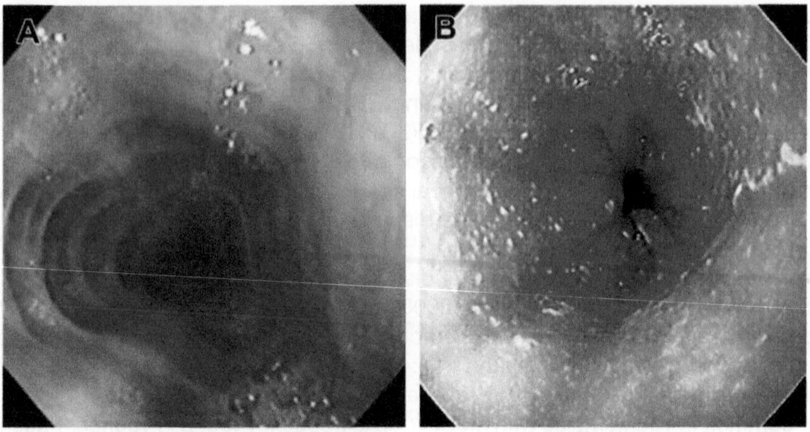

Fig. 8. Endoscopic findings associated with eosinophilic esophagitis (EE). (*A*) Mucosal rings representative of transient contractions or fixed strictures, also referred as trachealization or concentric rings. (*B*) Whitish exudates scattered across the mucosal surface; these represent rests of eosinophilic purulence bursting through the mucosa. (*From* Furata GT, Liacouras CA, Collins MH, et al. Eosinophilic esophagitis in children and adults: a systemic review and consensus recommendations for diagnosis and treatment. Gastroenterology 2007;133(4): 1342–63; with permission.)

by skin testing for foods or inhalants.[141,159] Multiple food allergies tend to be the rule rather than the exception. There are 6 major food groups that seem to be involved most commonly:

1. Wheat
2. Fish
3. Nuts
4. Bread
5. Milk
6. Eggs.

Avoidance, either by determining which foods the patient is allergic to (by skin-prick and patch testing) and removing them from the diet or complete removal of all 6 groups, has led to success in treatment.[160,161] In severe, recalcitrant cases, an elemental diet is instituted. Unfortunately, in many cases patients may require an enteral feeding tube.

Skin allergy may also play a role in the development of EE. Atopic dermatitis is believed to "prime" the patient for the development of respiratory-induced EE.[147] Many of the patients with EE report having a preceding episode of atopic dermatitis. Aeroallergens or food allergens induce T-helper (Th) cells to secrete interleukin-13 (IL-13) (**Fig. 9**). IL-13 induces hyperplastic epithelial cells in the esophagus to produce eotaxin-3.[162] Eotaxin-3 is a chemoattractant for the eosinophils in the bone marrow. IL-13 also induces overproduction of periostin.[163] Periostin is an extracellular matrix molecule that regulates eosinophil adhesion and assists in eotaxin-3 stimulated recruitment. IL-13 also downregulates flaggrin production. Flaggrin is a skin structure protein. Underexpression of this protein causes an increase in skin permeability and an increased susceptibility to atopic dermatitis. An increase in permeability results in further inflammation, which may enable acid to further erode the cell's defenses, thus allowing more antigen uptake into the esophageal epithelial cell and activating

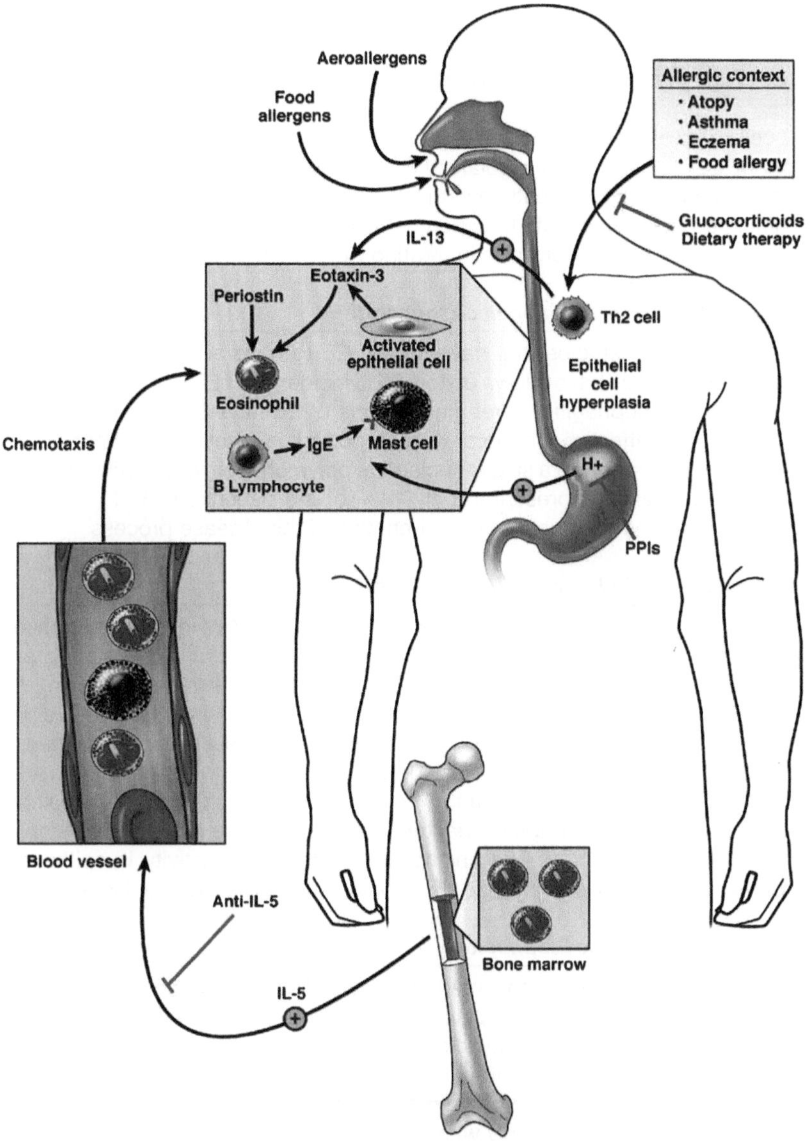

Fig. 9. Pathogenesis and treatment of EE. Aeroallergens, food allergens, and skin sensitization have been implicated in the pathogenesis of EE. Therapies such as an elemental diet, systemic glucocorticoids, and anti–interleukin-5 (IL-5) improve the microscopic features of EE, acting at different steps of pathogenesis. Determining the response to proton pump inhibitors (PPIs), which reduce gastric acidity, is important in the diagnosis of EE; inflammation is still present in patients following administration of these drugs. Allergens induce Th2 cells to produce interleukin-13 (IL-13), which can cause hyperplasic epithelial cells of the esophagus to overexpress eotaxin-3, and fibroblasts to overexpress periostin and downregulate filaggrin. Eotaxin-3 and periostin overexpression cooperatively chemoattract $CCR3^+$ cells (Th2 cells). Activated Th2 cells also produce IL-5, which regulates eosinophil numbers and their response to eotaxin-3. Inheritance studies indicate that there is a genetic component to EE; a single-nucleotide polymorphism in *eotaxin-3* has been associated with the disease. In addition to eosinophils, mast cells and lymphocytes (including B cells) accumulate in the esophagus to contribute to the local inflammatory responses observed in patients with EE. (*From* Rothenberg M. Biology and treatment of eosinophilic esophagitis. Gastroenterology 2009;137(4):1238–49; with permission.)

the B cells and mast cells. In situ production of immunoglobulins has been noted in EE patients.[164–167]

Th2 cells also express interleukin-5 (IL-5), which has been implicated in the pathogenesis of EE. IL-5 helps to regulate the eosinophil and increase its sensitivity to eotaxin-3. In animal experiments, overproduction or added IL-5 causes EE. Blocking IL-5 eliminates allergen, and IL-13 experimentally induced EE in mice. Anti–IL-5 medications have shown some promise in treating EE.[168–171]

Genetic Predilection for Eosinophilic Esophagitis

There are numerous studies that have shown EE to have a familial relationship.[141] Some pediatric studies have shown up to a 25% incidence of EE in a sibling or a parent with eosinophilic esophagitis. Three generations of EE have been reported in some studies.[172] Three affected brothers were reported in another.[173] Blanchard and colleagues[164] have reported a single-nucleotide polymorphism of eotaxin-3 in patients with EE, but this allele is present in only 14% of the patients with EE. Much more research needs to be conducted on the genetics of this disease process.

Eosinophil Function in Eosinophilic Esophagitis

Eosinophils are pleiotropic cells that participate in the adaptive immune response and propagate the inflammatory reaction.[174] The eosinophil contains secretory granules that contain 4 primary cationic proteins: EDN (eosinophil derived neurotoxin), major basic protein (MBP), eosinophil cationic protein (ECP), and eosinophilic derived peroxidase (EPO).[175] Eosinophils secrete cytokines (many interleukins), chemokines, lipid mediators, and neuromodulators. Eosinophils can directly present antigen to and regulate T-cell activities by modulating the release of its chemokines. Eosinophils can release mitochondrial traps for bacteria and can release tumor growth factor-β, which causes fibrosis.[176–178] The end result of eosinophil activity is epithelial cell hyperplasia, cell cytotoxicity, muscle dysmotility, and fibrosis of the tissue.

Treatment of Eosinophilic Esophagitis

Avoidance diets, anti-inflammatory medications, and surgical dilation are the mainstay of treatment. Patients are usually placed on anti-GERD medications. If they do not improve with these medications (histologically), patients are placed on selective diets to avoid the specific allergens that affect them. An elemental (amino acid based) diet can be used as well. Unfortunately, these diets are not very palatable and often require feeding-tube placement to comply with the nutritional needs of the patient. Selective diets may be difficult to determine because of the many food groups that patients may be sensitive to. Patch testing and skin-prick testing are used to make the allergic diagnosis.[139] Spergel and colleagues[160,179] demonstrated 77% resolution of the disease in their biopsy specimens after treatment with diets determined by both tests. A resolution of 98% was achieved in patients treated with an elemental diet.[148]

Corticosteroids, both systemic and topical, have been used to treat EE. Systemic steroid therapy is only necessary when urgent relief of symptoms is required. Severe dysphagia, dehydration, weight loss, or strictures are conditions that may warrant treatment. In 1998 Liacouras and colleagues[180] presented findings of clinical symptom relief (in 7 days) and histologic improvement (in 4 weeks) in 20 of 21 children with EE. Reported doses are 1 to 2 mg/kg/d (maximum 60 mg/d). Typically when the medicine was discontinued, the disease returned. Because of the long-term side effects and risk factors, systemic steroid treatment is not recommended unless deemed absolutely necessary.

Faubion and colleagues[181] were the first to describe the use of topical steroids to treat EE. Other studies showed improvement with topical steroid treatment. Complete resolution occurred in 75% of the patients. About 25% recurred after discontinuation of the treatment.[156,165,182,183] Reported doses are 440 to 880 μg fluticasone per day in children and 880 to 1760 μg in adults, in divided dosing 2 to 4 times a day for 4 to 6 weeks.

Dilation of the esophagus in these patients is tricky and is associated with mucosal tears, significant pain, and rare perforation.[184–187] A 7% to 50% recurrence rate was noted 2 to 24 months later.[184,185,188,189]

Antibody therapy, such as anti–IL-5, and anti–IL-13, has promising results for treating experimental EE.[162,169,190–192] Anti-IgE therapy may also be of benefit to reduce inflammation.[193] Human studies are ongoing, and future research will determine their effectiveness.

SUMMARY

There are many different diagnostic mimics of allergy. A thorough history and physical examination usually enables the clinician to avoid the various pitfalls that may complicate making an accurate diagnosis. An allergic diagnosis is made after ruling out a vast myriad of conditions. This article presents some of the most common conditions encountered in clinical practice.

REFERENCES

1. Cincik H, Ferguson BJ. The impact of endoscopic cultures on care in rhinosinusitis. Laryngoscope 2006;116(9):1562–8.
2. Daly KA, Hunter LL, Giebink GS. Chronic otitis media with effusion. Pediatr Rev 1999;20:85–93 [quiz: 4].
3. Rosenfeld RM, Culpepper L, Doyle KJ, et al. Clinical practice guideline: otitis media with effusion. Otolaryngol Head Neck Surg 2004;130(Suppl 5):S95–118.
4. Ziehuis GA, Rach GH, van der Broek P. Predisposing factors for otitis media with effusion in young children. Adv Otorhinolaryngol 1988;40:65–9.
5. Williamson IG, Dunleavey J, Bain J, et al. The natural history of otitis media with effusion—a three year study of the incidence and prevalence of abnormal tympanograms in four South West Hampshire infant and first schools. J Laryngol Otol 1994;108:930–4.
6. Thomsen J, Tos M. Spontaneous improvement of secretory otitis media: a long-term study. Acta Otolaryngol 1981;92:493–9.
7. Zelhuis GA, Rach GH, van der Broek P. Screening for otitis media with effusion in preschool children. Lancet 1989;1:311–4.
8. Bondy J, Berman S, Glazer J, et al. Direct expenditures related to otitis media diagnoses: extrapolations from a pediatric Medicaid cohort. Pediatrics 2000; 105:E72.
9. Hurst DS, Venge P. The presence of eosinophil cationic protein in middle ear effusion. Otolaryngol Head Neck Surg 1993;108:711–22.
10. Tomonaga K, Kurono Y, Mogi G. The role of nasal allergy in otitis media with effusion: a clinical study. Acta Otolaryngol 1988;458:S41–7.
11. Bernstein JM. The role of IgE-mediated hypersensitivity in the development of otitis media with effusion. Otolaryngol Clin North Am 1992;25:197–211.
12. Bernstein J, Lee J, Conboy K, et al. Further observations on the role of IgE mediated hypersensitivity in recurrent otitis media with effusion. Otolaryngol Head Neck Surg 1985;93:611–5.

13. Daly KA, Brown JE, Lindgren BR, et al. Epidemiology of otitis media onset by six months of age. Pediatrics 1999;103(6 Pt 1):1158–66.
14. McCaig LF, Besser RE, Hughes JM. Trends in antimicrobial prescribing rates for children and adolescents. JAMA 2002;287(23):3096–102.
15. Teele DW, Klein JO, Rosner B. Epidemiology of otitis media during the first years of life in children in Greater Boston: a prospective, cohort study. J Infect Dis 1989;160(1):83–94.
16. Coker TR, Chan LS, Newberry SJ, et al. Diagnosis, microbial epidemiology, and antibiotic treatment of acute otitis media in children: a systematic review. JAMA 2010;304(19):2161–9.
17. Baraibar R. Incidence and risk factors for acute otitis media. Clin Microbiol Infect 1997;3(Suppl 3):S13–22.
18. Uhari M, Mantysaari K, Niemela M. A meta-analytical review of the risk factors for acute otitis media. Clin Infect Dis 1996;22:1079–83.
19. Bluestone CD, Doyle WJ. Anatomy and physiology of the eustachian tube and middle ear related to otitis media. J Allergy Clin Immunol 1988;81(5 Pt 2): 997–1003.
20. Janfaza P, Nadol LB. Temporal bone and ear. In: Janfaza P, editor. Surgical anatomy of the head and neck. 1st edition. Philadelphia: Lippincott Williams & Wilkins; 2001. p. 420–79.
21. Fireman P. Otitis media and eustachian tube dysfunction: connection to allergic rhinitis. J Allergy Clin Immunol 1997;99:787–97.
22. Lazo-Saenz LG, Galvan-Aguilera AA, Martinez–Ordaz VA, et al. Eustachian tube dysfunction: in allergic rhinitis. Otolaryngol Head Neck Surg 2005;132: 626–31.
23. Takahashi H, Hayashi M, Sato H, et al. Primary deficits in eustachian tube function in patients with otitis media with effusion. Arch Otolaryngol Head Neck Surg 1989;115:581–4.
24. Miller GF Jr. Eustachian tube function in normal and diseased ears. Arch Otolaryngol 1965;81:41–8.
25. Bernstein JM. Role of allergy in eustachian tube blockage and otitis media with effusion: a review. Otolaryngol Head Neck Surg 1996;114:562–8.
26. Bernstein JM, Doyle WJ. Role of IgE-medicated hypersensitivity in otitis media with effusion, pathophysiologic considerations. Ann Otol Rhinol Laryngol Suppl 1994;16:15–9.
27. Bernstein JM. Allergic disease in the middle ear. In: Krouse JH, editor. Allergy and immunology: an otolaryngic approach. 1st edition. Philadelphia: Lippincott, Williams and Wilkins; 2002. p. 192–200.
28. Miller JJ, Osguthorpe JD. Physical examination of the allergic patient. In: Krouse JH, editor. Allergy and immunology: an otolaryngic approach. 1st edition. Philadelphia: Lippincott, Williams and Wilkins; 2002. p. 87–98.
29. King HC, Mabry RL, Mabry CS. Allergy in ENT practice: a basic guide. New York: Thieme Medical; 1998.
30. Dereberry MJ, Berliner KI. Allergy for the otologist: external canal to inner ear. Otolaryngol Clin North Am 1998;31:157–73.
31. Nurse LA, Duncavage JA. Surgery of the inferior and middle turbinates. Otolaryngol Clin North Am 2009;42:295–309.
32. Younger RA, Denton AB. Controversies in turbinate surgery. Facial Plast Surg Clin North Am 1999;7:311–7.
33. Belsito DV. Mechanisms of allergic contact dermatitis. Immunol Allergy Clin North Am 1989;9:579–95.

34. Zeiss CR. Reactive chemicals as inhalant allergens. Immunol Allergy Clin North Am 1989;9:235–44.
35. Frischer T, Kuehr J, Meinert R, et al. Maternal smoking in early childhood: a risk factor for bronchial hyperresponsiveness to exercises in primary school children. J Pediatr 1992;121:17–22.
36. Jindal SK, Gupta D, Singh A. Indices of morbidity and control of asthma in adult patients exposed to environmental tobacco smoke. Chest 1994;106:746–9.
37. Shusterman D. Toxicology of nasal irritants. Curr Allergy Asthma Rep 2010;3(3): 258–65.
38. Cometto-Muniz JE, Cain WS. Sensory irritation: relation to indoor air pollution. Ann N Y Acad Sci 1992;641:137–51.
39. Hendry KM, Cole EC. A review of mycotoxins in indoor air. J Toxicol Environ Health 1993;38:183–98.
40. Dykewicz MS, Fineman S, Skoner DP. Diagnosis and management of rhinitis: complete guidelines of the Joint Task Force on Practice Parameters in Allergy, Asthma, and Immunology. American Academy of Allergy, Asthma, and Immunology. Ann Allergy Asthma Immunol 1998;81:478–518.
41. Settipane RA, Lieberman P. Update on nonallergic rhinitis. Ann Allergy Asthma Immunol 2001;86:494–508.
42. Settipane RA, Klein DE. Nonallergic rhinitis: demography of eosinophils in nasal smear, blood total eosinophil counts and IgE levels. N Engl Reg Allergy Proc 1985;6:363–6.
43. Joe SA, Patel S. Nonallergic rhinitis. Chapter 46. In: Flint PW, Cummings CW, editors. Otolaryngology, head and neck surgery. 5th edition. Philidelphia: Mosby; 2010.
44. Mullarkey MF, Hill JS, Webb DR. Allergic and nonallergic rhinitis: their characterization with attention to the meaning of nasal eosinophilia. J Allergy Clin Immunol 1980;65:122–6.
45. Connell JT. Nasal mastocytosis. J Allergy 1969;43:182.
46. McKenna EL. Nasal mastocytosis. Laryngoscope 1974;84:112–5.
47. NIAID Task Force. Asthma and other allergic diseases. Washington, DC: N.I.A.I.D. Task Force Report; 1979. p. 23–31. US Dept. Of Health, Education and Welfare, National Institutes of Health Publication 79–387.
48. Toppozada H, Michaels L, Toppozada M, et al. The human respiratory nasal mucosa in pregnancy. An electron microscopic and histochemical study. J Laryngol Otol 1982;96:613–26.
49. Sorri M, Bortikanen-Sorri AL, Kanja J. Rhinitis during pregnancy. Rhinology 1980;18:83–6.
50. Schatz M, Hoffman CP, Zeiger RS, et al. The course and management of allergic diseases during pregnancy. In: Middleton E, Reed CE, Ellis EF, et al, editors. 4th edition, Allergy principles and practice, vol. 2. St Louis (MO): Mosby; 1997. p. 1301–42.
51. Olsen KD, Neel HB, DeRemee RA, et al. Nasal manifestations of allergic granulomatosis and angiitis (Churg-Strauss syndrome). Otolaryngol Head Neck Surg 1980;88:85–9.
52. Reiter D, Myers AR. Asymptomatic septal perforations in systemic lupus erythematosus. Ann Otol Rhinol Laryngol 1980;89:78.
53. Hughes RA, Berry CL, Seifert M, et al. Relapsing polychondritis. Three cases with a clinico-pathological study and literature review. Q J Med 1972;41:363–80.
54. Henkin RI, Talal N, Larson AL, et al. Abnormalities of taste and smell in Sjögren's syndrome. Ann Intern Med 1972;76:375–83.

55. Wilson R, Lund V, Sweatman M, et al. Upper respiratory tract involvement in sarcoidosis and its management. Eur Respir J 1988;1:269–72.
56. Fauci AS, Haynes BF, Katz P, et al. Wegener's granulomatosis: prospective clinical and therapeutic experience with 85 patients for 21 years. Ann Intern Med 1983;98:76–85.
57. Bachert C. Persistent rhinitis—allergic or nonallergic? Allergy 2004; 59(Suppl 76):11–5.
58. Schatz M. The safety of asthma and allergy medications during pregnancy. J Allergy Clin Immunol 1983;2:242.
59. Moore GF, Freeman TJ, Ogren FP, et al. Extended follow-up of total inferior turbinate resection for relief of chronic nasal obstruction. Laryngoscope 1985; 95:1095.
60. Naclerio RM, Proud D, Kagey-Sobotka A, et al. Cold dry air-induced rhinitis: effect of inhalation and exhalation through the nose. J Appl Physiol 1995;79:467.
61. Togias AG, Naclerio RM, Proud D, et al. Nasal challenge with cold, dry air results in the production of inflammatory mediators: possible mast cell involvement. J Clin Invest 1985;76:1375–81.
62. Proud D, Bailey GS, Naclerio RM, et al. Tryptase and histamine as markers to evaluate mast cell activation during the responses to nasal challenge with allergen, cold, dry air, and hyperosmolar solutions. J Allergy Clin Immunol 1992;89:1098–110 76.
63. Raphael GD, Hauptschein-Raphael M, Kaliner MA. Gustatory rhinitis. Am J Rhinol 1989;3:145.
64. Fokkens WJ. Thoughts on the pathophysiology of nonallergic rhinitis. Curr Allergy Asthma Rep 2002;2:203.
65. Raphael G, Raphael MH, Kaliner M. Gustatory rhinitis: a syndrome of food induced rhinorrhea. J Allergy Clin Immunol 1989;83:110.
66. Bascom R. Air pollution. In: Mygind N, Naclerio RM, editors. Allergic and nonallergic rhinitis. Copenhagen (Denmark): Munksgaard; 1993. p. 33.
67. Graham D, Henderson F, House D. Neutrophil influx measured in nasal lavages of humans exposed to ozone. Arch Environ Health 1988;43:228–33.
68. Olsen JH, Jensen SP, Hink M, et al. Occupational formaldehyde exposure and increased nasal cancer risk in man. Int J Cancer 1984;34:639–44.
69. Baraniuk JN, Kaliner MA. Functional activity of upper-airway nerves. In: Busse W, Holgate S, editors. Asthma and rhinitis. Cambridge (MA): Blackwell Scientific; 1995. p. 652.
70. Bardana EJ. Occupational asthma and related respiratory disorders. Dis Mon 1995;41:143–99.
71. Bernstein DI. Clinical assessment and management of occupational asthma. In: Bernstein IL, Chan-Yeung M, Malo JL, editors. Asthma in the workplace. New York: Marcel Dekker; 1993. p. 103–23.
72. Meggs WJ. Neurogenic inflammation and sensitivity to environmental chemicals. Environ Health Perspect 1993;48:14.
73. Darrow DH, Siemens C. Indications for tonsillectomy and adenoidectomy. Laryngoscope 2002;112:6–10.
74. Macy E, Melton M, Schatz M, et al. Drug allergy. In: Adelman D, Casale T, Corren J, editors. Manual of allergy and immunology. 4th edition. Philadelphia: Lippincott Williams & Wilkins; 2002. p. 208–18.
75. Brown NJ, Snowden M, Griffin MR. Recurrent angiotension-converting enzyme inhibitor-associated angioedema. JAMA 1997;278:232–3.

76. Coulter DM, Edwards IR. Cough associated with captopril and enalapril. Br Med J (Clin Res Ed) 1987;296:1521–3.
77. Abdi R, Dong VM, Lee CJ, et al. Angiotension II receptor blocker-associated angioedema on the heels of ACE inhibitor associated angioedema. Pharmacotherapy 2002;22:1173–5.
78. Gaynor EB. Otolaryngologic manifestations of gastroesophageal reflux. Am J Gastroenterol 1991;86:801.
79. Giacchi RJ, Sullivan D, Rothstein SG. Compliance with anti-reflux therapy in patients with otolaryngologic manifestations of gastroesophageal reflux disease. Laryngoscope 2000;110:19.
80. Gumpert L, Kalach N, Dupont C, et al. Hoarseness and gastroesophageal reflux in children. J Laryngol Otol 1998;112:49.
81. Hogan WJ, Shaker R. Management issues in supraesophageal complication of GERD. First Multi-Disciplinary International Symposium on Supraesophageal Complications of Gastroesophageal Reflux Disease. Workshop Consensus Reports. Am J Med 1997;103:149S.
82. Shaker R, Lang IM. Reflux mediated airway protective mechanisms against retrograde aspiration. Am J Med 1997;103:64S.
83. Sontag SJ. The medical management of reflux esophagitis, role of antacids and acid inhibition. Gastroenterol Clin North Am 1990;19:683.
84. Toohill RJ, Kuhn JC. Role of refluxed acid in pathogenesis of head and neck disorders. Am J Med 1997;103:100S.
85. Koufman JA, Amin MR, Panetti M. Prevalence of reflux in 113 consecutive patients with laryngeal and voice disorders. Otolaryngol Head Neck Surg 2000;123:364.
86. Ford CN. GERD related chronic laryngitis: Pro. Arch Otolaryngol Head Neck Surg 2010;136(9):910–4.
87. Belafsky PC, Postma GN, Amin MR, et al. Symptoms and findings of laryngopharyngeal reflux. Ear Nose Throat J 2002;81(Suppl 2):10 2002.
88. Belafsky PC, Postma GN, Koufman JA. The validity and reliability of the reflux finding score (RFS). Laryngoscope 2001;111:1313.
89. Belafsky PC, Postma GN, Koufman JA. The association between laryngeal pseudosulcus and laryngopharyngeal reflux. Otolaryngol Head Neck Surg 2002;126:649.
90. Belafsky PC, Postma GN, Koufman JA. Laryngopharyngeal reflux symptoms improve before changes in physical findings. Laryngoscope 2001;111:979.
91. Hickson C, Simpson CB, Falcon R. Laryngeal peudosulcus as a predictor of laryngopharyngeal reflux. Laryngoscope 2001;111:1742.
92. Beaver ME, Stasney CR, Weitzel E, et al. Diagnosis of laryngopharyngeal reflux disease with digital imaging. Otolaryngol Head Neck Surg 2003;128:103.
93. Branski RC, Bhattacharyya N, Shapiro J. The reliability of the assessment of endoscopic findings associated with laryngopharyngeal reflux disease. Laryngoscope 2002;112:1019.
94. Aviv JE, Liu H, Parides M, et al. Laryngopharyngeal sensory deficits in patients with laryngopharyngeal reflux and dysphagia. Ann Otol Rhinol Laryngol 2000; 109:1000–6.
95. Zalzal GH, Tran LP. Pediatric gastroesophageal reflux and laryngopharyngeal reflux. Otolaryngol Clin North Am 2000;33:151.
96. Aviv J, Pandes M, Fellowes J, et al. Endoscopic evaluation of swallowing as an alternative to 24 hr pH monitoring for diagnosis of extraesophageal reflux. Ann Otol Rhinol Laryngol 2000;109:S25.

97. Merati AL, Lim HJ, Ulualp SO, et al. Metaanalysis of upper probe measurements in normal subjects and patients with laryngopharyngeal reflux. Ann Otol Rhinol Laryngol 2005;114(3):177–82.
98. Postma GN. Ambulatory pH monitoring methodology. Ann Otol Rhinol Laryngol 2000;109:S10.
99. Postma GN, Belafsky PC, Aviv JE, et al. Laryngopharyngeal reflux testing. Ear Nose Throat J 2002;81(Suppl 2):14.
100. Hanson DG, Conley D, Jiang J, et al. Role of esophageal pH recording in management of chronic laryngitis: an overview. Ann Otol Rhinol Laryngol 2000;109:54.
101. Shaw GY. Application of ambulatory 24-hour multiprobe pH monitoring in the presence of extraesophageal manifestations of gastroesophageal reflux. Ann Otol Rhinol Laryngol 2000;109:S15.
102. Vincent DA Jr, Garrett JD, Radionoff SL, et al. The proximal probe in esophageal pH monitoring: development of a normative database. J Voice 2000;14:247.
103. Shaker R, Milbrath M, Ren J, et al. Esophagopharyngeal distribution of refluxed gastric acid in patients with reflux laryngitis. Gastroenterology 1995;109:1575.
104. Ulualp SO, Toohill RJ, Hoffman R, et al. Pharyngeal pH monitoring in patients with posterior laryngitis. Otolaryngol Head Neck Surg 1999;120:673.
105. Contencin P, Narcy P. Gastropharyngeal reflux in infants and children: a pharyngeal pH monitoring study. Arch Otolaryngol Head Neck Surg 1992;118:1028.
106. Koufman JA. The otolaryngologic manifestations of gastroesophageal reflux disease (GERD): a clinical investigation of 225 patients using ambulatory 24 hr pH monitoring and an experimental investigation of the role of acid and pepsin in the development of laryngeal injury. Laryngoscope 1991;101:S1.
107. Shaker R. Functional relationship of the larynx and upper GI tract. Dysphagia 1993;8:326–30.
108. Jadcherla S, Gupta A, Coley D, et al. Esophago-glottal closure reflex in human infants: a novel reflex elicited with concurrent manometry and ultrasonography. Am J Gastroenterol 2007;102(10):2286–93.
109. Chotiprashidi P, Liu J, Carpenter S, et al. ASGE Technology Status Evaluation Report: wireless esophageal pH monitoring system. Gastrointest Endosc 2005;62:485–7.
110. Marchese M, Spada C, Iacopini F, et al. Nonendoscopic transnasal placement of a wireless capsule for esophageal pH monitoring feasibility, safety, and efficacy of a monometry-guided procedure. Endoscopy 2006;38(8):813–8.
111. Ward EM, Devault KR, Bouras EP. Successful oesophageal pH monitoring with a catheter-free system. Aliment Pharmacol Ther 2004;19:449–54.
112. Wenner J, Johnsson F, Johansson J, et al. Wireless esophageal pH monitoring is better tolerated than the catheter-based technique: results from a randomized cross-over trial. Am J Gastroenterol 2007;102:239–45.
113. Johnson N, Dettmar PW, Bishwokarma B, et al. Activity/stability of human pepsin: implications for reflux attributed laryngeal disease. Laryngoscope 2007;117(6):1036–9.
114. Gill GA, Johnson N, Buda A, et al. Laryngeal epithelial defenses against laryngopharyngeal reflux. Ann Otol Rhinol Laryngol 2005;114:913–21.
115. Samuels TL, Handler E, Johnson N, et al. Mucin gene expression in human laryngeal epithelia: effect of laryngopharyngeal reflux. Ann Otol Rhinol Laryngol 2008;117:688–95.
116. Johnson N, Knight J, Dettmar PW, et al. Pesin and carbonic anhydrase isoenzyme III as diagnostic markers for laryngopharyngeal reflux disease. Laryngoscope 2004;114(12):2129–34.

117. Sasaki CT, Marotta J, Hundal J, et al. Bile-induced laryngitis: is there a basis in evidence? Ann Otol Rhinol Laryngol 2005;114(3):192–7.
118. Knight RE, Wells JR, Parrish RS. Esophageal dysmotility as an important co-factor in extraesophageal manifestations of gastroesophageal reflux. Laryngoscope 2000;110:1462.
119. Dickman R, Fass R. Ambulatory esophageal pH monitoring: new directions. Dig Dis 2006;24:313–8.
120. Mainie I, Tutuian R, Agrawal A, et al. Fundoplication eliminates chronic cough due to non-acid reflux identified by impedance monitoring. Thorax 2005;60: 521–3.
121. Orr WC, Craddock A, Goodrich S. Acidic and non-acidic reflux during sleep under conditions of powerful acid suppression. Chest 2007;131:460–5.
122. Tutuian R, Castell DO. Review article: complete gastro-oesophageal reflux monitoring-combined pH and impedance. Aliment Pharmacol Ther 2006; 24(Suppl 2):27–37.
123. Tack J. The role of bile and pepsin in the pathophysiology and treatment of gastro-oesophageal reflux disease. Aliment Pharmacol Ther 2006;24(Suppl 2): 10–6.
124. Naef AP, Savary M, Ozzello L. Columnar-lined lower esophagus: an acquired lesion with malignant predisposition: report on 140 cases of Barrett's esophagitis with 12 adenocarcinomas. J Thorac Cardiovasc Surg 1975;70:826–35.
125. Kocher HM, Patel S, Linklater K, et al. Increase in incidence of oesophagogastric carcinoma in the south Thames region: an epidemiological study. Br J Surg 2000;87:362–73.
126. Brock MV, Gou M, Akiyama Y, et al. Prognostic importance of promoter hypermethylation of multiple genes in esophageal adenocarcinoma. Clin Cancer Res 2003;9:2912–9.
127. Lund O, Kimose HH, Aagard MT, et al. Risk stratification and long-term results after surgical treatment of carcinoma of the thoracic esophagus and cardia: a 25-yr retrospective study. J Thorac Cardiovasc Surg 1990;99(2):200–9.
128. Reavis KM, Morris CD, Gopal DV, et al. Laryngopharyngeal reflux symptoms better predict the presence of esophageal adenocarcinoma than typical gastroesophageal reflux symptoms. Ann Surg 2004;239:849–56.
129. Chan MF. Complications of upper gastrointestinal endoscopy. Gastrointest Endosc Clin N Am 1996;6:287–303.
130. Bini EJ, Firoozi B, Choung RJ, et al. Systematic evaluation of complications related to endoscopy in a training setting: a prospective 30-day outcomes study. Gastrointest Endosc 2003;57:8–16.
131. Chadwick SJ. Allergy and the contemporary laryngologist. Otolaryngol Clin North Am 2003;36:957–88.
132. Corey JP, Gungor A, Kamell M. Allergy for the laryngologist. Otolaryngol Clin North Am 1998;31:189–205.
133. Dworkin JP, Reidy P, Stachler RJ, et al. Effects of sequential dermatophagoides pteronyssinus antigen stimulation on the anatomy and physiology of the larynx. Ear Nose Throat J 2009;88(2):793–9.
134. Alimov AL. The clinical symptomatology in the diagnosis of allergy in acute and chronic laryngitis. Vestn Otorinolaringol 1968;30:71–5 [in Russian].
135. Baroody FM. Allergic rhinitis: broader disease effects and implications for management. Otolaryngol Head Neck Surg 2003;128:616–31.
136. Naito K, Baba R, Ishii G, et al. Laryngeal allergy: a commentary. Eur Arch Otorhinolaryngol 1999;256:455–7.

137. Corey JP. Allergy for the laryngologist. Otolaryngol Clin North Am 1998;31: 422–6.
138. Krouse JH, Dworkin JP, Carron MA, et al. Baseline laryngeal effects among individuals with dust mite allergy. Otolaryngol Head Neck Surg 2008;139(1):149–51.
139. Furuta GT, Liacouras CA, Collins MH, et al. Eosinophilic esophagitis in children and adults: a systemic review and consensus recommendations for diagnosis and treatment. Gastroenterology 2007;133:1342–63.
140. Dahms BB. Reflux esophagitis: sequelae and differential diagnosis in infants and children including eosinophilic esophagitis. Pediatr Dev Pathol 2004;7: 5–16.
141. Noel RJ, Putnam PE, Rothenberg ME. Eosinophilic esophagitis. N Engl J Med 2004;351:940–1.
142. Straumann A, Simon HU. Eosinophilic esophagitis: escalating epidemiology? J Allergy Clin Immunol 2005;115:418–9.
143. Veerappan GR, Perry JL, Duncan TJ, et al. Prevalence of eosinophilic esophagitis in an adult population undergoing upper endoscopy: a prospective study. Clin Gastroenterol Hepatol 2009;7:420–6, e1–2.
144. Kapel RC, Miller JK, Torres C, et al. Eosinophilic esophagitis: a prevalent disease in the United States that affects all age groups. Gastroenterology 2008;134:1316–21.
145. Spergel JM, Brown-Whitehorn TF, Beausoleil JL, et al. 14 years of eosinophilic esophagitis: clinical features and prognosis. J Pediatr Gastroenterol Nutr 2009;48:30–6.
146. Orenstein SR, Shalaby TM, Di Lorenzo C, et al. The spectrum of pediatric eosinophilic esophagitis beyond infancy: a clinical series of 30 children. Am J Gastroenterol 2000;95:1422–30.
147. Walsh SV, Antonioli DA, Goldman H, et al. Allergic esophagitis in children: a clinicopathological entity. Am J Surg Pathol 1999;23:390–6.
148. Liacouras CA, Spergel JM, Ruchelli E, et al. Eosinophilic esophagitis: a 10-year experience in 381 children. Clin Gastroenterol Hepatol 2005;3:1198–206.
149. Noel RJ, Rothenberg ME. Eosinophilic esophagitis. Curr Opin Pediatr 2005;17: 690–4.
150. Desai TK, Stecevic V, Chang CH, et al. Association of eosinophilic inflammation with esophageal food impaction in adults. Gastrointest Endosc 2005;61: 795–801.
151. Mackenzie SH, Go M, Chadwick B, et al. Eosinophilic oesophagitis in patients presenting with dysphagia–a prospective analysis. Aliment Pharmacol Ther 2008;28:1140–6.
152. Ruchelli E, Wenner W, Voytek T, et al. Severity of esophageal eosinophilia predicts response to conventional gastroesophageal reflux therapy. Pediatr Dev Pathol 1999;2:15–8.
153. Rothenberg ME, Mishra A, Collins MH, et al. Pathogenesis and clinical features of eosinophilic esophagitis. J Allergy Clin Immunol 2001;108:891–4.
154. Shah A, Kagalwalla AF, Gonsalves N, et al. Histopathologic variability in children with eosinophilic esophagitis. Am J Gastroenterol 2009;104:716–21.
155. Collins MH. Histopathologic features of eosinophilic esophagitis. Gastrointest Endosc Clin N Am 2008;18:59–71, viii–ix.
156. Noel RJ, Putnam PE, Collins MH, et al. Clinical and immunopathologic effects of swallowed fluticasone for eosinophilic esophagitis. Clin Gastroenterol Hepatol 2004;2:568–75.

157. Fox VL, Nurko S, Teitelbaum JE, et al. High-resolution EUS in children with eosinophilic "allergic" esophagitis. Gastrointest Endosc 2003;57:30–6.
158. Dahshan A, Rabah R. Correlation of endoscopy and histology in the gastroesophageal mucosa in children: are routine biopsies justified? J Clin Gastroenterol 2000;31:213–6.
159. Fox VL, Nurko S, Furuta GT. Eosinophilic esophagitis: it's not just kid's stuff. Gastrointest Endosc 2002;56:260–70.
160. Spergel JM, Andrews T, Brown-Whitehorn TF, et al. Treatment of eosinophilic esophagitis with specific food elimination diet directed by a combination of skin prick and patch tests. Ann Allergy Asthma Immunol 2005;95:336–43.
161. Spergel JM. Eosinophilic esophagitis in adults and children: evidence for a food allergy component in many patients. Curr Opin Allergy Clin Immunol 2007;7: 274–8.
162. Blanchard C, Mingler MK, Vicario M, et al. IL-13 involvement in eosinophilic esophagitis: transcriptome analysis and reversibility with glucocorticoids. J Allergy Clin Immunol 2007;120:204–14.
163. Blanchard C, Mingler MK, McBride M, et al. Periostin facilitates eosinophil tissue infiltration in allergic lung and esophageal responses. Mucosal Immunol 2008;1: 289–96.
164. Blanchard C, Wang N, Stringer KF, et al. Eotaxin-3 and a uniquely conserved gene-expression profile in eosinophilic esophagitis. J Clin Invest 2006;116: 536–47.
165. Teitelbaum JE, Fox VL, Twarog FJ, et al. Eosinophilic esophagitis in children: immunopathological analysis and response to fluticasone propionate. Gastroenterology 2002;122:1216–25.
166. Lucendo AJ, Navarro M, Comas C, et al. Immunophenotypic characterization and quantification of the epithelial inflammatory infiltrate in eosinophilic esophagitis through stereology: an analysis of the cellular mechanisms of the disease and the immunologic capacity of the esophagus. Am J Surg Pathol 2007;31: 598–606.
167. Vicario M, Blanchard C, Stringer KF, et al. Local B cells and IgE production in the esophageal mucosa in oeosinophilic esophagitis. Gut 2010;59(1):12–20.
168. Garrett JK, Jameson SC, Thomson B, et al. Anti-interleukin-5 (mepolizumab) therapy for hypereosinophilic syndromes. J Allergy Clin Immunol 2004;113: 115–9.
169. Stein ML, Collins MH, Villanueva JM, et al. Anti-IL-5 (mepolizumab) therapy for eosinophilic esophagitis. J Allergy Clin Immunol 2006;118:1312–9.
170. Stein ML, Villanueva JM, Buckmeier BK, et al. Anti-IL-5 (mepolizumab) therapy reduces eosinophil activation ex vivo and increases IL-5 and IL-5 receptor levels. J Allergy Clin Immunol 2008;121:1473–83, e1–4.
171. Straumann A, Conus S, Kita H, et al. Mepolizumab, a humanized monoclonal antibody to IL-5, for severe eosinophilic esophagitis in adults: a randomized placebo-controlled double-blind trial. J Allergy Clin Immunol 2008;121:S44.
172. Zink DA, Amin M, Gebara S, et al. Familial dysphagia and eosinophilia. Gastrointest Endosc 2007;65:330–4.
173. Patel SM, Falchuk KR. Three brothers with dysphagia caused by eosinophilic esophagitis. Gastrointest Endosc 2005;61:165–7.
174. Rothenberg M. Biology and treatment of eosinophilic esophagitis. Gastroenterology 2009;137:1238–49.
175. Rothenberg ME, Hogan SP. The eosinophil. Annu Rev Immunol 2006;24:147–74.

176. Nizet V, Rothenberg ME. Mitochondrial missile defense. Nat Med 2008;14: 910–2.
177. Jacobsen EA, Ochkur SI, Pero RS, et al. Allergic pulmonary inflammation in mice is dependent on eosinophil-induced recruitment of effector T cells. J Exp Med 2008;205:699–710.
178. Walsh ER, Sahu N, Kearley J, et al. Strain-specific requirement for eosinophils in the recruitment of T cells to the lung during the development of allergic asthma. J Exp Med 2008;205:1285–92.
179. Spergel JM, Beausoleil JL, Mascarenhas M, et al. The use of skin prick tests and patch tests to identify causative foods in eosinophilic esophagitis. J Allergy Clin Immunol 2002;109:363–8.
180. Liacouras C, Wenner W, Brown K, et al. Primary eosinophilic esophagitis in children: successful treatment with oral corticosteroids. J Pediatr Gastroenterol Nutr 1998;26:380–5.
181. Faubion WA Jr, Perrault J, Burgart LJ, et al. Treatment of eosinophilic esophagitis with inhaled corticosteroids. J Pediatr Gastroenterol Nutr 1998;27:90–3.
182. Remedios M, Campbell C, Jones DM, et al. Eosinophilic esophagitis in adults: clinical, endoscopic, histologic findings, and response to treatment with fluticasone propionate. Gastrointest Endosc 2006;63:3–12.
183. Arora AS, Perrault J, Smyrk TC. Topical corticosteroid treatment of dysphagia due to eosinophilic esophagitis in adults. Mayo Clin Proc 2003;78:830–5.
184. Morrow JB, Vargo JJ, Goldblum JR, et al. The ringed esophagus: histological features of GERD. Am J Gastroenterol 2001;96:984–9.
185. Straumann A, Spichtin HP, Grize L, et al. Natural history of primary eosinophilic esophagitis: a follow-up of 30 adult patients for up to 11.5 years. Gastroenterology 2003;125:1660–9.
186. Vasilopoulos S, Murphy P, Auerbach A, et al. The small-caliber esophagus: an unappreciated cause of dysphagia for solids in patients with eosinophilic esophagitis. Gastrointest Endosc 2002;55:99–106.
187. Nurko S, Teitelbaum JE, Hussain K, et al. Association of Schatzki ring with eosinophilic esophagitis in children. J Pediatr Gastroenterol Nutr 2004;38:436–41.
188. Langton DE. Response to Straumann et al: primary eosinophilic esophagitis. Gastroenterology 2004;127:364–5.
189. Straumann A, Rossi L, Simon HU, et al. Fragility of the esophageal mucosa: a pathognomonic endoscopic sign of primary eosinophilic esophagitis? Gastrointest Endosc 2003;57:407–12.
190. Mishra A, Hogan SP, Brandt EB, et al. An etiological role for aeroallergens and eosinophils in experimental esophagitis. J Clin Invest 2001;107:83–90.
191. Mishra A, Hogan SP, Brandt EB, et al. Interleukin-5 promotes eosinophil trafficking to the esophagus. J Immunol 2002;168:2464–9.
192. Blanchard C, Mishra A, Saito-Akei H, et al. Inhibition of human interleukin-13-induced respiratory and oesophageal inflammation by anti-human-interleukin-13 antibody (CAT-354). Clin Exp Allergy 2005;35:1096–103.
193. Stone KD, Prussin C. Immunomodulatory therapy of eosinophil associated gastrointestinal diseases. Clin Exp Allergy 2008;38:1858–65.

Immunology of Allergy

Minka Schofield, MD[a], Karen H. Calhoun, MD[b,*]

KEYWORDS

- Immunology • Allergy • Immune system • T cells
- Regulatory cells • Chemical mediators

Key Points: Immunology of Allergy

- Understanding of the roles of the white blood cells in allergic reactions is continually expanding.
- T-regulatory (Treg) cells are recently described as immune modulators that probably play a key role in allergy immunotherapy.
- Basophils and eosinophils, originally thought to be mainly reactive cells, are proving to have extensive input in the developing balance between helper T cells T_h1 and T_h2 influences.
- Multiple chemical mediators play a role in modulating the allergic response, including histamine, cytokines, prostaglandins (PGs), leukotrienes (LTs), and chemokines.
- T_h2 cells are dominant in the allergic response and release interleukin (IL)-4, IL-5, IL-9, IL-13, IL-25, and IL-31 predominantly to promote T_h2 proliferation and recruitment of other inflammatory cells as well as IgE class switching.
- IL-17 family originates from a unique T_h17 cell and has a role in inducing chemokines, cytokines, PGE_2, neutrophil recruitment, and fibroblast activation. This family serves as a potential target for future therapies.
- PGE_2 is the most abundant PG with inflammatory effects dependent on receptor binding consisting of bronchoconstriction, bronchodilation, mast cell stabilization, and activation.
- LTB_4 and LTC_4 are the predominant LTs resulting in bronchoconstriction, vascular leakage, edema, and mast cell proliferation as well as cytokine generation.
- Chemokines are small proteins that function via a G protein–coupled receptor that serve as inducers of chemotaxis for various cell types with key roles identified in allergic disorders.
- IL-10, IL-35, transforming growth factor (TGF-), lipoxins, resolvins, IL receptor antagonist (IL-1ra), and suppressors of cytokine signaling (SOCS) molecules play a key role in down-regulating the immune response by decreasing the secretion of chemical mediators and promoting apoptosis of inflammatory cells.

[a] The Eye and Ear Institute, Department of Otolaryngology – Head and Neck Surgery, The Ohio State University Medical Center, 915 Olentangy River Road, Suite 4A, Columbus, OH 43212, USA
[b] Department of Otolaryngology – Head and Neck Surgery, The Ohio State University Medical Center, 915 Olentangy River Road, Suite 4A, Columbus, OH 43212, USA
* Corresponding author.
E-mail address: karen.calhoun@osumc.edu

Otolaryngol Clin N Am 44 (2011) 591–601
doi:10.1016/j.otc.2011.03.002
oto.theclinics.com
0030-6665/11/$ – see front matter

Knowledge of the immune system is advancing rapidly. Thirty years ago it was taught that specific immunotherapy for allergies worked by creating IgG antibodies that blocked incoming antigens before they had a chance to meet the IgE on mast cells and cause degranulation. Since then, it has been found that induction of allergen-specific, IL-10–producing Treg cells is a major mechanism driving the immune changes that occur during immunotherapy. This review provides an update on the allergy players—the cells and major mediators—and the form and function of each; discusses how these cells and mediators weave together in the elegant but destructive dance of allergy; and details how specific immunotherapy can cure allergy.

INFLAMMATORY CELLS

The cells of the immune system all begin as bone marrow stem cells. The initial differentiation is into either a common lymphoid progenitor cell or common myeloid progenitor cell (CMP). Common lymphoid progenitor cells become lymphocytes: T cells, B cells, or natural killer (NK) cells. CMPs become erythrocytes, monocytes, and granulocytes. B cells and T cells along with dendritic cells (DCs) or antigen-presenting cells (APCs) play major roles in starting an allergic response.[1]

Dendritic Cells

DCs (APCs) are the first stop for a new antigen entering a human body. DCs originate in the bone marrow and circulate peripherally as monocyte-like cells before entering tissue to become DCs. They station themselves mainly near skin and mucosa, the places where human tissue interacts with the outside world. Their primary job is to process pathogen or antigen for presentation to and activation of T cells. Monocytes and macrophages can also function as APCs.

When needed, this immature APC is activated, either by cytokines from other leukocytes of the innate immune system or by pattern recognition. Pattern recognition receptors, such as toll-like receptors, allow an immature DC to recognize incoming pathogens.

On activation, these DCs take up samples of pathogen or antigen from their local environment. The activated DC with antigen inside then travels via lymph to a nearby lymph node. The antigen phagocytized by the DC is broken up enzymatically into short polypeptide fragments. These fragments are loaded onto major histocompatibility complex (MHCs) molecules for display on the surface of the cell.

T Cells

T cells, in the meantime, travel from the bone marrow to the thymus. After acquiring T-cell–specific surface markers, they travel back out into the bloodstream and thence to lymph nodes. Some are $CD4^+$ (often called helper T cells), some are $CD8^+$ (often called cytotoxic T cells), and a few are T cells, which are CD4/CD8. They can also become Treg cells (formerly named suppresser T cells). NK cells are non–B-cell, non–T-cell lymphocytes.

Digested peptide fragments from within DCs in the lymph node can be loaded on major histocompatibility complex class 1 (MHC1) or major histocompatibility complex class 2 (MHC2) molecules. Peptide fragments plus MHC1 molecules present to $CD8^+$ T cells (cytotoxic T lymphocytes [CTLs]). Polypeptides with MHC2 molecules on the cell surface are meant to be read by naive $CD4^+$ cells. The DC with MHC_2 and peptide fragment sits in the lymph node, waiting to see if a naive T cell with its cognate comes by. Cognate means that the unactivated T cell is looking for exactly the same protein as is displayed on the APC's surface. If this match occurs and a second signal also occurs—in this case usually B7 on the APC surface plugging into a CD28 on the T-cell surface—activation of the T helper ($CD4^+$) cell occurs. These antigen-activated T cells then proceed with proliferation, making many copies of themselves.

Exactly which type of T cell develops depends on the local cytokines and other chemical mediators in the immediate environment. Traditional T_h1 cytokines—IL-2, TGF-, interferon (IFN)-, and IL-12—drive these naive T cells to become T_h1 cells. Similarly, IL-4 drives development of T_h2 cells; IL-23, TGF-, and IL-6 help drive development of T_h17 cells[2]; thymic stromal lymphopoietin (TSLP) influences DCs toward making more T_h2 cells.

Cytokines produced by T cells make an interwoven determination of immune responses, each dependent on many other cells and mediators. T cells are morphologically identical, differing in the cytokines they produce. T_h1 cells produce IFN- and tumor necrosis factor (TNF)-. T_h2 cells produce IL4, IL-5, IL-9, IL-13, IL-25, and IL-31. Both T_h1 cells and T_h2 cells make TNF-, granulocyte-macrophage colony-stimulating factor (GM-CSF), IL-2, IL-3, and IL-10. T_h17 cells make IL-17A and IL-17F, IL-21, and IL-22. T_h3 cells make TGF- and IL-10, and Treg cells and Tr1 cells make only IL-10.[3]

Treg cells suppress both T_h1 and T_h2 immune responses and help regulate self-tolerance and prevent autoimmunity. Naturally occurring Treg cells are $CD4^+CD25^+Foxp3^+$. T_h3 cells are active in gastrointestinal mucosal tolerance, and Treg suppression of gastrointestinal T cells helps maintain tolerance to commensal gut bacteria.[4] Induction of $CD4^+$ cells producing IL-10 is one mechanism by which immunotherapy may be effective.[5]

B Lymphocytes

In the bone marrow, the pre–B cell becomes a mature naive B cell. This part of the maturation is antigen independent and these cells all express IgM and IgD on the surface. These B cells are incredibly diverse in the antigens they are capable of recognizing—but each cell can only recognize a single antigen. The total universe of unactivated B cells can probably recognize just about any antigen the body might encounter. Each unactivated B cell roams through the lymph, hoping to meet up with the antigen it can recognize. If this unactivated B cell never meets its cognate, it dies unactivated.

This unactivated B cell has IgD and IgM on its surface. These are the same immunoglobulins the cells eventually secrete, with the addition of an amino acid sequence at the tip of the heavy chain that anchors it to the surface of the B cell, making a B-cell receptor. Once this B cell becomes activated, it produces both forms—immunoglobulin with the anchor to continually repopulate the cell surface and immunoglobulin without the anchor for external secretion.

Activation of the B cell requires more than just meeting up with its cognate antigen. It requires costimulation. Once the B cell meets its cognate, the still-unactivated B cell takes that antigen within the cell and then places it back on the cell surface with its own MHC2. This is recognized and joined by the appropriate $CD4^+$ T cell. In addition, the CD40 on the B-cell surface joins with the CD40L on the T-cell surface. These contacts initiate many actions and changes, including cytokine production and gene expression. The end result is activation of the B cell into an antibody-producing plasma cell. A few of these cells become B memory cells, which facilitate a quick response (rapid buildup of antibody production) if that particular antigen is encountered again in the future.

After activation, the B cells can also undergo isotype switching by somatic hypermutation. This changes the heavy chain DNA sequence so the cell can make IgA,

IgG, or IgE. Each individual cell, however, responds only to one antigen, and this does not change through the lifespan of the cell. Thus, a mature unactivated B cell with IgM and IgD on its surface that recognizes a specific amino acid sequence that becomes an activated IgE-producing plasma cell still makes only antibody to that original specific amino acid sequence.

These antibodies circulate looking for their antigen. When encountered, the typical antibody joins with the antigen to make an antigen-antibody complex, which is eliminated by complement or in the spleen or liver. IgE, however, mostly populates the surface of cells that express IgE receptors, such as basophils, mast cells, eosinophils, and others cells.

Mast Cells

Mast cells are granulocytes developing from bone marrow–derived progenitor cells under the influence of IL-3. They leave the bone marrow as immature cells, travel through the vascular system, out into tissue, where differentiation is completed.[1,6] As with DCs, they live primarily in skin and mucosa, the locations where contact with antigens occurs.

Once IgE antibodies are formed, they circulate in the blood for a short while before going into tissue and attaching to IgE receptors on mast cells, among others cells. When the appropriate antigen comes along, it can cause cross-linking of the surface IgEs, triggering release of preformed granules containing histamine and other allergic mediators. These include eosinophil chemotactic factors, bringing a concentration of eosinophils and release of their preformed mediators.

Increasing numbers of IgE molecules on a mast cell increase its sensitivity to antigen, requiring a lower dose to trigger degranulation. Anti-IgE therapy (omalizumab [Xolair]) takes advantage of this. The omalizumab combines with free serum IgE, making it incapable of binding onto mast cells, basophils, and other cells. This gradually reduces each cell's IgE surface population, making degranulation signals more difficult and thus less common.[7]

Eosinophils

Eosinophils are also granulocytes that develop from CMPs. They develop fully in the bone marrow and exit into the vasculature as mature eosinophils. They evolved originally to help bodies respond to parasitic infections.[1,6] They stain deep pink on hematoxylin-eosin stain. Eosinophils also express the high affinity IgE receptor, Fc-epsilon R1. When this receptor is activated, they release their granules containing peroxidases, lysozymes, major basic protein and eosinophil cationic protein. These cells increase in number during allergic inflammation and contribute to tissue damage.

The IL-5 produced by T_h2 cells is critical in the esoinophil life cycle, assisting with differentiation and maturation. Recent work suggests that eosinophils also have a role in initiating the T_h2 response and are present from early in this response cycle, rather than just responding after mast cell degranulation.[8]

Monocytes and Macrophages

Monocytes originate in the bone marrow and exit into the vasculature. Typically they circulate for a few days and then move out into the tissue where they mature into macrophages. These form an important part of the innate immune system. *Macro* means large and *phage* refers to eating. This big eater destroys pathogens by engulfing or phagocytizing them.

Macrophages express on their surfaces receptors for IgE and IgG. They can function as APCs. Mediators expressed by macrophages influence what type of T cell is expressed after activation. Monocytes and macrophages express both MHC1 and MHC2 molecules, so they can present antigen to both CTL and helper T cells.

Basophils

Basophils are the least common leukocytes in the peripheral blood, making up less than 1% of circulating white blood cells.[1,6] They are histologically nearly identical to mast cells and were for many years considered the circulating poor relation of the tissue-based mast cell. Both cells stain deep purple on hematoxylin-eosin stain. Both also express high-affinity IgE receptors, enabling cross-linking to initiate release of preformed inflammatory mediators. Unlike mast cells, basophils complete their maturation in the bone marrow, then enter the peripheral circulation for their lifespan of approximately 60 hours.

Basophils were formerly regarded as primarily responder cells, meaning they released mediators in response to various stimuli. It now seems that these have a much larger role in the allergic response.[9] They produce large amounts of IL-4, IL-13, platelet-activating factor, and TSLP, setting the stage for a T_h2 slant to helper T-cell activation. IL-3 is required by basophils for optimal productivity.[1,6,10] Basophils can also serve as APCs.[11]

Neutrophils

Like eosinophils, mast cells, and basophils, neutrophils contain preformed granules, with inflammatory mediators. Neutrophils are the most numerous circulating white blood cells and are the first responding cells to any injury or inflammatory challenge. They live predominantly within the vascular system, going out into tissue in response to specific chemotactic and other mediator signals. These cells make up the majority of pus.

CHEMICAL MEDIATORS

The allergic response is a complex orchestration of these inflammatory cells and chemical mediators. The inflammatory mediators function to regulate the inflammatory response in many ways, such as promoting the migration of additional inflammatory cells, promoting the release of other chemical mediators, and modifying vascular permeability, mucus secretion, and bronchial smooth muscle tone.

Histamine

Histamine is probably the most commonly associated mediator of the allergic response and serves as a therapeutic target for controlling the inflammatory reaction via histamine blockers, such as antihistamines or H_2 blockers. Derived from the Greek word for tissue, *histos*, histamine can be found in various tissues of the body, including the lung, liver, and brain. It is a low-molecular-weight amine synthesized from L-histidine and serves as a rapid, potent vasodepressor and smooth muscle constrictor. Mast cells, basophils, histaminergic neurons, and gastric enterochromaffin cells are the predominant source of histamine but mononuclear phagocytes, DCs, platelets, T lymphocytes, and B lymphocytes can also produce histamine. Histamine effects are primarily initiated by binding of histamine to various histamine receptors (HRs). Four histamine receptor types have been identified (HR_1, HR_2, HR_3, and HR_4), present on nerve cells, airway and vascular smooth muscles, hepatocytes, chondrocytes, endothelial cells, epithelial cells, neutrophils, eosinophils, monocytes/macrophages, B lymphocytes and T lymphocytes, DCs, and other organs of the body, such as the heart, colon, and lung.[12] Histamine effects on HR_1 are responsible for the development of allergic rhinitis, atopic dermatitis, asthma, and anaphylaxis. HR_2primarily functions as a negative feedback control of histamine release.

Cytokines

Cytokines are secreted proteins that modulate the immune response on multiple levels determining the onset of the response as well as the type of immune response. Through genomic studies, further classification and identification of new cytokines have been outlined and at least 70 cytokines have been proposed. **Table 1** outlines the various cytokine families and the associated members.[13] These proteins can function as proinflammatory, anti-inflammatory, or both.

Cytokines released by monocytes/macrophages predominantly include TNF, IL-1, IL-6, IL-12, IL-15, IL-18, IL-23, and IL-27. TNF is a potent activator of neutrophils, increases vascular permeability, and interacts with endothelial cells to induce intercellular adhesion molecule-1 and vascular cell adhesion molecule-1, promoting the migration of granulocytes. Lipopolysaccharide (LPS) is a potent activator of its release from monocytes. The IL-1 family consists of 5 types: IL-1α, IL-1β, IL-1ra, IL-18, and IL-33. IL-1 has an important role in activating T lymphocytes by enhancing IL-2 production and expression of IL-2 receptors (**Table 2**). IL-33 has been shown to have several proinflammatory functions in the allergic response, such as enhancing basophil adhesion, activation of eosinophils, attracting T_h2 cells, and promotion of IL-5 and IL-13 release from T_h2 cells.[14,15]

IL-6 has proinflammatory actions by promoting B-lymphocyte differentiation, secretion of immunoglobulins, and differentiation of T_h17 lymphocytes while inhibiting IL-1 and TNF synthesis and stimulating IL-1ra to down-regulate the immune response.

Table 1
Cytokine families

Family	Members
Hematopoietic	—
Common γ chain	IL-2, IL-4, IL-7, IL-9, IL-15, IL-21
Shared β chain (CD131)	IL-3, IL-5, GM-CSF
Shared	IL-2, IL-15
IL-2 β chain (CD122)	—
Other Hematopietic	IFN-γ, IL-7, IL-13, IL-21, IL-31, TSLP
IL-1 Family	IL-1α, IL-1β, IL-1ra, IL-18, IL-33
gpl30-Utilizing	IL-6, IL-11, IL-27, IL-31, ciliary neurotrophic factor, cardiotrophin-1, leukemia inhibitory factor, oncostatin M, osteopontin
IL-12	IL-12, IL-23, IL-35
IL-10 Superfamily	IL-10, IL-19, IL-20, IL-22, IL-24, IL-26, IL-28, IL-29
IL-17	IL-17A-F, IL-25 (IL-17E)
Interferons	—
Type I	INF-α, IFN-β, IFN-ω
Type II	IFN-γ
Type III	IFN-λ1 (IL-29), IFN-λ2 (IL-28A), IFN-λ3 (IL-28B)
TNF Superfamily	TNF-α, TNF-β, a proliferation-inducing signal (APRIL), B-cell activation factor from the TNF family (BAFF)

Data from Commins S, Borish L, Steinke J. Immunologic messenger molecules: cytokines, interferons, and chemokines. J Allergy Clin Immunol 2010;125:S53–72.

IL-6 signals through an IL-6R and signal transducer gp130 (CD30) along with other IL-6–like cytokines involved in the allergic response, such as IL-11, IL-31, and osteopontin.[13]

T cells also release specific cytokines key to the allergic response, which include IL-2, IL-17, and newly identified IL-34. IL-2 release promotes IL-2R expression and IL-2 production by effector T cells, resulting in T-cell proliferation specific to an antigen along with activation of Treg cells. The IL-17 family consists of IL-17A–D and IL-17F, which originate from a unique T cell, T_h17. Evidence suggests that IL-17E is derived from T_h2 cells rather than T_h17 cells, resulting in renaming this cytokine IL-25.[13] Biologic functions of this family include inducing the production of chemokines (CXCL8 and CXCL10), cytokines (GM-CSF, IL-1, IL-6, and TGF-β), and PGE_2 along with neutrophil recruitment and fibroblast activation.[13,14] Park and Lee[16] describe therapeutic strategies to modify IL-17 to control asthma via inhibitors of IL-17, IL-23, IL-1, and IL-6; agonists of IL-4 and IFN-; inhibitors of phosphodiesterase 4; vascular endothelial growth factor inhibitors; p13 and p38 kinase inhibitors; statins; steroids; PPAR and STAT3 transcription factor inhibitors; and omega-3 fatty acid products, such as resolvin E1.

IL-4, IL-5, IL-9, IL-13, IL-25, and IL-31 are predominantly released by T_h2 lymphocytes in the allergic response driving the inflammatory response by inducing cell adhesion molecules and chemokines. IL-4 is key to the initiation of the T_h2 response but also works with IL-13 to induce immunoglobulin class switching to IgE. IL-5 is key to eosinophil development and maintenance and also promotes histamine release from basophils. IL-25 stimulates the release if IL-4, IL-5, and IL-13 from Th cells and nonlymphoid cells, resulting in T_h2 proliferation, IgE secretion, and eosinophilia.[13,17] IL-31 induces chemokines involved in recruitment of neutrophils, monocytes, and T cells.

Table 2
Cytokine production from various cell types

Cell Type	Cytokine Produced
Mast Cells	IL-1, IL-3, IL-4, TNF-α, IL-5, IL-6, IL-10, IL-13, GM-CSF, TGF-β
Monocytyes/Macrophages	IL-1, IL-6, IL-10, IL-12, IL-15, IL-18, IL-23, IL-27, TNF-α, IFN-α, lesser degree IFN-γ, lesser degree TGF-β
DCs	IL-1, IL-12, IL-18, IL-23, IL-27, TNF-α,
Neutrophils	IL-1, IL-12, TNF-α, GM-CSF
Basophils	IL-4, IL-10, IL-13
Eosinophils	IL-1, IL-2, IL-3, IL-4, IL-5, IL-6, IL-9, IL-10, IL-12, IL-13, IL-16, GM-CSF, TGF-β, TNF
B Lymphocytes	IL-12, IL-10
T Lymphocytes	—
T_h1	IFN-γ, TNF-α, TGF-β, GM-CSF, IL-2, IL-3
T_h2	IL-2, IL-3, IL-4, IL-5, IL-9, IL-13, IL-25, IL-31 TNF-α, GM-CSF
T_h3	IL-10, TGF-β
T_h17	IL-17, IL-21, IL-22
Treg Cells	IL-10, TGF-β, IL-35
NK Cells	IL-4, IL-5, IFN-γ, TNF-α

IL-3 is released predominantly by T lymphocytes and is an important stimulator of hematopoietic cells, especially basophils. GM-CSF seems to have a key function along with IL-3 and IL-5 in prolonging eosinophil survival and promoting activation.

Chemokines

Chemokines are a special group of small 8- to 12-kDa proteins that induce chemotaxis in many cell types. They function via binding to receptors that are 7-transmembrane-spanning, G protein–coupled receptors. Various cell types produce these proteins, including leukocytes, platelets, endothelial cells, and epithelial cells. Approximately 52 types of chemokines have been identified and most are within 2 subfamilies, the CXC family, which targets primarily neutrophils, and the CC family, which targets eosinophils, monocytes, and T cells.[13] Other subfamilies include C family and CX3C. Several chemokines have been identified as playing a role in allergic disorders. Increased levels of CCL2, CCL3, CCL5, CCL7, CCL11, CCL13, CCL24, CXCL8, and CXCL10 have been demonstrated in asthmatic patients.[13,18,19] CCL5 and CCL11 seem the most important eosinophil chemoattractants in allergic inflammation. CXCL8 is one of the most potent chemoattractants for neutrophils in addition to stimulating neutrophil respiratory burst and adherence. CXCL10 seems to be released in the early phase of allergen exposure whereas CXCL13 is released after secondary or subsequent exposures.

Eicosanoids

Lipid-based mediators originate from the cell membrane and are known as eicosanoids. They originate from a cell-membrane precursor called arachidonic acid, which is converted to eicosanoids on cell perturbation from an infection, allergen, or injury. Once arachidonic acid has been released from the cell membrane, it is then converted by enzymes to various eicosanoids.

Prostaglandins

PGs originate from arachidonic acid conversion to PGH_2 by the cyclooxgenase (COX) enzymes. COX-1 is expressed in most cells and tissues and is primarily responsible for maintaining a static PG production whereas COX-2 is up-regulated by a wide range of inflammatory stimuli, resulting in enhanced production of PGs. $PGH_2$is further acted on by enzymes to result in various PG products, such as thromboxane A_2, PGD_2, PGE_2, and PGI_2. The major product of macrophages and bronchial surface cells is PGE_2 whereas mast cells primarily produce PGD_2. PGE_2 is the most abundant PG and has both anti-inflammatory and proinflammatory effects depending on the situation and the receptor, such as bronchoconstriction E-prostanoid-1; bronchodilation and mast cell stabilization E-prostanoid-2; and mast cell activation and inhibition of pulmonary inflammation E-prostanoid-3.[20] PGD_2 is predominantly released from mast cells and is associated with the inflammatory component of allergic asthma. PGI_2 is predominantly expressed by endothelial cells and has a major role in vascular homeostasis via a single receptor, IP. Its major function is to inhibit bronchconstriction and T_h2 cell cytokine production.

Leukotrienes

LTs result from arachidonic acid conversion to LTA_4 by 5-lipoxygenase enzyme. Further enzymatic actions result in multiple LTs with the 2 major classes of LTs being LTB_4 and LTC_4. LT production is restricted to cells of the myeloid lineage. Cys-LT receptor binding by LTC_4 and other LTs results in bronchoconstriction, vascular leakage and edema, mast cell proliferation, inflammation, and cytokine generation.[21]

LTB_4 receptor binding (BLT1 and BLT2) results in recruitment of neutrophils, eosinophils, $CD8^+$ effector/memory cells, and mast cell progenitors.[20,22,23]

Lipoxins and resolvins represent another group of eicosanoids, which serve to reduce the inflammatory response.[20,23] They are produced via various transcellular interactions occurring in endothelial cells, epithelial cells, and neutrophils.

Anti-Inflammatory Mediators

Suppression or down-regulation of the inflammatory response is essential to avoid excessive effects of the proinflammatory mediators. Previous anti-inflammatory factors have been discussed, in this article including lipoxins and certain PGs. IL-1ra, TGF-β, IL-12, IL-35, and IL-10 have been implicated in this control as well.

IL-1ra production is induced by IL-4, IL-6, IL-13, and TGF-β, limiting the effects of IL-1. IL-35 is a dimer of IL-12p35 and IL-27p28 (IL-30) chains secreted by Treg cells and suppresses the inflammatory response by causing proliferation of Treg cells while reducing T_h17 cells.[13] TGF-β is largely inhibitory for B lymphocytes and T lymphocytes promoting apoptosis, with the exception of promoting both T_h17 producing T_h2 cells and IL-9 producing T_h2 cells.

The IL-10 family consists of IL-10, IL-19, IL-20, IL-22, IL-2, IL-26, IL 28, and IL29, which are produced by T_h1 and T_h2 cells, cytotoxic T cells, B lymphocytes, mast cells, mononuclear phagocytic cells, and DCs. IL-10 is predominantly produced by B lymphocytes and monocytes in humans but Treg cells serve as the most common type of T-lymphocyte–producing IL-10. IL-10 inhibits the production of IFN-γ and IL2 by T_h1 cells; IL-4, IL-5 by T_h2 cells; IL-1β, IL-6, IL-8 (CXCL8), IL-12, TNF- by mononuclear phagocytes; and TNF- by NK cells and LPS.[12,21,24] IL-10 also has direct effects on T cells to inhibit cytokine production. Its overall effects function to inhibit cellular immunity and allergic inflammation. In B lymphocytes, IL-10 stimulates cell proliferation and immunoglobulin secretion, thereby promoting the humoral response.[24,25]

SOCS molecules have been identified as critical regulators of the cytokine response. There are 8 members of the SOCS family, SOCS1–7 and cytokine-induced SH2-containing protein. SOCS1 is the most studied molecule and is induced by various mediators, including IFN-α and IFN- , IL-2, IL-3, IL-4, IL-6, IL-7, IL-9, IL10, IL-13, IL-15, TNF-, and LPS, and seems to regulate these same mediators via negative feedback.[26]

Other chemical mediators, such as platelet-activating factor, kinins, growth factors (eg, platelet-derived growth factor and vascular endothelial growth factor), adhesion molecules, and transcription factors are also key players in the inflammatory response.[27]

SPECIFIC IMMUNOTHERAPY

Immunotherapy is the only actual cure for allergies, initiating a permanent change in the immune system. All other therapies are temporary, causing symptom improvement only when actively in use. It also decreases the risk of developing future allergies and, at least for children, the risk of following the allergic march from rhinitis to asthma.[28]

Immunotherapy involves administering small doses of the actual antigen itself, usually by subcutaneous injection or sublingual hold and swallow. This dose is administered at intervals ranging usually from daily to weekly, and the dose is slowly increased up to a known or extrapolated effective dose. Administration of these doses for a total of 3 to 5 years seems effective at decreasing allergy/asthma symptoms and need for medication. This effect continues for several years after stopping immunotherapy.[29]

When pollen immunotherapy, for example, is begun, there is an initial bump upward in the specific IgE level, similar to that seen during pollen season. This gradually over months settles down to below initial baseline level. Next, antigen-specific IgG1 increases, followed by IgG4. These IgG4 molecules may or may not act as blocking antibodies, but developing concensus seems to be that they do not.[29]

After a course of immunotherapy, there are more antigen-specific Treg cells and increased IL-10. An allergen challenge results in less T-cell and eosinophil recruitment. There are more T_h1 cells and fewer T_h2 cells suggesting a general shift toward a T_h1 (nonallergic) response.[29] Nasal mucosal biopsies after immunotherapy show increased production of IFN- and IL-10, also decreasing allergic inflammation.[30]

SUMMARY

Every month, medical journals report discovery of new cell types, new mediatiors, or new interactions or influences among known cells and mediators. Perhaps something about to be reported holds the key for a safe, rapid, and effective cure for allergies and asthma. Or perhaps the key pieces of information are already known but the right way to fit them together is not. Either way, the immunology of the allergic response and how it can be modified is a fascinating field. Stay tuned for future updates!

REFERENCES

1. Sullivan BM, Locksley RM. Basophils: a non-redundant contributor to host immunity. Immunity 2009;30:12–20.
2. Khader SA, Gopal R. IL-17 in protective immunity to intracellular pathogens. Virulence 2010;1:423–7.
3. Borish L, Rosenwasser LJ. Cytokines in allergic inflammation. In: Middleton's allergy: principles and practice. 7th edition. Philadelphia: Mosby Elsevier; 2009. p. 172.
4. Park SG, Mathur R, Long M, et al. T regulatory cells maintain intestinal homeostasis by suppressing gamma delta T cells. Immunity 2010;33(5):791–803.
5. Francis JN, Till SJ, Durham SR. Induction of IL-10+CD4+CD25+ T cells by grass pollen immunotherapy. J Allergy Clin Immunol 2003;111:1255–61.
6. Nakanishi K. Basophils as APC in Th2 response in allergic inflammation and parasite infection. Curr Opin Immunol 2010;22:814–20.
7. Xolair website. Available at: http://www.xolairhcp.com/xolairhcp/. Accessed January 2, 2011.
8. Spencer LA, Weller PF. Eosinophils and Th2 immunity: contemporary insights. Immunol Cell Biol 2010;88:250–6.
9. Karasuyama H, Mukai K, Obata K, et al. Nonredundant roles of basophils in immunity. Annu Rev Immunol 2010. [Epub ahead of print].
10. Min B. Basophils induce Th2 immunity: is this the final answer? Virulence 2010;1:399–401.
11. Weaver CT, Harrington LE, Mangan PR, et al. Th17: an effector CD4 T cell lineage with regulatory T cell ties. Immunity 2006;24:677–88.
12. Jutel M, Akdis M, Akdis C. Histamine and histamine receptors and their role in immune pathology. Clin Exp Allergy 2009;39:1786–800.
13. Commins S, Borish L, Steinke J. Immunologic messenger molecules: cytokines, interferons, and chemokines. J Allergy Clin Immunol 2010;125:S53–72.

14. D'Acquisto F, Maione F, Pederzoli-Ribeil M. From IL-5 to IL-33: the never-ending list of new players in inflammation. Is it time to forget the humble aspirin and move ahead. Biochem Pharmacol 2010;79:525–34.
15. Yamaguchi M, Koketsu R, Suzukawa M, et al. Human basophils and cytokines/chemokines. Allergol Int 2009;58:1–10.
16. Park S, Lee Y. Interleukin-17 regulation: an attractive therapeutic approach for asthma. Respir Res 2010;11:1–11.
17. Rosenwesser L. New insights into the pathophysiology of allergic rhinitis. Allergy Asthma Proc 2007;28:10–5.
18. Medoff B, Sauty A, Tager A, et al. IFN-γ-inducible protein 10 (CXCL10) contributes to airway hyperactivity and airway inflammation in a mouse model of asthma. J Immunol 2002;168:5278–86.
19. Gonzalo J, Lloyd C, Peled A, et al. Critical involvement of the chemotactic axis CXCR4/stromal cell-derived factor-1a in the inflammatory component of allergic airway disease. J Immunol 2000;165:499–508.
20. Boyce J. Eicosanoids in asthma, allergic inflammation, and host defense. Curr Mol Med 2008;8:335–49.
21. Steinke J, Borish L. Cytokines and chemokines. J Allergy Clin Immunol 2006;117: S441–5.
22. Ohnishi H, Miyahara N, Gelfand E. The role of leukotrienes B4 in allergic diseases. Allergol Int 2008;57:291–8.
23. Nauta A, Engels F, Knippels L, et al. Mechanisms of allergy and asthma. Eur J Pharmacol 2008;585:354–60.
24. Commins S, Steinke J, Borish L. The extended IL-10 superfamily:IL-10, IL-19, IL-20, IL-22, IL-24, IL-26, IL-28, and IL-29. J Allergy Clin Immunol 2008;121:1108–11.
25. Ogawa Y, Duru E, Ameredes B. Role of IL-10 in the resolution of airway inflammation. Curr Mol Med 2008;8:437–45.
26. Cassel S, Rothman P. Role of SOCS in allergic and innate immune responses. Adv Immunol 2009;103:49–76.
27. Barnes P. Pathophysiology of allergic inflammation. In: Adkinson NF, Yunginger JW, Busse WW, et al, editors. Middleton's allergy: principles and practice, vol. 1. 7th edition. Philadelphia: Mosby Elsevier; 2009. p. 455–72.
28. Till SJ, Durham SR. Immunological responses to allergen immunotherapy. In: Lockey RF, Bukantz SC, Bousquet J, editors. Allergens and allergen immunotherapy. 3rd edition. New York: Marcel Dekker; 2004. p. 95.
29. Frew AJ. Allergen immunotherapy. J Allergy Clin Immunol 2010;125:S306–16.
30. Krishna MT, Huissoon AP. Clinical immunology review series: an approach to desensitization. Clin Exp Immunol 2011;163(2):131–46.

Physical Findings in Allergy

Kristin Woodbury, DO[a,*], Berrilyn J. Ferguson, MD[b]

KEYWORDS

• Physical exam • Allergy diagnosis • Allergic rhinitis • Atopy

Nearly one-third of the population in the United States reports nasal and ocular symptoms of allergy.[1] As ear, nose, and throat physicians, we have a unique role in helping these patients. Many allergic symptoms manifest in the head and neck. The term allergic rhinitis is used as a diagnosis for patients with nose and eye symptoms secondary to IgE-mediated, or type 1 hypersensitivity reactions to various antigens.[2] Atopic IgE-mediated allergic reactions can occur throughout the body; however, inhalant allergy is usually limited to the nose, eyes, and lungs.

A thorough history of a patient's symptoms will often include symptoms both localized in areas such as the eyes or throat as well as systemic symptoms. History alone is often sufficient to make the diagnosis of allergic rhinitis. Confirmation can be obtained in the form of skin or in vitro testing for better-guided avoidance measures as well as appropriate institution of immunotherapy. Though arguably not as important as history, the physical examination can also be a helpful adjunct in diagnosing allergy. The authors present several head and neck physical examination findings the otolaryngologist will likely encounter in the examination of the allergic patient.

NASAL EXAMINATION

Optimal nasal examination for an allergic evaluation includes the use of a nasal speculum and headlight as well as inspection of the nasal skin and the patient's behavior. Nose blowing, wiping, sneezing, and sniffing are commonly seen in the allergic patient with acute symptom exacerbation.

Nasal Drip and Nasal Crease

Clear nasal secretions can be copious in allergic rhinitis (**Figs. 1** and **2**). Some patients develop a pattern of wiping the nose with the palm of their hand leading to the term the

The authors have nothing to disclose.

[a] Department of Otolaryngology, University of Pittsburgh Medical Center, 1400 Locust Street Building D, Suite 2100, Pittsburgh, PA 15219, USA
[b] Division of Sinonasal Disorders and Allergy, Department of Otolaryngology, University of Pittsburgh Medical Center, 1400 Locust Street Building D, Suite 2100, Pittsburgh, PA 15219, USA
* Corresponding author.
E-mail address: woodburykw@upmc.edu

Otolaryngol Clin N Am 44 (2011) 603–610
doi:10.1016/j.otc.2011.03.018 oto.theclinics.com

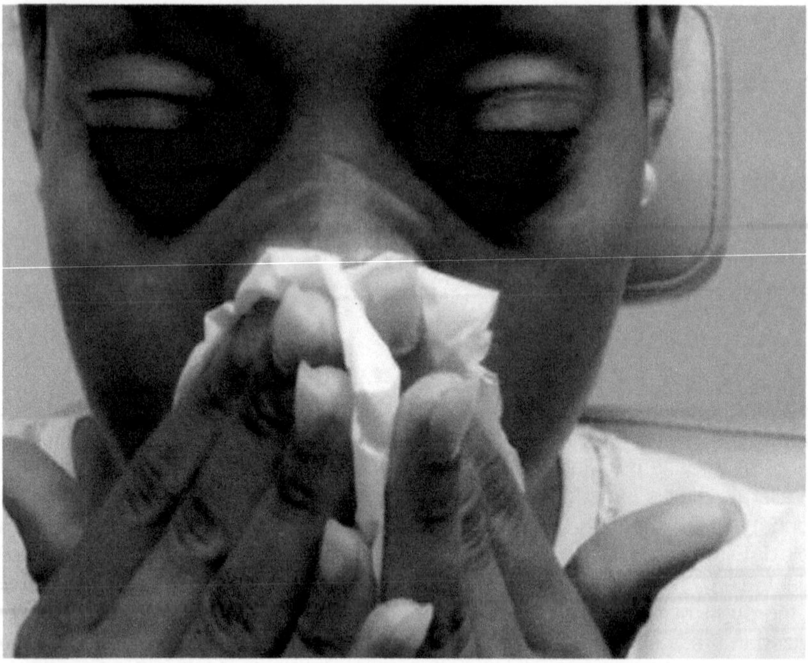

Fig. 1. Patient with nasal drip and modified "allergic salute" leading to the creation of a nasal crease.

"allergic salute." These patients may also develop a horizontal crease in the nasal supratip area called an allergic nasal crease.[2]

Pale and Boggy Inferior Turbinates

The nasal mucosa of the inferior turbinates often becomes edematous without erythema after inhalant allergen exposure leading to a pale or blue appearing surface (**Fig. 3**). The turbinates can become significantly swollen and obstruct the nasal airway and are typically surrounded by copious clear mucus.[3]

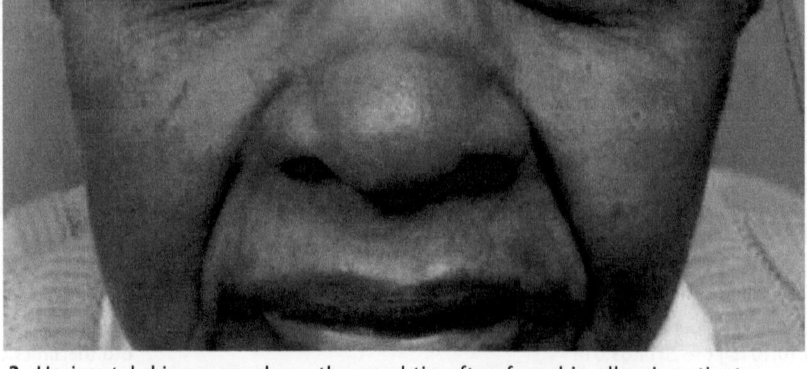

Fig. 2. Horizontal skin crease above the nasal tip often found in allergic patients.

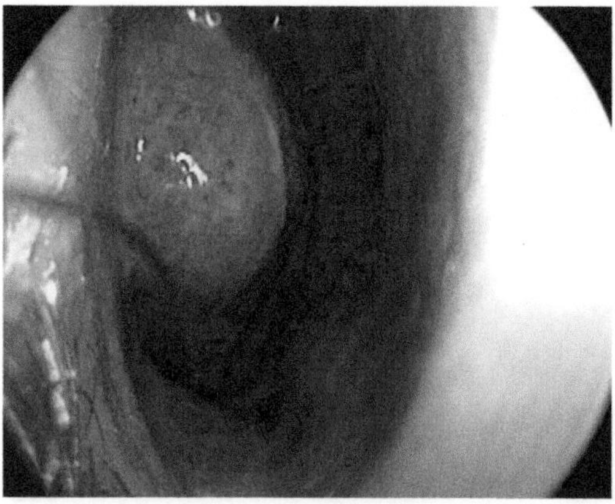

Fig. 3. Example of a pale, boggy inferior turbinate and associated clear rhinorrhea.

Red Inferior Turbinate

Reddened nasal mucosa is less frequently associated with inhalant allergy (**Fig. 4**). The differential diagnosis for red turbinates includes exposure to cigarette smoke (either active or second hand), overuse of topical decongestants, or (in the senior author's experience) food allergy.

Nasal Polyposis

Whereas atopy alone as the cause of nasal polyp development is controversial, the presence of IgE to various antigens has certainly been identified in nasal polyp specimens (**Fig. 5**). Many patients with nasal polyps also exhibit positive skin testing or in vitro IgE to inhalant allergens. Wise and colleagues[4] discussed a population of patients with high nasal-IgE levels and nasal polyps and negative skin or in vitro allergy testing. The higher sensitivity of detecting local IgE production in the nose may allow better treatment of truly allergic nasal polyp patients with negative conventional testing.

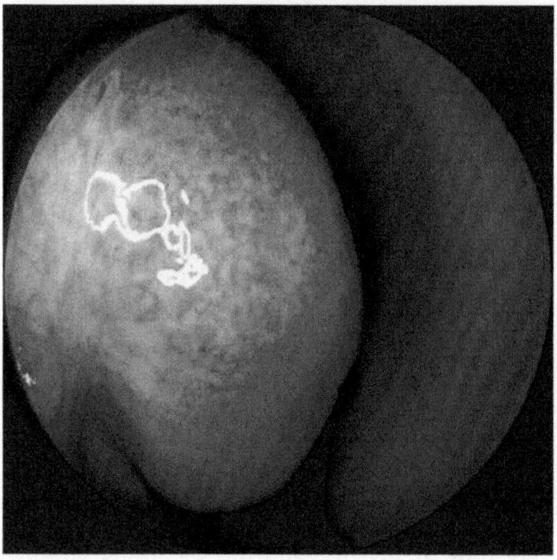

Fig. 4. Red inferior turbinate often associated with food allergy and sensitivity.

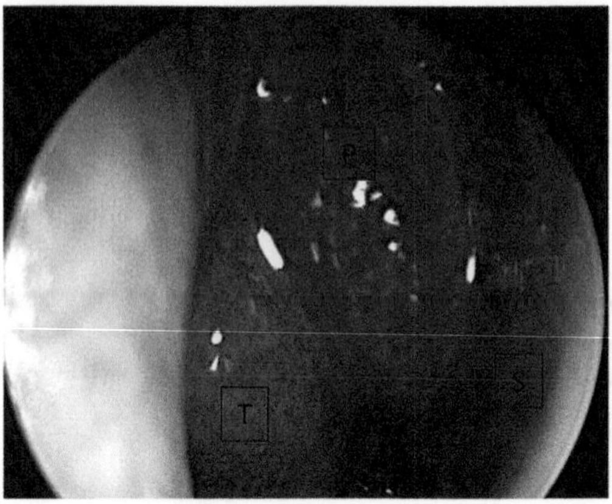

Fig. 5. Classic nasal polyp (P) appearance visualized between the septum (S) and an allergic-looking inferior turbinate (T) in a right nasal cavity.

Adenoid Hypertrophy

Inflammatory mediators in nasal secretions of the allergic patient can lead to enlargement of the lymphoid tissue within the nasopharynx also known as adenoid tissue (**Fig. 6**). This is more common in the pediatric patient and can be a significant source of nasal obstruction, sleep disordered breathing, and bacterial rhinosinusitis in untreated allergic children.[5]

EAR EXAMINATION

The ears can display a few different types of allergic pathology. Whether inflammation and edema in the nose and nasopharynx lead to eustachian tube blockage or whether a systemic allergic pathology is the cause, recognizing and appropriately treating these entities by control of underlying condition is important.

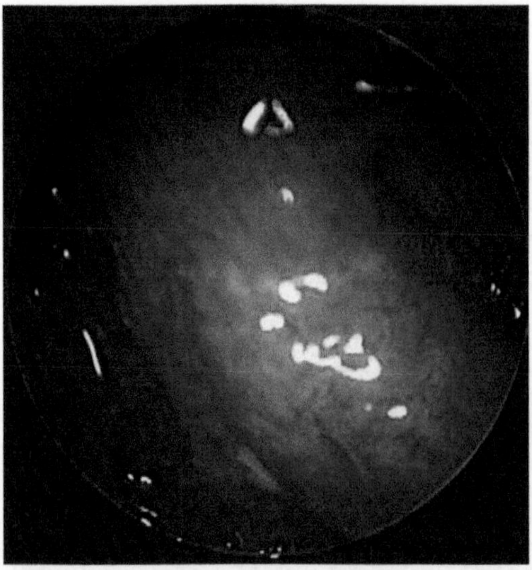

Fig. 6. Nasal endoscopic view of the nasopharynx exhibiting an enlarged and inflamed appearing adenoid.

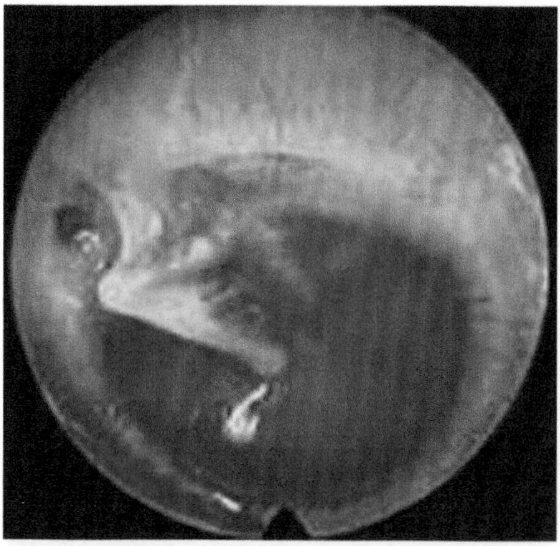

Fig. 7. Serous middle ear effusion filling the middle ear space with the classic amber appearance.

Serous Otitis Media

Eustachian tube dysfunction resulting from allergic rhinitis is thought to contribute to the formation of a middle ear effusion without evidence of infection (**Fig. 7**).[6] Middle ear mucosa is also thought to be a target organ for inflammation associated with the allergic process and subsequent development of fluid in the middle ear space.[7]

External Ear Canal Dermatitis

The dry, flaky skin of IgE-mediated atopic dermatitis can manifest in most any area of the body (**Fig. 8**). The external auditory canal is the only skin-lined invagination of the body, which lends itself to unique complications with interruptions in the skin barrier

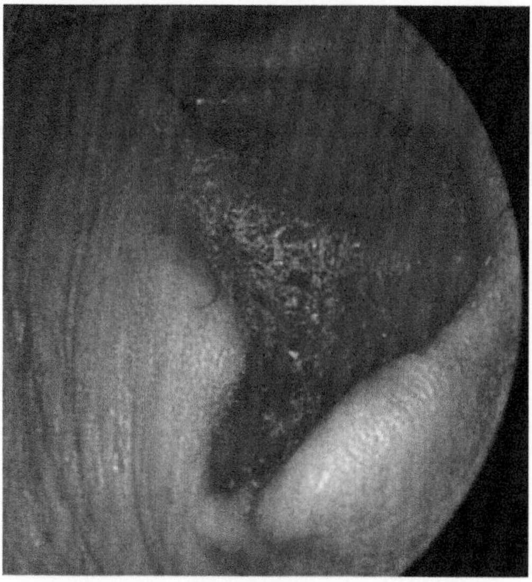

Fig. 8. External auditory canal and conchal bowl atopic dermatitis.

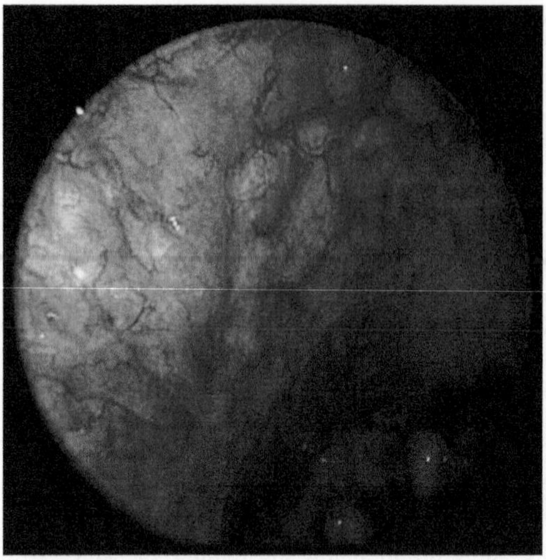

Fig. 9. Posterior pharyngeal submucosal lymphoid tissue hypertrophy and cobblestoning appearance with the arytenoids in view inferiorly.

and skin debris that result from dermatitis allowing secondary bacterial and fungal infections. Recognizing and treating this allergic entity with antiinflammatory topicals can significantly contribute to control of bacterial colonization.[8]

THROAT EXAMINATION

The oropharynx can be the site of a few physical examination findings that are seen in the allergic population. Nasal secretions can drain in a postnasal fashion and elicit irritation or lymphoid response from the tissues that are contacted.

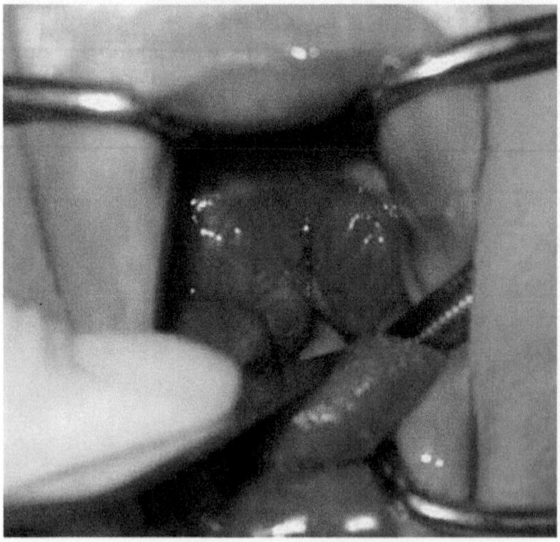

Fig. 10. Tonsillar hypertrophy in a pediatric patient undergoing tonsillectomy.

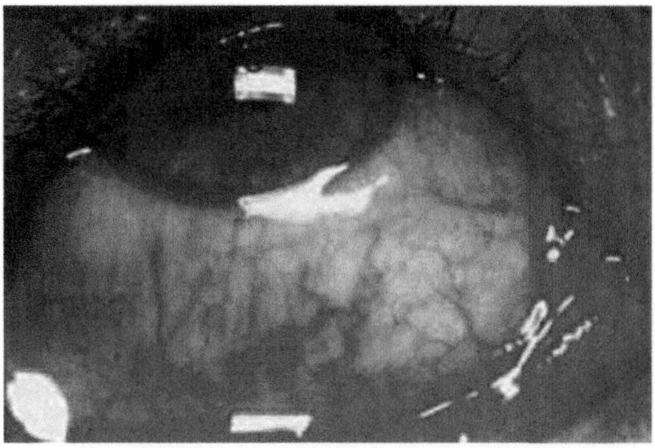

Fig. 11. Conjunctival injection and mild edema or chemosis in allergic conjunctivitis.

Posterior Pharyngeal Cobblestoning

The lateral pharyngeal tissue, where nasal secretions drain, may exhibit hypertrophy or lymphoid banding (**Fig. 9**). When the submucosal lymphoid tissues of the posterior pharynx are chronically exposed to inflammatory mediators of allergy in secretions, the development of cobblestoning is seen.[9]

Tonsillar Hypertrophy

Lymphoid hypertrophy of the upper airway from allergic rhinitis includes the palatine tonsils (**Fig. 10**). Children with tonsillar hypertrophy and sleep disordered breathing are significantly more likely to have allergic rhinitis than those with small tonsils.[5]

EYE EXAMINATION

Although detailed ocular examinations are outside of most otolaryngologists' field of practice, there are some aspects of evaluating the eyes that are simply observational and can provide helpful information. The periorbital skin can exhibit several classic patterns important to be aware of when caring for the allergic population.

Conjunctivitis

Unlike most of the other regions in the head and neck, the eye lacks a protective barrier to allergen exposure (**Fig. 11**). The mucosal surface of the eyelid and globe or conjunctiva may exhibit redness and swelling as well as inflammatory follicles or bumps.[10] These are nonspecific findings, but may be confirmatory to a history suggesting allergy.

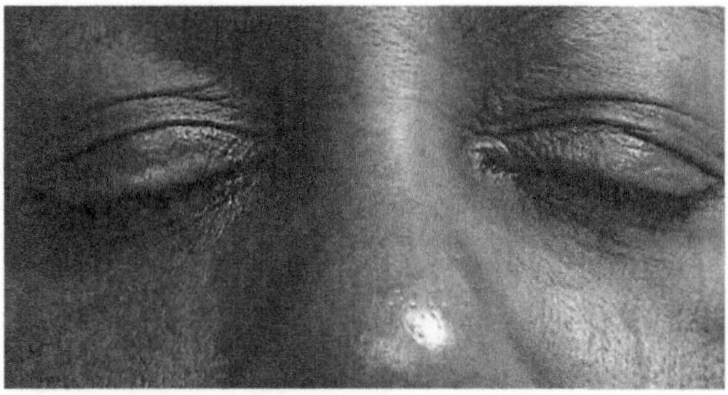

Fig. 12. Allergic shiner or dark circles in the lower eyelids of a patient with chronic nasal obstruction associated with allergic rhinitis.

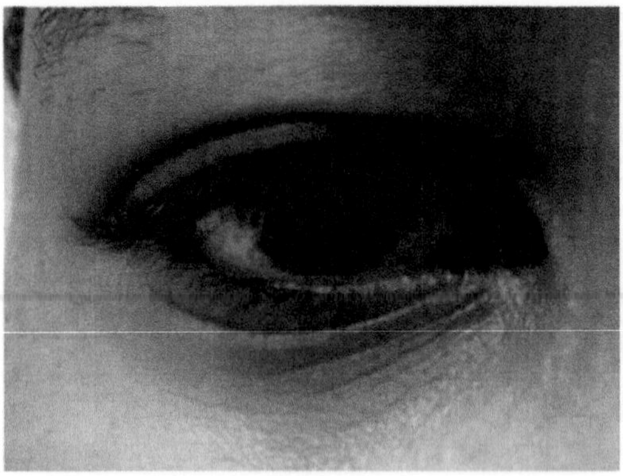

Fig. 13. Dennie-Morgan (or Dennie's) lines. Creases paralleling the inferior eyelid margin thought to arise from Mueller muscle spasms.

Allergic Shiner

Discoloration of the loose lower eyelid skin results in the characteristic dark circles or allergic shiner (**Fig. 12**). This is thought to be the result of venous stasis and hemosiderin deposition in the skin resulting from chronic nasal congestion.[9]

Dennie-Morgan Lines

Typically slightly less prominent than the allergic shiner, these ocular findings are thought to result from similar pathology (**Fig. 13**). Vascular congestion of the nose and subsequently the periorbital tissue leads to the hypoxic spasms of the Muller muscle and, subsequently, creases in the lower eyelid parallel to the lid margin.[2]

REFERENCES

1. Singh K, Axelrod S, Bielory L. The epidemiology of ocular and nasal allergy in the United States, 1988–1994. J Allergy Clin Immunol 2010;126:778–83.
2. Franzese CB, Burkhalter NW. The patient with allergies. Med Clin North Am 2010; 4:891–902.
3. Skoner DP. Allergic rhinitis: definition, epidemiology, pathophysiology, detection, and diagnosis. J Allergy Clin Immunol 2001;108:S2–8.
4. Wise SK, Ahn CN, Scholsser RJ. Localized immunoglobulin E expression in allergic rhinitis and nasal polyposis. Curr Opin Otolaryngol Head Neck Surg 2009;17:216–22.
5. Lack G. Pediatric allergic rhinitis and comorbid disorders. J Allergy Clin Immunol 2001;108:S9–15.
6. Friedman RA, Doyle WJ, Casselbrandt ML, et al. Immunologic-mediate eustachian tube obstruction: a double-blind crossover study. J Allergy Clin Immunol 1983;71:442–7.
7. Bernstein JM. The role of IgE-mediated hypersensitivity in the development of otitis media with effusion: a review. Otolaryngol Head Neck Surg 1993;109: 611–20.
8. Niebuhr M, Werfel T. Innate immunity, allergy and atopic dermatitis. Curr Opin Allergy Clin Immunol 2010;10:463–8.
9. Mabry RL, Ferguson BJ, Krouse JH. Allergy: the otolaryngologist's approach. Washington, DC: American Academy of Otolaryngologic Allergy; 2005.
10. Bielory L. Allergic diseases of the eye. Med Clin North Am 2006;90:129–48.

Diagnosis of Inhalant Allergies: Patient History and Testing

Christine Franzese, MD

KEYWORDS

- Allergy • Atopy • Allergic rhinitis • In-vitro testing
- Intradermal testing • Prick testing • Skin testing
- Modified quantitative testing

Key Points: Diagnosis of Inhalant Allergies

- Allergic disease affects multiple systems through one common immunologic mechanism of IgE-mediated response, and its symptoms can range from annoying to life threatening.
- A thorough exploration of symptoms, including timing, patient location when symptomatic, and duration/onset of symptoms, will help the physician determine if allergic disease is present and which possible antigens are potentially responsible.
- Testing for the presence of IgE-mediated disease is performed by either skin testing or in vitro testing.
- Both types of testing methods are valid and the choice of testing methods is influenced by a number of different factors.
- Patient history should guide the selection of antigens for testing and support clinical decision making.

In the United States, roughly 20% to 25% of the general adult population is afflicted by some form of chronic allergic respiratory disease, making allergy one of the most commonly diagnosed disorders.[1] Among children, allergic disease is more common, with some sources estimating that it affects up to 40% of children.[2] The social and economic burden of allergic disease is substantial, with allergic rhinitis alone responsible for 3.5 million missed days of work[3] and more than $6 billion spent on prescription medications alone for its treatment in 2000.[4] This does not take into account loss of productivity, physician office visits, over-the-counter medications, or other costs associated with additional manifestations of allergic disease.

The author has nothing to disclose and had no funding support for this work.
Department of Otolaryngology and Communicative Sciences, University of Mississippi Medical Center, 2500 North State Street, Jackson, MS 39216, USA
E-mail address: cfranzese@umc.edu

Otolaryngol Clin N Am 44 (2011) 611–623
doi:10.1016/j.otc.2011.03.003 oto.theclinics.com

Allergic disease affects all ages, ethnicities, and socioeconomic classes, and occurs throughout the United States, accounting for a large number of physician visits annually. Basically, allergy is the undesirable clinical manifestation of an exaggerated immunologic response to an otherwise harmless antigen. These responses also are known as hypersensitivity reactions and are classified further into several different types, depending on the immunologic mechanism of the reaction. The focus of this article involves making the diagnosis of the most familiar and best understood of the hypersensitivity reactions, type 1 hypersensitivity, also termed immediate hypersensitivity. This diagnosis is made through a combination of eliciting symptoms from the patient's history, noting physical examination findings, and testing for evidence of immunoglobulin E (IgE)-mediated disease by either some form of skin testing or in vitro testing.

Type 1 hypersensitivity reactions are IgE mediated, and the process of IgE production in response to exposure to an allergen is termed atopy. Although type 1 hypersensitivity can be caused by ingestion of food antigens or pharmaceuticals, this article focuses on IgE-mediated allergic disease caused primarily by inhalant allergens. In addition to allergic disease and allergic rhinitis, there are other types of rhinitis and disorders that may be similar or confused with true allergic disease, and should be included in the physician's differential diagnosis. These are discussed in other articles within this publication.

Inhalant allergic diseases can manifest in a variety of organ symptoms, but, generally, complaints are focused on the head and neck and upper airways. All types of allergic complaints tend to be grouped together under the term "allergic rhinitis," as the myriad of symptoms all result from a single common pathogenesis. Much of the allergy literature centers around the diagnosis and management of allergic rhinitis, although the disease manifestations typically are not isolated or restricted to the nose.

At the beginning of taking a patient's allergy history, the patient may state on questioning that he or she "has allergies." This self-diagnosis may or may not be accurate and a patient's self-diagnosis should not be passively accepted without further query to establish the likelihood of allergic disease. Nonallergic triggers may cause symptoms that are identical to allergic disease; however, it is just as common for patients to be completely unaware that the main cause of their complaints is allergy. A good example is the patient with frequent sinus complaints who often feels ill from repeated infections. Many times, the cause is an underlying allergic pathology, not sinusitis. History taking and testing for evidence of IgE-mediated disease are important steps in determining whether or not the diagnosis of allergic disease is appropriate for each patient.

HISTORY: INHALANT ALLERGIES

For any patient with chronic or recurrent upper respiratory complaints, the diagnosis of allergic disease should be considered. Food allergy or hypersensitivity has some crossover manifestations similar to inhalant allergic disease but this article focuses on inhalant allergic disease. For all types of allergy, though, the patient's history is the single most important source of information in making the diagnosis of atopy.[5] Additionally, there are various inflammatory conditions of the head and neck for which allergy may be a contributing factor to the underlying disease process. For some patients with head and neck symptoms, complete improvement may not occur unless the associated allergic issues also are addressed.

For the allergic history, the history of present illness can be broken down into 3 essential components: symptoms (ie, what they are), timing (ie, onset, duration, seasonality), and location/environment (ie, types of exposures, geography). In reality, a discussion of the patient's symptoms will not occur in isolation; that is to say, the patient will not generally relate a history of itchy eyes (ie, symptom) without mentioning when this occurs (ie, timing) or where (ie, location). If the patient does not, the physician will promptly question the patient at that point about timing and location for that particular symptom, rather than elicit all possible symptoms before moving on to discover the timing and location of each. Although the performance of the patient interview will be more fluid in actuality than what is described here, the mechanics of the patient history have been isolated into the essential components as an aid in understanding. Family history and past medical history are also very important to elicit but come later in the patient interview.

Common and Important Aspects of History for Inhalant Allergies

The potential number and kinds of questions that could be asked of the patient during the allergy history are almost infinite. The purpose of this portion is not to present an exhaustive list of all questions that should be considered. Rather, for practicality's sake, the most common and important aspects of the history are covered. However, the reader should keep in mind that an allergic history is like a detective story or a murder mystery. Not all the facts or clues are presented in the initial setting, but are discovered over a period of time and not all are relevant or completely accurate. Information vital to identifying the culprit allergen may be missing and the physician will need to further investigate areas outside what is most commonly encountered. The history of the allergic patient is an ongoing process, not just an occurrence at the initial visit, and continues over the course of the physician-patient relationship.[5] This becomes very important if the patient develops recurrence of allergic symptoms or onset of new allergic symptoms. The detective must remember his magnifying glass and begin to search for more clues.

Patient Symptoms in Allergy

The first type of "clue" to consider is the patient's specific symptoms. Sneezing; itchy, red, or watery eyes; and clear rhinorrhea are common, well-known allergic symptoms. Wheezing, particularly expiratory wheezing, coughing, urticaria, complaints of increased mucus, and shortness of breath are more potential allergic symptoms. However, other less specific symptoms may indicate allergy, such as complaints of nasal congestion; frequent sinus infections; change in hearing, ear pressure, or pain; the feeling of ears being stopped up; itchy throat; hoarseness; heartburn; and gastrointestinal upset.[6,7] In addition, other disease processes, such as obstructive sleep apnea, eustachian tube dysfunction, asthma, and chronic rhinosinusitis can be exacerbated by inhalant allergies, so it is critical that the practitioner investigate the presence of allergic symptoms.[6,7]

Timing of Symptoms in Allergy

The timing of symptoms is helpful to establish in diagnosing allergy. Timing includes onset of symptoms (ie, both age at onset and duration of symptoms), fluctuation or seasonality (ie, only in the spring vs year round), and symptom pattern. The age of onset is important because onset of true inhalant allergies is rare in the infant and geriatric populations, but more common in the teen and young adult ages, peaking at around age 30.[5] Duration of symptoms includes not only the time frame of onset (ie, How many years have you had this complaint?) but also time course of symptoms (ie, I only sneeze for a week or my eyes itch most of the year). Questions about the time course of symptoms overlap somewhat with questions about fluctuation or seasonality, but the key thing to identify is if the symptom occurs periodically, associated with a season or location, or perennially. Whether the symptoms are present year-round or only during certain seasons is very helpful in diagnosing perennial versus seasonal allergic disease. **Fig. 1** demonstrates examples of the seasonal pattern and distribution by geographic location of a few common inhalant allergens. This type of information can be very helpful in the investigation of allergic symptoms. Establishing any symptom patterns is crucial as well. If multiple symptoms are elicited, do they all occur together or only certain ones? This helps the physician track down potential suspect allergens and aids in identification of which allergen is causing which symptom or symptom pattern.

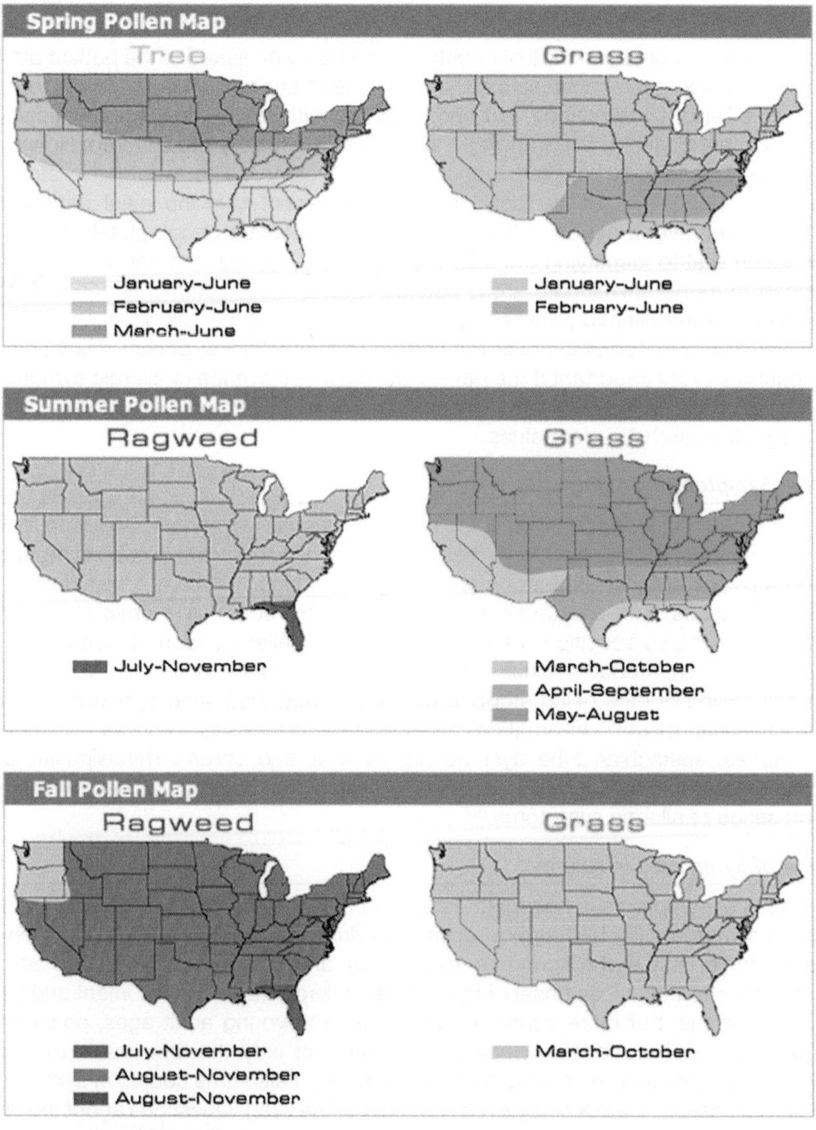

Fig. 1. Seasonal pollen map of the contiguous United States. (*From* the American Academy of Otolaryngic Allergy Web site, www.aaoaf.org; with permission.)

Location and Environment in Allergies

Location and environment complete the critical elements of information to obtain in the history of present illness. The current geographic location helps establish what potential aeroallergens the patient is exposed to, but previous locations where the patient has lived are also important. A significant change in environment, such as a cross-country move, with exposure to new allergens, can be factor in the development of allergies in the adult population, so it is important to elicit this history when seeing a new patient with allergic-type symptoms.[5] Questions of timing overlap with location and environment as the patient's fluctuations in symptoms may not necessarily be seasonal but related to local exposures at work or home. The list of environmental exposures can be exhaustive when considering home, outdoor, and occupational environments, but key things to inquire about are the presence of pets (indoor or outdoor) or livestock, tobacco use, hobbies, stuffed animals, carpeting or draperies in the domicile, type of heating or air conditioning, indications of mold or humidity, and nearby landscaping. Certainly it is impossible during one session to investigate all possible exposures, but if the allergic patient is not improving with appropriate treatment, it can be highly beneficial to review additional environmental exposures.

Past Medical History and Family History in Allergies

Additional components of the allergic history are past medical history and family history. Past medical history should include a review of any previous treatments or testing, surgeries, particularly past sinus surgery, and medications. Previous treatment includes not only treatment the patient may have received from a physician, such as previous skin or in vitro testing or immunotherapy, but also self-administered medications, such as over-the-counter antihistamines and cold preparations. The effectiveness of any previous treatment should be documented. A thorough review of medications is important, as certain medications, like tricyclic antidepressants and antihistamines, can effect skin reactivity or increase the risk of certain testing and treatment options, such as beta-blockers or angiotensin-converting enzyme (ACE) inhibitors. Family history is also key historical information. Allergic disease is hereditary, and other family members usually will be affected by the same or similar complaints as the patient.

DIAGNOSTIC TESTING

Not all patients with allergic rhinitis or atopic disease require confirmatory diagnostic testing. The patient's history and physical examination are sufficient to make the diagnosis of allergic disease in most cases. If appropriate medical therapy is instituted and it controls the patient's symptoms, then no further workup or testing is needed. However, if medical therapy fails or incompletely resolves the patient's symptoms, the patient wishes to implement environmental control measures and wants guidance on what to avoid, or wishes to receive allergy immunotherapy, then proceeding with diagnostic testing is appropriate. It is important to note that although diagnostic testing does not necessarily mean that the patient must proceed with immunotherapy, immunotherapy cannot commence without the evidence of IgE-mediated disease that diagnostic testing provides. A patient who undergoes diagnostic allergy testing with negative results is not a candidate for immunotherapy.

Diagnostic allergy testing for inhalant allergens includes selecting a type of in vivo testing (ie, skin testing) or in vitro testing. The decision as to which testing method the physician chooses to use can be a complex one and is influenced by a number of factors. Some of these factors are discussed in the following paragraphs with each different type of testing method and are also discussed toward the end of the article. The following described testing methods are all considered acceptable standard medical practice and the author does not espouse one technique over the other.

Skin Testing in Allergies

Skin testing generally involves prick testing, intradermal testing, or a combination of the two testing methods, such as modified quantitative testing (MQT).[8,9] For all types of skin testing, appropriate types of positive histamine controls and negative controls must be placed at the start of testing to confirm the validity of any positive or negative skin tests. The type of negative control used will depend on any diluents used in the antigen testing vials.[8] If an antigen is presented in a mixture containing 50% glycerin, then 50% glycerin should be used as the negative control and so forth. Skin testing has the advantage of providing the patient with an immediate answer as to which allergens do or do not potentially cause his or her symptoms but it can be time consuming, carries the risk of a systemic reaction or anaphylaxis, and involves some discomfort. Its accuracy is also subject to medication effects and skin disorders, so not all patients may be eligible candidates for skin testing. Patients with dermatographism or active eczema, who are actively taking antihistamines or antihistamine-containing over-the-counter cold preparations, or who are on beta-blockers are just a few examples of patients who are more appropriate for an alternative method of allergy testing, such as in vitro allergy testing.

Prick Testing in Allergies

Prick testing can be used to confirm clinical sensitivity to inhalant and other types of allergens and can be done in a number of ways with different devices.[10] Prick testing is a type of epicutaneous test and involves placing an antigen concentrate on the patient's skin after small, superficial punctures have been made to the epidermis, placing the antigen concentrate on the skin, and making a small puncture through the concentrate, or using a device that applies the antigen concentrate to the skin at the same time the puncture is made (**Fig. 2**). These devices can be either a single-prong device or a multiprong device (**Fig. 3**) or the testing can be done with needles or lancets. There are no objective data comparing devices that support a clear-cut advantage of using one type of device over another and good results

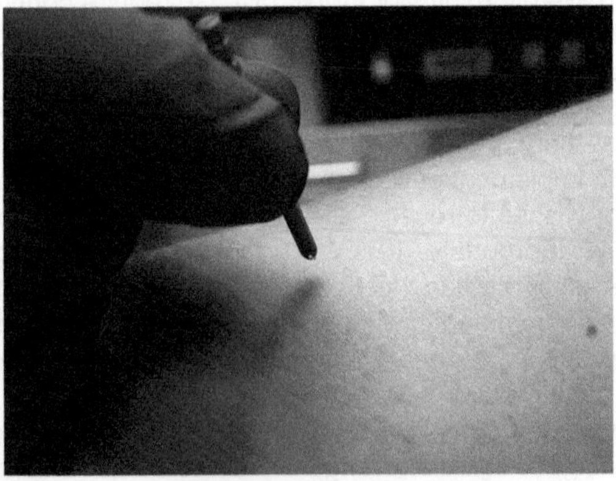

Fig. 2. Skin-prick testing with a single-prick device.

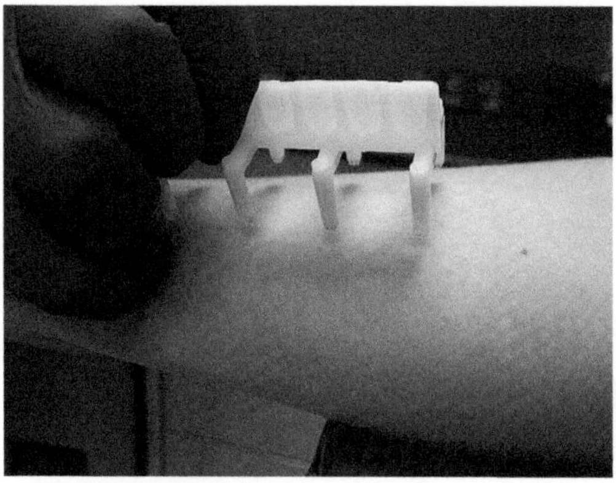

Fig. 3. Skin testing with a multiprick device.

can be achieved with any device, as long as there is consistency in its use and proper training.[10]

After a period of time, generally 15 to 20 minutes, any resulting wheals are noted and measured.[8,10] Assuming appropriate responses to control tests, the size of any resulting wheals can be graded, termed "qualitative scoring," and used to confirm presence of allergic disease or can be used to guide placement of an intradermal test, if a blended technique like MQT is used. There are a variety of wheal-grading systems and scales that categorize size of the resulting wheal and erythema (ie, flare reaction); an example of one such grading system for classifying wheals is in **Table 1**. Many practitioners no longer grade wheals because of the demonstrated variability between physicians, and solely judge wheals as positive or negative.[11] If a grading scale is used, which scale or system is used is not so important as the consistency of its application.[8] Depending on the system or scale used, +3-sized or +4-sized wheals are considered positive and a wheal smaller than 3 mm is considered negative.

Intradermal Testing in Allergies

Intradermal testing involves injecting dilute solutions of antigenic material into the patient's dermis. This can be a single intradermal injection placed after a negative prick test, as part of a blended testing method, or as a part of a progressively stronger series of dilutions, such as intradermal dilutional testing (IDT).[8,9] Intracutaneous tests, such as intradermal tests and the various intradermal testing techniques, are more sensitive and will identify a large number of patients with lower skin sensitivity than epicutaneous tests, like skin-prick testing.[10]

Table 1
Sample grading scale for skin-prick testing

Grade	Wheal Size
0 or Negative	Less than 3 mm
+1	3 mm to 5 mm
+2	6 mm to 10 mm
+3	11 mm to 15 mm
+4	Greater than 15 mm or pseudopods

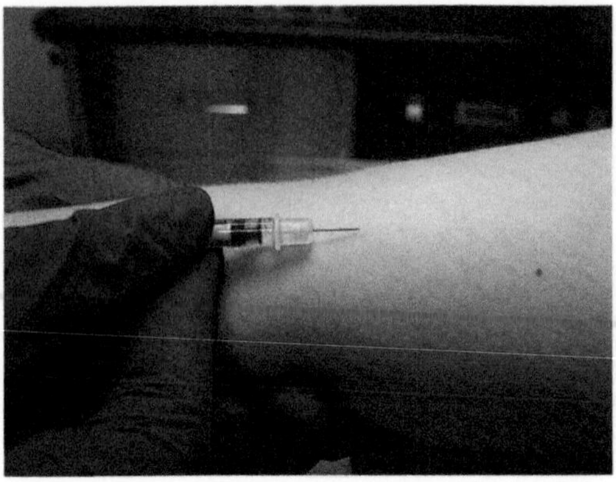

Fig. 4. An intradermal injection is performed with a very small amount of antigenic material.

In general, a small needle is used to inject a dilute quantity of antigen into the superficial dermis, raising a wheal of roughly 3 to 4 mm in size (**Figs. 4** and **5**). Appropriate positive and negative controls are placed for intradermal tests as well. If a positive control has been placed for prick testing, then a subsequent positive control for intradermal testing is not necessarily needed if the prick test positive control was positive and the prick test negative control was negative. It is important to note, however, that if no positive control was previously placed, an intradermal positive histamine control is placed, which is different from that placed for prick testing. This type is generally an aqueous form of histamine in a more dilute strength.[8] A negative control is almost always placed, as the diluents used for intradermal testing are different from those used in prick testing and, depending on the concentration of the intradermal dilution used, an intradermal glycerin control or controls may need to be placed if there are suspicions of glycerin sensitivity.

After a period of time, usually 10 to 15 minutes, any resulting wheals are measured, assuming appropriate responses to the positive and negative controls.[10] Overall, for an inert liquid substance or nonantigen material injected intradermally, physical spreading in and of itself will cause the initially placed 4-mm wheal to enlarge to

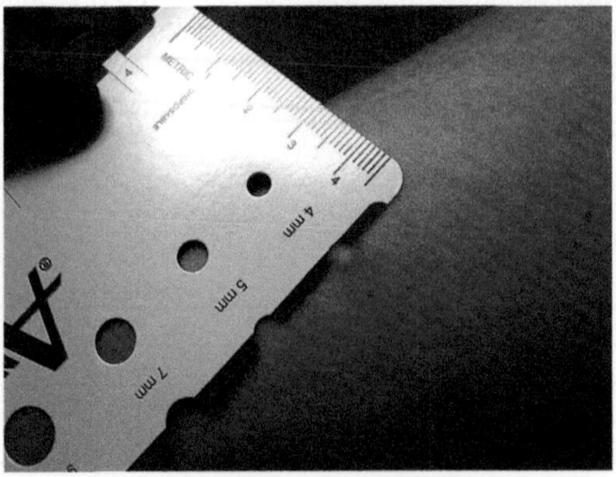

Fig. 5. An intradermal injection should raise a 4-mm wheal.

roughly 5 mm in size, so wheals of this size can be considered negative. Inflammation would cause the wheal to enlarge further beyond the 5-mm size, so wheals are usually considered positive when they are 2 mm larger than what is expected from a negative wheal.[8,9] The size of the resultant wheal can be graded alone with a variety of scales similar to that of **Table 1**, or if part of technique, such as IDT or MQT, the size of the wheal is used to guide the next step in testing or is in itself graded as the end result.[8,9] When an intradermal injection is used as part of a series (IDT) or as a blended method, its purpose is to try to "quantify" how sensitive that patient is to that a particular antigen. The purpose of this quantification is to provide the physician with a way to potentially adjust the starting dose of immunotherapy. Not all skin-testing methods will provide the practitioner with such a quantification. IDT and MQT are examples of skin-testing methods that have the ability to do so. However, even when such information is available, it is the practitioner's choice as to whether the test results are used to adjust the immunotherapy dosage or not.

In IDT, several different concentrations of an antigen have been previously mixed that are part of a treatment or testing board of dilute antigen solution vials. Depending on the method used, the different concentrations are mixed as 1:5 dilutions of 6 different strengths, with dilution #1 being the most concentrated and dilution #6 being most dilute.[8] These dilutions are introduced into the dermis in a series, starting from weakest to strongest. The purpose of IDT is to not only demonstrate if the patient is sensitive, but also attempt to quantify how sensitive the patient is to the test antigen by introducing progressively stronger concentrations of the test antigen until either sensitivity is demonstrated or the highest concentration of antigen that is safe for intradermal use is reached. IDT has been demonstrated to be equivalent to prick/puncture testing for both positive and negative predictability of clinical allergy when both are compared with nasal challenge.[12]

A full discussion on the exact procedure for IDT, its nuances, and testing variations is beyond the scope of this article. In general, dilutions of increasing strength are placed one at a time until there is no reaction to a #2 dilution, a confirmatory wheal is reached, or one of several possible uncommon to rare variant reactions happen that preclude making a positive diagnosis of IgE-mediated disease to that specific antigen. If there is no positive wheal response to a dilution #2 intradermal injection, then the patient is graded as having a negative response, or no allergy to that particular antigen. In general practice, a #1 dilution is not placed after a negative response to a #2 dilution, as the false positive rate for that concentration of antigen is much higher and no confirmatory wheal would be available to validate it, as this would require intradermal injection of antigenic concentrate that is considered unsafe.[8,10] A #1 dilution is rarely placed, except in the case where a confirmatory wheal is required to validate a #2 dilution end point.

A confirmatory wheal occurs at a point when there is demonstrated definite sensitivity to an antigen, and can be defined by certain wheal size and positioning criteria. A patient who has a confirmatory wheal can be said to demonstrate IgE-mediated sensitivity to that antigen, and the adjacent wheal(s) can be used to determine a safe starting dose for immunotherapy, if the patient desires to proceed with allergy shots.[9] A confirmatory wheal is defined as a wheal (1) that is the first wheal 2 mm larger than the negative control wheal and (2) is followed by a second wheal that is at least 2 mm larger than the preceding one.[12] If an uncommon or rare variant reaction happens, testing for that antigen may cease and the patient may be brought back on another day for testing or, depending on the variant reaction, the patient may be able to be declared allergic or not allergic to that particular antigen.

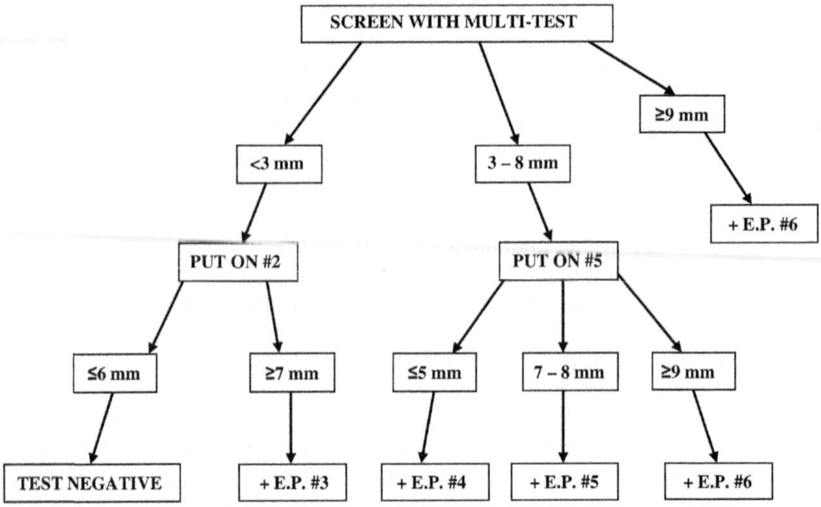

Fig. 6. Modified quantitative testing algorithm. (*From* Krouse JH, Mabry RL. Skin testing for inhalant allergy 2003: current strategies. Otolaryngol Head Neck Surg 2003;29(Suppl 4):S45; with permission.)

Modified Quantitative Testing for Allergies

MQT is a blending of prick and intradermal skin-testing techniques that also can be used to determine a starting dose for immunotherapy.[13] The technique begins with placing a series of prick tests, usually using a multiprong device. Any resulting wheals and their size are used to guide whether an intradermal injection is placed or not and what strength dilution the intradermal test should be. The MQT algorithm is shown in **Fig. 6**. If both prick and intradermal tests are negative, then the patient is confirmed to lack IgE-mediated disease to that particular antigen. Other results will classify the patient as belonging to a particular IDT equivalent end point. Whether that end point determined by MQT is truly equivalent to the end point determined by IDT has been questioned.[14] Still, MQT is a safe alternative to IDT and has been used to guide starting doses of immunotherapy.[15]

In Vitro Testing for Allergies

In vitro testing for inhalant allergens is an equally acceptable method of diagnostic testing. In vitro testing is performed using the patient's own blood and is either sent to a reference laboratory or can be done in the practitioner's office, if the office has the machinery and meets certain federal regulations. It has the advantages of no risk of anaphylaxis and much less discomfort, as only a single needle stick to draw blood is needed; however, many offices lack the capability to perform in vitro testing, so this generally requires the blood to be sent out to a laboratory for analysis, and so does not give the immediate answers that skin testing can give.

There are several variations on the actual testing technique used for in vitro testing and these variations either change how the amount of antigen-specific IgE is measured or how the test antigen is presented, but the general method does not change between each of these different forms of in vitro testing. The general overall method of in vitro testing involves attaching the test antigen in question to a surface, exposing that antigen-coated surface to the patient's blood or serum, then raising that away after a specified period of time. If the patient has IgE specific to the test antigen, it will remain behind attached to the antigen on the surface. Then IgG antibodies specific to human IgE antibodies are introduced into the testing area and washed away after a set period of time. These anti-IgE IgG antibodies are labeled in some measureable fashion so that the amount of IgE in the patient's serum can be quantified.

Variations in technique in how the antigen-specific IgE is measured include what specifically is used to label the anti-IgE IgG antibodies so they can be measured and how the test antigen is presented in the testing chamber or area. Variations on how the antibodies are labeled include radioallergosorbant testing (RAST), enzyme-linked immunosorbent assay (ELISA), fluoroenzyme immunoassay (FEIA), and chemiluminescence. Variations in presenting the test antigen include presentation on a 2-dimensional surface, such as a disk, or 3-dimensional presentations, such as in a cellulose sponge, on beads, or threads. At this point in time, there is no definitive literature to support the use of one particular type of modality over another. Which type of in vitro test to use is generally influenced by other factors, such as availability of a clinical laboratory and its specific capabilities.

What these different testing techniques share is the ability to determine the presence of antigen-specific IgE in a patient's blood and quantify it based on comparison with a reference standard. When the amount of IgE in the patient's blood is compared with a reference standard, the amount of IgE is categorized as belonging to one of several different classes. In general, the higher the numerical class, the more antigen-specific IgE is present in the patient's blood and the more sensitive the patient is to that antigen, theoretically. In contrast, the lower the numerical class, the less antigen-specific IgE is present and the less sensitive the patient is to that antigen, theoretically. It is important for the practitioner to keep in mind that each laboratory will have its own quantification scheme as to what result (ie, how much antigen-specific IgE is present) corresponds to which class and that the results from one laboratory cannot be categorized using another's testing classification. In vitro testing has been shown to correlate well with skin testing, but not necessarily with clinical sensitivity, and it has been shown to be a useful determinant in setting the starting dose for immunotherapy.[16]

Allergy Testing Modalities: Considerations

Whether the physician decides to pursue one type of testing modality over the other, be it skin testing or in vitro testing, will be influenced by a myriad of factors and should include a discussion of patient preferences. The testing modalities themselves are, for the most part, equivalent and the decision to use one over another can be based on other factors.[12,16] Certain skin conditions, such as eczema, or medications may make the patient ineligible for accurate skin testing, or patient preferences (a fear of needles) may influence the decision. The physician's familiarity and expertise with skin testing may also affect which type of testing is chosen. The important thing for any practitioner to keep in mind is that no testing modality is 100% sensitive and specific. If a patient has negative testing with one method and continues to have symptoms and history strongly suggesting a positive history of allergy, consideration should be given to retesting the patient with a testing method different from that first used or testing for antigens not on this initial testing battery.

One last consideration is the number and types of antigens tested when ordering or performing diagnostic allergy testing. Testing the patient for all possible antigens, especially ones where there is not sufficient evidence that the patient is even exposed to them, is unnecessary and inappropriate; routine use of large screening panels without significant clinical indication is not justified.[10] The patient's history can be used to help guide the physician in choosing which antigens to test, and the number and type selected should be determined based on the patient's age, history, environment and living conditions (ie, region of the country), occupation, and activities.[10] In general practice, many physicians start with a diagnostic screening battery of between 10 and 14 antigens, although this varies, with some screening as many as 20 to 40 antigens.

Screens can be created to test for outdoor/seasonal allergens only, for indoor/perennial allergens only, or a combination of both. Screens for outdoor or seasonal antigen can include between 1 and 3 trees, between 1 and 3 weeds, and between 2 and 3 grass families native to the area. Which species of grasses, trees, and weeds are most common in a given location can be discovered through a large number of resources. Inquiries can be made to different antigen-manufacturing companies, which usually have lists of antigens by geographic location, to local colleges or universities that have botany divisions or departments, and even online resources, such as the National Allergy Bureau Web site (www.aaaai.org) or www.pollen.com. Other local allergy practitioners may be helpful in selecting appropriate local antigens to test. Indoor or perennial screening panels usually include 1 or 2 species of house dust mite, 1 or a mix of cockroach species, and at least 1 epidermal antigen, the most common being cat. Molds can also be included on these types of panels or a separate screening panel can be created solely with mold antigens. If molds are included as part of another screening panel, at least 1 or 2 of the more common indoor species (ie, *Alternaria* and *Aspergillus* species) should be considered for inclusion.[10]

Which antigens used in a screen or selected for testing will usually not be affected by the choice of testing modality, although there are more antigens available for skin testing at present than there are for in vitro testing. In vitro tests can be ordered as part of a preset panel determined by the laboratory or can be part of a panel tailored to the individual practitioner's requests. Additionally, tests for only one or a few antigens can be ordered. Skin testing, either prick, intradermal, or other techniques, can also be performed using a screening panel or panels the practitioner has created or only a single or few antigens may be tested if the patient's history supports the clinical decision making.

The important point is that the patient's history should guide the selection tests or support the application of a particular screening battery. Annual repeat testing of allergens is not supported by literature, unless there is specific clinical indication in the patient's history.[10] If a patient develops new allergy symptoms, in addition to further investigation in clinical history and changes in the patient's environment, consideration can be given to retesting a patient to see if new allergies have developed or to testing antigens that were not initially tested.

REFERENCES

1. Sibbald B, Rink E. Epidemiology of seasonal and perennial rhinitis: clinical presentation and medical history. Thorax 1991;46:895–905.
2. Dykewicz MS, Fineman S, Skoner DP, et al. Diagnosis and management of rhinitis: complete guidelines of the Joint Task Force on Practice Parameters in Allergy, Asthma, and Immunology. Ann Allergy Asthma Immunol 1998;81:478–518.
3. Kay GG. The effects of antihistamines on cognition and performance. J Allergy Clin Immunol 2000;105:S622–7.
4. Stempel DA, Woolf R. The cost of treating allergic rhinitis. Curr Allergy Asthma Rep 2002;2:223–30.

5. King HC, Mabry RL, Mabry CS, et al. Interaction with the patient. In: Allergy in ENT practice: the basic guide. 2nd edition. New York: Thieme Medical Publishers; 2005. p. 67–104.
6. Friedman RA, Doyle WJ, Casselbrant ML, et al. Immunologic-mediated eustachian tube obstruction: a double-blind crossover study. J Allergy Clin Immunol 1993;71:442.
7. Fireman P. Otitis media and eustachian tube dysfunction: connection to allergic rhinitis. J Allergy Clin Immunol 1997;99:S787–97.
8. King HC, Mabry RL, Mabry CS, et al. Testing methods for inhalant allergy. In: Allergy in ENT practice: the basic guide. 2nd edition. New York: Thieme Medical Publishers; 2005. p. 105–54.
9. Seshul M, Pillsbury H 3rd, Eby T. Use of intradermal dilutional testing and skin prick testing: clinical relevance and cost efficiency. Laryngoscope 2006;116(9): 1530–8.
10. Bernstein IL, Li JT, Bernstein DI, et al. Allergy diagnostic testing: an updated practice parameter. Ann Allergy Asthma Immunol 2008;100(3 Suppl 3):S1–122.
11. McCann WA, Ownby DR. The reproducibility of the allergy skin test scoring and interpretation by board-certified/board-eligible allergists. Ann Allergy Asthma Immunol 2002;89(4):368–71.
12. Gungor A, Houser SM, Aquino BF, et al. A comparison of skin endpoint titration and skin-prick testing in the diagnosis of allergic rhinitis. Ear Nose Throat J 2004;83(1):54–60.
13. Krouse JH, Mabry RL. Skin testing for inhalant allergy 2003: current strategies. Otolaryngol Head Neck Surg 2003;29(Suppl 4):S33–49.
14. Simons JP, Rubinstein EN, Kogut VJ, et al. Comparison of multi-test II skin prick testing to intradermal dilutional testing. Otolaryngol Head Neck Surg 2004; 130(5):536–44.
15. Peltier J, Ryan MW. Comparison of intradermal dilutional testing, skin prick testing, and modified quantitative testing for common allergens. Otolaryngol Head Neck Surg 2007;137(2):246–9.
16. Corey JP, Mamikoglu B, Akbar I, et al. ImmunoCAP and HY*TEC enzyme immunoassays in the detection of allergen-specific IgE compared with serial skin endpoint titration by receiver operating characteristic analysis. Otolaryngol Head Neck Surg 2000;122(1):64–7.

Role of Allergy in Sleep-Disordered Breathing

Ryan J. Soose, MD

KEYWORDS

• Snoring • Sleep apnea • Allergic rhinitis • Nasal obstruction
• Hypersomnia

Key Points: Allergy and Sleep-Disordered Breathing

- Allergic rhinitis significantly contributes to sleep-disordered breathing through multiple mechanisms, with the greatest impact mediated primarily through nasal obstruction
- Sleep impairment is very common in patients with allergic rhinitis, chronic rhinosinusitis, and nasal polyposis, and has a significant impact on disease-specific and general health quality of life measures
- The degree of sleep disturbance is directly related to the severity of the allergic disease at a given time
- Nasal obstruction also demonstrates circadian rhythm and positional variability, with worsening in the overnight hours and in the supine position
- Nasal obstruction increases the likelihood of snoring, obstructive sleep apnea, and intolerance to medical device therapies for sleep apnea.

ALLERGIC RHINITIS AND SLEEP IMPAIRMENT

Scope of the Problem

Sleep-related symptoms are extremely common in patients with allergic rhinitis. Sleep impairment is likely a major contributor to the overall disease morbidity, direct and indirect health care costs, and the loss of work productivity associated with allergic rhinitis. The association between allergic rhinitis and sleep, and the subsequent impact on disease-specific and general health quality of life measures, is well documented in large epidemiologic studies as well as controlled clinical trials.[1,2] In a survey of allergy patients, 48% with seasonal allergic rhinitis (SER) and 68% with perennial allergic rhinitis (PER) reported that their condition interfered with their sleep.[3] In

The author has no conflicts of interest to disclose.

Division of Sleep Surgery, Department of Otolaryngology, University of Pittsburgh School of Medicine, UPMC Mercy Building B, Suite 11500, 1400 Locust Street, Pittsburgh, PA 15219, USA
E-mail address: sooserj@upmc.edu

Otolaryngol Clin N Am 44 (2011) 625–635
doi:10.1016/j.otc.2011.03.020 oto.theclinics.com

another population survey by Craig and colleagues,[4] of the more than 2000 allergy patients surveyed, approximately half reported difficulty falling asleep or staying asleep as a result of their allergic condition (**Fig. 1**).

In a large cross-sectional epidemiologic study, Leger and colleagues[1] showed that allergic rhinitis can affect multiple aspects of sleep, with numerous consequences on daytime function. Sleep-related breathing disorders, insomnia, as well as daytime somnolence, morning headaches, and cognitive dysfunction, were all more common in the allergic rhinitis patients than in controls. Furthermore, the degree of sleep impairment and associated symptoms appears to be directly related to the severity of the allergic rhinitis. In patients with seasonal allergic rhinitis, subjective and objective sleep measures correlate with the severity of their sinonasal disease at the time, that is, patients with predominant tree pollen allergy may have noticeable worsening in their sleep during the spring pollen season.[2] As such, sleep disturbance is one of the key factors in the Allergic Rhinitis and its Impact on Asthma (ARIA) guidelines that distinguishes between mild and moderate-severe disease.[5]

Pathophysiology

The pathophysiology of disrupted sleep in patients with allergic rhinitis is likely complex and multifactorial. Upper airway resistance, increased work of breathing, obstructive respiratory events, sleep-onset and sleep-maintenance insomnia, anxiety, depression, confounding effects of allergy medication and sedative drugs, as well as other biochemical and hormonal effects all may play a role in the negative impact on sleep quality. Clearly, however, one of the vital and well-established links between allergic rhinitis and sleep disturbance is nasal obstruction. In the large epidemiologic

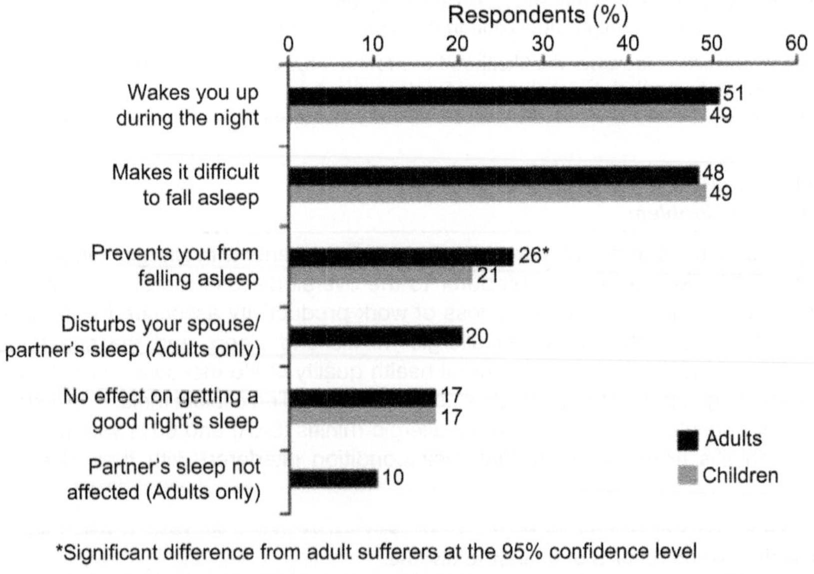

Fig. 1. Results of a survey of 2355 allergic rhinitis patients and the subjective impact of nasal congestion on sleep. Note that approximately half of the respondents reported that their allergy-related nasal congestion makes it difficult to both fall and stay asleep. (*Reproduced from* Craig TJ, Ferguson BJ, Krouse JH. Sleep impairment in allergic rhinitis, rhinosinusitis, and nasal polyposis. Am J Otolaryngol 2008;29:211; with permission from Elsevier Health Sciences.)

survey by Craig and colleagues,[4] nasal congestion was the most commonly reported symptom of allergic rhinitis patients (**Fig. 2**).

Several mechanisms have been proposed to explain how nasal obstruction negatively affects breathing during sleep (**Table 1**). Nasal obstruction may result in decreased stimulation of nasal receptors that are critical to control of breathing during sleep. Abolishment of the nasal receptor reflexes with topical lidocaine appears to increase airway obstruction and depress the central respiratory drive.[6] In a controlled crossover study, patients were evaluated with in-laboratory polysomnography and randomized to either (1) topical nasal saline with decongestant or (2) topical nasal lidocaine (4%) with decongestant, and then subsequently crossed over to the other group for a second night. The mean apnea-hypopnea index (AHI) increased from 6.4 with nasal saline to 25.8 with topical lidocaine. Of note, the increased apneic events observed with topical nasal lidocaine were split between both central and obstructive events, leading the investigators to conclude that nasal receptor stimulation is critical for central respiratory control of ventilation as well as maintenance of pharyngeal muscle tone.

These findings have been supported by additional studies comparing the nasal and oral routes of breathing. Oral breathing appears to have a detrimental effect on sleep, leading to loss of protective pharyngeal muscle activity and loss of control of breathing. The nasal route of breathing, however, has been shown to improve minute

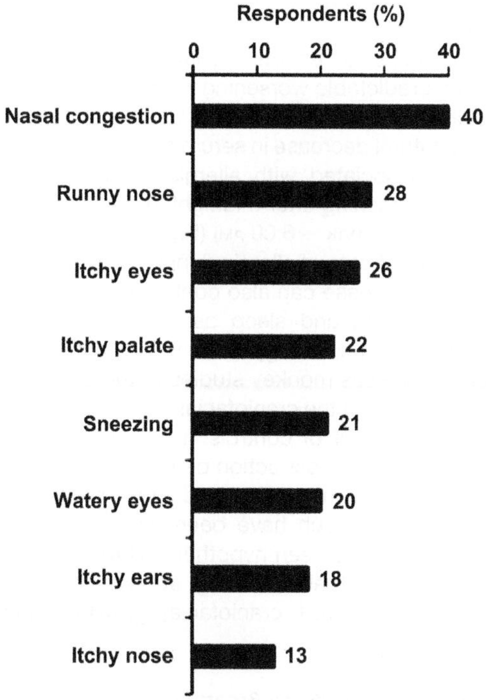

Fig. 2. Nasal congestion is the most commonly reported "severe" symptom of patients with allergic rhinitis and is likely the primary mechanism linking allergic rhinitis and sleep-disordered breathing. (*Reproduced from* Craig TJ, Ferguson BJ, Krouse JH. Sleep impairment in allergic rhinitis, rhinosinusitis, and nasal polyposis. Am J Otolaryngol 2008;29:211; with permission from Elsevier Health Sciences.)

Table 1
Pathophysiologic mechanisms of nasal obstruction and sleep-disordered breathing

Acute	Chronic
• Decreased nasal receptor mediated control of pharyngeal muscle activity and central respiratory drive • Increased negative inspiratory pressure in the pharynx • Increased velocity and turbulence of airflow and palatal flutter • Shift to oral breathing and posterior displacement of the mandible	• Maxillary hypoplasia • Inferior displacement of the mandible • Narrowing of dental arches • Anterior crossbite • Maxillary overjet • Increased anterior facial height (elongated face)

ventilation and increase pharyngeal muscle activity.[7,8] In a randomized single-blind placebo and sham-controlled crossover study, McLean and colleagues[9] compared the impact of the fraction of oral breathing on objective sleep measures. With polysomnography, they demonstrated that patients with lower nasal resistance and a normal nasal route of breathing had decreased light sleep (stage 1), increased deep sleep (slow-wave), increased rapid eye movement sleep (REM), and improved sleep efficiency. Multiple human studies of experimental nasal occlusion support these findings as well, demonstrating abnormal sleep continuity, abnormal sleep architecture, and increased respiratory events in normal patients with experimentally induced nasal obstruction.[10–12]

Further contributing to the sleep effects of allergic rhinitis is the diurnal variation of nasal congestion, with a predictable worsening overnight in most patients. This physiology is also likely multifactorial, and attributable to the gravity effect of the dependent sleeping position and a natural decrease in serum cortisol levels overnight. In addition, inflammatory mediators associated with allergic rhinitis demonstrate a circadian rhythm with progressive worsening after midnight in most individuals, peaking in the early morning hours (average peak ~6:00 AM) (**Fig. 3**).[4]

Besides the acute nightly effects of allergic rhinitis on sleep, chronic nasal obstruction and persistent allergic disease can also contribute to long-term, potentially irreversible, changes in breathing and sleep as well. These long-term effects are particularly concerning in pediatric allergy patients in whom the craniofacial skeleton is still rapidly developing. Rhesus monkey studies at the University of California, San Francisco in the 1970s compared the craniofacial development in animals with experimental nasal occlusion with that of controls. The studies showed that over time, young animals with chronic nasal obstruction developed maxillary deficiency, posterior/inferior displacement of the mandible, and other severe maladaptive skeletal changes (see **Table 1**), all of which have been associated with sleep-disordered breathing in adulthood.[13,14] It has been hypothesized that a vicious cycle evolves in some patients in whom nocturnal breathing abnormalities cause unstable oral breathing and secondary impaired craniofacial growth, which then reinforces abnormal breathing.

Nasal Obstruction and Sleep-Disordered Breathing

Several large population-based studies have analyzed the association of nasal obstruction and subjective sleep measures, snoring, and sleep apnea. In the Wisconsin cohort of almost 5000 patients, patients with chronic rhinitis symptoms were more likely to report habitual snoring, nonrestorative sleep, and daytime sleepiness.[15]

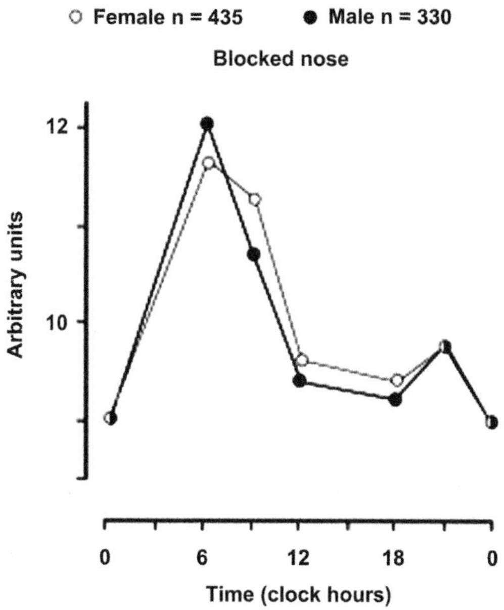

Fig. 3. Circadian variation of nasal congestion demonstrates progressive worsening overnight with an average peak in nasal resistance at approximately 6 AM. Proposed mechanisms for the observed circadian fluctuation include the gravity effect of the dependent sleeping position, normal nocturnal decline in serum cortisol levels, and upregulation of inflammatory cytokines overnight. (*Reproduced from* Craig TJ, Ferguson BJ, Krouse JH. Sleep impairment in allergic rhinitis, rhinosinusitis, and nasal polyposis. Am J Otolaryngol 2008;29:211; with permission from Elsevier Health Sciences.)

Patients with nasal congestion due to allergy were 1.8 times more likely to have moderate to severe obstructive sleep apnea (OSA) compared with allergy patients without nasal congestion. Other epidemiologic studies have confirmed that across a large population, nasal obstruction is an independent risk factor for both snoring and OSA.[16–18]

On the spectrum of sleep-related breathing disorders, nonapneic snoring is a very common condition. In the Wisconsin cohort, patients with chronic nasal congestion had a threefold increased risk of habitual snoring, even after controlling for OSA.[16] Snoring is often the chief sleep complaint in many patients, and subjectively is more important to most patients than daytime sleepiness.[19] Snoring has been shown to disrupt bed-partner sleep and have a negative impact on marital relationships. Further, treatment of snoring not only improves the patient's sleep but has also been documented to improve the bed-partner's sleep, with a reduction in the bed-partner's arousal index and improvement in sleep duration and efficiency.[20]

Recent evidence also suggests that vibratory trauma from snoring may cause direct endothelial injury and may be an independent risk factor for carotid atherosclerosis.[21] Researchers in Australia[22,23] have developed a rabbit model to evaluate the effects of snoring on the carotid artery. These investigators conclude that significant vibrational energy is transmitted to the carotid arterial wall during snoring, and may provide a link to carotid atherogenesis and cerebrovascular risk. Even in pediatric populations, primary snoring has been directly linked to elevated nocturnal diastolic blood pressure, even after controlling for other clinical factors.[24] In summary, reports of snoring in patients with allergic rhinitis should not be overlooked. What was previously considered "benign" or "simple" snoring may actually have significant psychosocial and physical health consequences.

The Impact of Medical Therapy

It is clear that nasal obstruction can have significant negative effects on both subjective and objective sleep measures as well as on the risk of sleep-disordered breathing. Until recently, however, it has been less clear as to what effect treatment of the nose has on these parameters. If nasal obstruction is the driving force behind much of the sleep disturbance in patients with allergic rhinitis, it would stand to reason that treatment of nasal obstruction and lowering of the nasal resistance would improve sleep in these patients.

Much of the research into medical therapy for allergic rhinitis and sleep-disordered breathing has focused on the role of nasal steroids. In a group of allergic rhinitis patients with subjective nasal congestion and sleep disturbance, Craig and colleagues[25] demonstrated that topical nasal steroid therapy improved subjective sleep quality and daytime function. Pediatric patients with symptomatic nasal obstruction and OSA have also been shown to respond favorably to nasal steroid therapy. Brouillette and colleagues[26] reported a reduction in the AHI from 10.7 to 5.8 with fluticasone nasal spray in a selected group of pediatric patients. Nevertheless, long-term adherence to nasal steroids may be suboptimal and difficult to monitor, particularly in pediatric patients with parental concerns about side effects.

Although treatment of allergic rhinitis and associated nasal obstruction can improve sleep, some of the medical therapy, notably antihistamines, may actually cause sleep-related symptoms. As such, the medical evaluation of allergy patients with nocturnal and daytime sleepiness must also take into account the side effects of the medications used to treat the underlying condition. Oral decongestants (ie, pseudoephedrine) and inhaled β-agonists (ie, albuterol) have been associated with insomnia symptoms in some patients. Conversely, oral antihistamines, particularly first-generation drugs, commonly cause sedation and may, at least in part, contribute to a patient's complaints of hypersomnia.

The Impact of Surgical Therapy

In many patients with allergic rhinitis, the symptomatic nasal obstruction and sleep-disordered breathing may be attributable to a combination of both inflammatory and structural pathology (**Table 2**). The management approach to the patient generally involves first identifying and medically treating any underlying inflammatory process that may be present. For structural anatomic problems, surgical therapy can be very effective, but the specific procedures indicated vary from patient to patient and depend on the specific anatomic problem. Benninger and colleagues[27] recently reported that subjective sleep quality improved significantly following endoscopic sinus surgery in patients with chronic rhinosinusitis (**Fig. 4**).

Structural causes of increased nasal resistance may not be confined to the nasal cavity alone. It is well known, particularly in pediatric patients, that adenoid hypertrophy contributes significantly to nasal obstruction and sleep-disordered breathing, and that adenoidectomy can dramatically improve sleep and breathing. The impact of tonsillar hypertrophy on nasal resistance, however, may be vastly underestimated. In 2007, Nakata and colleagues[28] showed that OSA patients with 3 to 4+ tonsils had significantly higher nasal resistance. Furthermore, simple tonsillectomy alone not only improved subjective and objective sleep measures but also greatly lowered nasal resistance.

Table 2
Examples of causes of symptomatic nasal obstruction and associated sleep-disordered breathing

Medical	Structural
• Allergic rhinitis	• Deviated nasal septum
• Vasomotor rhinitis	• Inferior turbinate hypertrophy
• Atrophic rhinitis	• Acquired nasal deformity
• Rhinitis medicamentosa	• Nasal valve collapse
• Nonallergic rhinitis with eosinophilia syndrome (NARES)	• Concha bullosa
• Medications (eg, antihypertensives, aspirin, oral contraceptives)	• Nasal polyps
• Infection (eg, common cold, chronic rhinosinusitis)	• Adenoid hypertrophy
• Hormonal (eg, pregnancy, hypothyroidism)	• Tonsillar hypertrophy
• Autoimmune (eg, lupus, Wegener, rheumatoid arthritis)	• Narrow pyriform aperture/hard palate
• Occupational (eg, chemicals, paint fumes, chalk dust, sawdust, perfumes)	• Inverting papilloma
• Smoking	• Neoplasm
	• Foreign body
	• Synechiae
	• Meningocele
	• Granulomatous disease

Although adenotonsillectomy alone often successfully treats the majority of children with OSA, many pediatric patients with allergic rhinitis may require concurrent treatment of turbinate hypertrophy. In a large retrospective study, Sullivan and colleagues[29] demonstrated that pediatric patients with enlarged inferior turbinates often had both subjective and polysomnographic evidence of persistent sleep-disordered breathing after adenotonsillectomy alone. These residual symptoms and AHI elevation were subsequently improved further with the addition of radiofrequency inferior turbinate reduction. Thus, overlooking treatment of nasal obstruction in children may lead to inadequate sleep apnea management.

Several recent studies have reported on the effect of surgically lowering nasal resistance on both subjective and objective measures of sleep-disordered breathing. In 2008, Li and colleagues[30] showed that for OSA patients with a deviated nasal septum

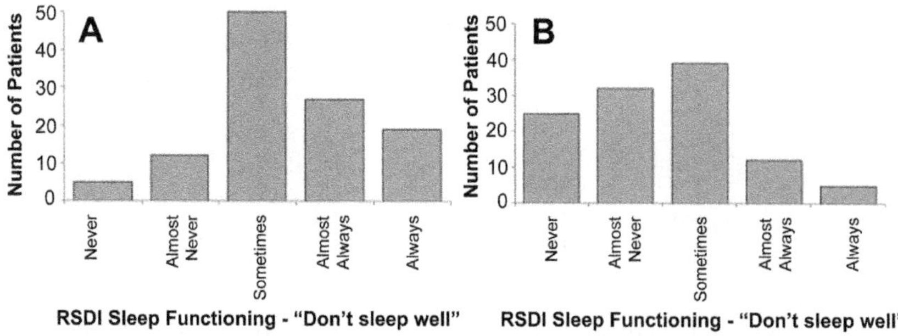

Fig. 4. Subjective sleep disturbance is commonly reported in patients with chronic rhinosinusitis (*A*: preoperative baseline), and may be significantly improved with treatment of the underlying structural and inflammatory disease (*B*: postoperative after endoscopic sinus surgery). RSDI, Rhinosinusitis Disability Index. (*Reproduced from* Benninger MS, Khalid AN, Benninger RM, et al. Surgery for chronic rhinosinusitis may improve sleep and sexual function. Laryngoscope 2010;120:1699; with permission from John Wiley & Sons.)

and symptomatic nasal obstruction, septoplasty lowered nasal resistance, increased mean cross-sectional area, and significantly improved snoring, as measured by both the Snore Outcomes Survey and Spouse/Bed Partner Survey.

Nakata also recently demonstrated that nasal surgery, in the setting of nasal obstruction and sleep apnea, improves nasal resistance, sleep architecture, and daytime sleepiness.[31] In these patients, the observed improvement in the Epworth Sleepiness Score (ESS) from 10.6 to 4.5 with nasal surgery is comparable with the improvement obtained with other forms of OSA therapy, including positive pressure. In a prospective longitudinal cohort study of patients with nasal obstruction and OSA, nasal surgery also significantly improved both disease-specific and general health (SF-36 Health Survey) quality of life measures.[32]

Despite the vast evidence of the beneficial impact of lower nasal resistance on sleep architecture, sleep efficiency, snoring, daytime sleepiness, and quality of life measures, the importance of treating nasal obstruction has been often overlooked because of its variable and sometimes negligible effect on the AHI. Although the AHI provides an important gauge of OSA severity in many patients, the AHI remains only one metric of the complex relationship between sleep and breathing. A critical opportunity to improve OSA patients' sleep may be lost by equating the AHI with the disease process itself and focusing treatment solely on lowering the AHI.

The current literature suggests that across a heterogeneous population, lowering nasal resistance has little overall effect on the AHI, which makes sense because it is in the pharynx, not the nose, where dynamic airway collapse occurs. Nevertheless, in selected OSA patients with a normal hypopharyngeal airway, as demonstrated by cephalometrics or physical examination, a clinically significant reduction in the AHI may be achieved. Findings that have been attributable to successful lowering of the AHI with nasal surgery alone include small tonsils, low modified Mallampati score,

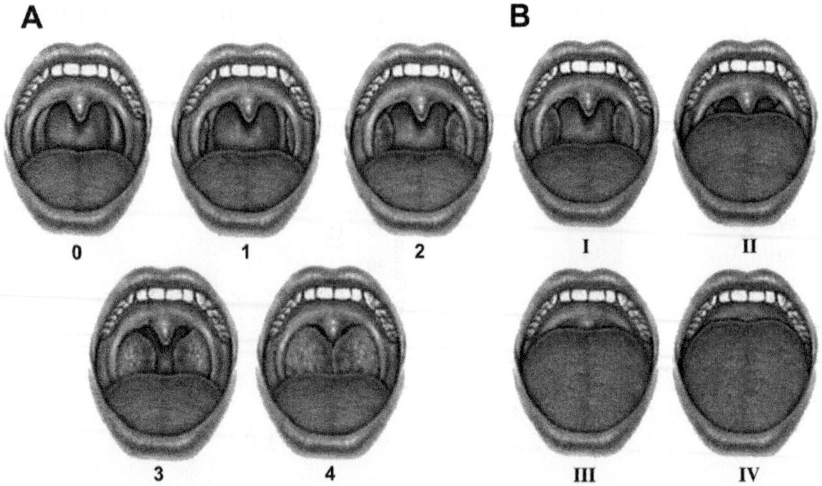

Fig. 5. Examination of the oropharynx. Examples of the methods used to stage and phenotype the oropharyngeal airway include (*A*) tonsil size, and (*B*) modified Mallampati or Friedman tongue/palate position. In OSA patients, higher tonsil stage (3 or 4+) and higher Friedman or modified Mallampati stage (III or IV) suggest minimal to no improvement in the AHI with treatment of nasal obstruction alone. (*Reproduced from* Friedman M, Ibrahim H, Joseph N. Staging of obstructive sleep apnea/hypopnea: a guide to appropriate treatment. Laryngoscope 2004;114:455; with permission.)

and a normal mandibular plane to hyoid distance on cephalometry. Conversely, large tonsils, modified Mallampati III/IV, and/or a low hyoid position suggest an unfavorable improvement in the AHI with nasal surgery alone (**Fig. 5**).[9,33,34]

Finally, treatment of nasal obstruction in OSA patients can significantly improve compliance and effectiveness of continuous positive airway pressure (CPAP) and oral appliance therapy. Mounting evidence suggests that increased nasal resistance negatively affects success rates and tolerance of medical therapy devices for OSA, which critically depend on regular usage to be effective. High nasal resistance has been associated with poorer treatment outcomes in OSA patients treated with mandibular advancement devices.[35] With logistic regression analysis, Suguira and colleagues[36] concluded that increased nasal resistance was one of only two factors associated with nonacceptance of CPAP. Further, in patients with poor CPAP compliance and nasal obstruction, lowering nasal resistance with surgical therapy has been shown to lower average CPAP pressures and improve compliance.[37]

SUMMARY POINTS

1. Sleep disorders, including insomnia and sleep-disordered breathing, are exceedingly common in patients with allergic rhinitis, and contribute greatly to the effects on daytime function and quality of life
2. The negative impact of allergic rhinitis on sleep is primarily mediated through nasal obstruction, which characteristically worsens in the overnight period
3. Nasal obstruction is associated with abnormal sleep efficiency, continuity, and architecture, as well as an increased risk of snoring and OSA
4. Treatment of nasal obstruction can significantly improve both subjective and objective measures of sleep disturbance, irrespective of the sleep apnea severity
5. Treatment of nasal obstruction can improve acceptance of and compliance with both positive pressure and oral appliance therapy for sleep apnea.

REFERENCES

1. Leger D, Annesi-Maesano I, Carat F, et al. Allergic rhinitis and its consequences on quality of sleep: an unexplored area. Arch Intern Med 2006;16:1744–8.
2. Stuck BA, Czajkowski J, Hagner AE, et al. Changes in daytime sleepiness, quality of life, and objective sleep patterns in seasonal allergic rhinitis: a controlled clinical trial. J Allergy Clin Immunol 2004;113:663–8.
3. Blaiss M, Reigel T, Philpot E. A study to determine the impact of rhinitis on sufferers' sleep and daily routine. J Allergy Clin Immunol 2005;115:S197.
4. Craig TJ, Ferguson BJ, Krouse JH. Sleep impairment in allergic rhinitis, rhinosinusitis, and nasal polyposis. Am J Otolaryngol 2008;29:209–17.
5. Mullol J, Maurer M, Bousquet J. Sleep and allergic rhinitis. J Investig Allergol Clin Immunol 2008;18(6):415–9.
6. White D, Cadieux R, Lomard R, et al. The effects of nasal anesthesia on breathing during sleep. Am Rev Respir Dis 1985;132:972–5.
7. McNicholas W, Coffey M, Boyle T. Effects of nasal airflow on breathing during sleep in normal humans. Am Rev Respir Dis 1993;147:620–3.
8. Basner R, Simon P, Schwartzstein R, et al. Breathing route influences upper airway muscle activity in awake normal adults. J Appl Physiol 1989;66:1766–71.
9. McLean HA, Urton AM, Driver HS, et al. Effect of treating severe nasal obstruction on the severity of obstructive sleep apnoea. Eur Respir J 2005;25:521–7.
10. Millman RP, Acebo C, Rosenberg C, et al. Sleep, breathing, and cephalometrics in older children and young adults. Chest 1996;109:673–9.

11. Carskadon MA, Bearpark HM, Sharkey KM, et al. Effects of menopause and nasal occlusion on breathing during sleep. Am J Respir Crit Care Med 1997; 155:205–10.
12. Fitzpatrick MF, McLean H, Urton AM, et al. Effect of nasal or oral breathing route on upper airway resistance during sleep. Eur Respir J 2003;22:827–32.
13. Harvold EP, Tomer BS, Vargervik K, et al. Primate experiments on oral respiration. Am J Orthod 1981;79(4):359–72.
14. Miller AJ, Vargervik K, Chierici G. Morphologic response to changes in neuromuscular changes experimentally induced by altered modes of respiration. Am J Orthod 1984;85(2):115–24.
15. Young T, Finn L, Kim H. Nasal obstruction as a risk factor for sleep-disordered breathing. The University of Wisconsin Sleep and Respiratory Research Group. J Allergy Clin Immunol 1997;99:S757–62.
16. Young T, Finn L, Palta M. Chronic nasal congestion at night is a risk factor for snoring in a population-based cohort study. Arch Intern Med 2001;161: 1514–9.
17. Stradling JR, Crosby JH. Predictors and prevalence of obstructive sleep apnea in 1001 middle-aged men. Thorax 1991;46:85–90.
18. Lofaso F, Coste A, d'Ortho MP, et al. Nasal obstruction as a risk factor for sleep apnoea syndrome. Eur Respir J 2000;16:639–43.
19. Woodson BT, Han JK. Relationship of snoring and daytime sleepiness as presenting symptoms in a sleep clinic population. Ann Otol Rhinol Laryngol 2005; 114(10):762–7.
20. McArdle N, Kingshott R, Engleman H, et al. Partners of patients with sleep apnoea/hypopnoea syndrome: effect of CPAP treatment on sleep quality and quality of life. Thorax 2001;56(7):513–8.
21. Lee SA, Amis TC, Byth K, et al. Heavy snoring as a cause of carotid artery atherosclerosis. Sleep 2008;31(9):1207–13.
22. Howitt L, Kairaitis K, Kirkness JP, et al. Oscillatory pressure wave transmission from the upper airway to the carotid artery. J Appl Physiol 2007;103:1622–7.
23. Amatoury J, Howitt L, Wheatley JR, et al. Snoring related energy transmission to the carotid artery in rabbits. J Appl Physiol 2006;100:1547–53.
24. Li AM, Au CT, Ho R, et al. Blood pressure is elevated in children with primary snoring. J Pediatr 2009;155:362–8.
25. Craig TJ, Teets S, Lehman EB, et al. Nasal congestion secondary to allergic rhinitis as a cause of sleep disturbance and daytime fatigue and the response to topical nasal corticosteroids. J Allergy Clin Immunol 1998;101:633–7.
26. Brouillette RT, Manoukian JJ, Ducharme FM, et al. Efficacy of fluticasone nasal spray for pediatric obstructive sleep apnea. J Pediatr 2001;138:838–44.
27. Benninger MS, Khalid AN, Benniger RM, et al. Surgery for chronic rhinosinusitis may improve sleep and sexual function. Laryngoscope 2010;120: 1696–700.
28. Nakata S, Miyazaki S, Ohki M, et al. Reduced nasal resistance after simple tonsillectomy in patients with OSA. Am J Rhinol 2007;21:192–5.
29. Sullivan S, Kasey Li, Guilleminault C. Nasal obstruction in children with sleep-disordered breathing. Ann Acad Med Singapore 2008;37:645–8.
30. Li HY, Lee AL, Wang PC, et al. Nasal surgery for snoring in patients with obstructive sleep apnea. Laryngoscope 2008;118:354–9.
31. Nakata S, Noda A, Yasuma F, et al. Effects of nasal surgery on sleep quality in obstructive sleep apnea syndrome with nasal obstruction. Am J Rhinol 2008; 22:59–63.

32. Li HY, Lin Y, Chen NH, et al. Improvement in QOL after nasal surgery alone for patients with OSA and NAO. Arch Otolaryngol Head Neck Surg 2008;134:429–33.
33. Series F, St Pierre S, Carrier G. Surgical correction of nasal obstruction in the treatment of mild sleep apnea: importance of cephalometry in predicting outcome. Thorax 1993;48:360–3.
34. Li HY, Lee LA, Wang PC, et al. Can nasal surgery improve obstructive sleep apnea: subjective or objective? Am J Rhinol Allergy 2009;23:1–5.
35. Zeng B, Ng AT, Qian J, et al. Influence of nasal resistance on oral appliance treatment outcome in obstructive sleep apnea. Sleep 2008;31(4):543–7.
36. Suguira T, Noda A, Nakata S, et al. Influence of nasal resistance on initial acceptance of CPAP in treatment of OSAS. Respiration 2007;74:56–60.
37. Nakata S, Noda A, Yagi H, et al. Nasal resistance for determinant factor of nasal surgery in CPAP failure patients with obstructive sleep apnea syndrome. Rhinology 2005;43:296–9.

The Role of Allergy in Otitis Media with Effusion

David S. Hurst, MD, PhD*

KEYWORDS

• Allergy • Otitis media with effusion • Immunotherapy • Atopy
• Eustachian tube

Key Points: Allergy in Otitis Media

- The middle ear, as part of the unified airway, can be a target organ of allergy.
- OME is frequently an IgE-mediated, late phase allergic disease.
- Allergy can cause eustachian tube dysfunction.
- SPT underestimates the incidence of allergy among patients with OME.
- Once patients are identified as being atopic, aggressive treatment of their allergies with immunotherapy can frequently resolve the underlying middle ear disease.

Otitis media with effusion (OME) is the major form of chronic relapsing inflammatory disease of the middle ear. It is a clinical disease defined as the presence of fluid in the middle ear behind an intact tympanic membrane with no active infection. For 70 years, the concept of the cause of this disease had been founded on clinical observation. The emergence of molecularly based diagnostic tools in genetics, cell biology, and immunology over the last decade has now enabled us to better understand the pathophysiology of OME and develop new therapies for OME based on the improved understanding.

Portions of this article were previously published in: Hurst DS. Efficacy of allergy immunotherapy as a treatment for patients with chronic otitis media with effusion. Int J Pediatr Otorhinolaryngol 2008;72(8):1215–23; with permission; and Hurst DS. The middle ear: the inflammatory response in children with otitis media with effusion and the impact of atopy. Clinical and histochemical studies. In: Comprehensive Summaries of Uppsala Dissertations from the Faculty of Medicine, Dept of Immunology and Clinical Chemistry #978. Uppsala (Sweden): Uppsala University Sweden; 2000; with permission.
Tufts University, Department of Otolaryngology/Head and Neck Surgery, 800 Washington Street, Box 850, Boston, MA 02111, USA
* Private Practice, 43 Carson Drive, Gorham, ME 04038.
E-mail address: meear43@gmail.com

Otolaryngol Clin N Am 44 (2011) 637–654
doi:10.1016/j.otc.2011.03.009
oto.theclinics.com

Chronic OME is associated with hearing loss and delayed speech development and may cause permanent middle ear damage with mucosal changes.[1] It is a disease of immense social and financial impact among families of young children, accounting for more than 16 million office visits a year at an annual cost of more than $3.5 billion (2003) in the United States alone.[2] Children with hearing loss secondary to OME constitute the largest group of people in the world with a reversible learning disorder. Among the 35% of preschool children who experience otitis media (OM), 50% maintain the effusion 14 days after initial treatment.[3] In another study the effusion was found to persist in 70% at 2 weeks, in 40% at 1 month, and in 20% beyond 2 months.[4] Chronic middle ear disease represents an entity with multiple contributing environmental factors interacting with a complex web of immunologic, genetic, mechanical, and inflammatory components.

Many otologists do not embrace a role of allergy in chronic middle ear disease. A recent clinical practice discussion and literature review states that "the relation between allergy and OME will remain controversial until well controlled clinical studies are conducted documenting that in select populations antiallergy therapy is efficacious in preventing or limiting the duration of OME."[5]

TERMINOLOGY AND DEFINITIONS

OM describes a symptom, not a disease. It is used to categorize a broad spectrum of middle ear abnormalities, which may involve recurrent acute infections occurring sporadically or extend to conditions of prolonged, ris intact, perforated, or draining.

Chronic suppurative OM (CSOM) refers to a chronic discharge through a perforation of the tympanic membrane. OME is defined by the current gGuidelines as "fluid in the middle ear without signs or symptoms of infection; OME is not to be confused with acute OM (inflammation of the middle ear with signs of infection)."[6] Confusion occurs when practitioners mistakenly equate inflammation with infection.

Allergy refers to symptoms of asthma, rhinitis, or otitis versus atopy, which is a sensitivity as reflected by elevated IgE antibody levels to various allergens without the patient necessarily having the symptoms.[7] There is little research on the role of allergy in OME. Of more than 10,570 articles published from 2001 to 2006 in the 2 major allergy journals (*Allergy* and *Journal of Allergy and Clinical Immunology*) and the 3 major ear, nose, and throat journals (*Otolaryngology, Head and Neck Surgery*; *Laryngoscope*; and *Annals of Otolaryngology*), only 16 articles addressed the link of allergy to middle ear disease.

IMMUNOLOGY OF ALLERGY

If the nomenclature published by both the European Academy of Allergy and Clinical Immunology and the American Academy of Allergy Asthma and Immunologyguidelines in 2001 and 2003, respectively,[7] for asthma or sinusitis as being either allergic or nonallergic, is extended to categorize inflammation in the middle ear, which is a direct extension of the mucosa-lined respiratory tract, allergic otitis inflammation could be divided into "IgE- or non–IgE-mediated" disease (**Fig. 1**).

All normal individuals, atopic or not, when exposed during an infection to bacterial antigen stimulate a cell-mediated T_H1 response that is activated by the cytokines interferon γ and interleukin (IL) 2.[8,9] In the T_H2 allergic reaction, allergens trigger the naive T cell to take a different pathway to become a T_H2 cell (**Fig. 2**). The immunology of IgE-mediated disease is detailed by Calhoun and Schofieldelsewhere in this issue. Although in summary, IgE-mediated disease is characterized by mast cell

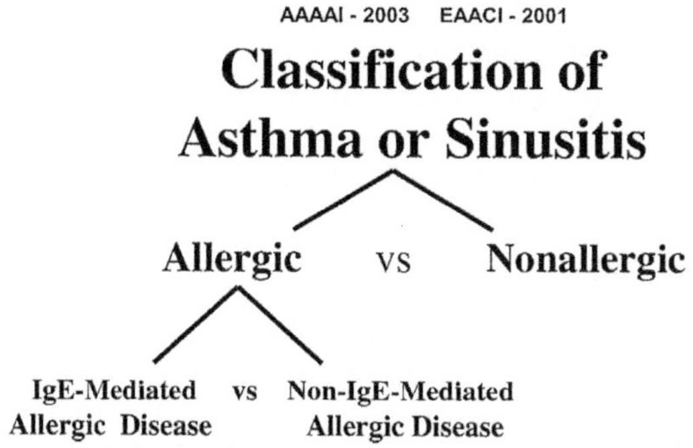

Fig. 1. AAAAI and EAACI classification of the inflammation of asthma or sinusitis. AAAAI, American Academy of Allergy Asthma and Immunology; EAACI, European Academy of Allergy and Clinical Immunology. (*From* Johansson SG, Bieber T, Dahl R, et al. Revised nomenclature for allergy for global use: report of the nomenclature review committee of the world allergy organization, October 2003. J Allergy Clin Immunol 2004;113(5):834; with permission.)

degranulation and a classic early phase of symptoms occurring within an hour of antigen exposure, the late phase occurs several hours later and is mediated by the recruitment of eosinophils attracted by IL-5 as well as other cytokines generated during the early phase response. This eosinophil response can be present chronically

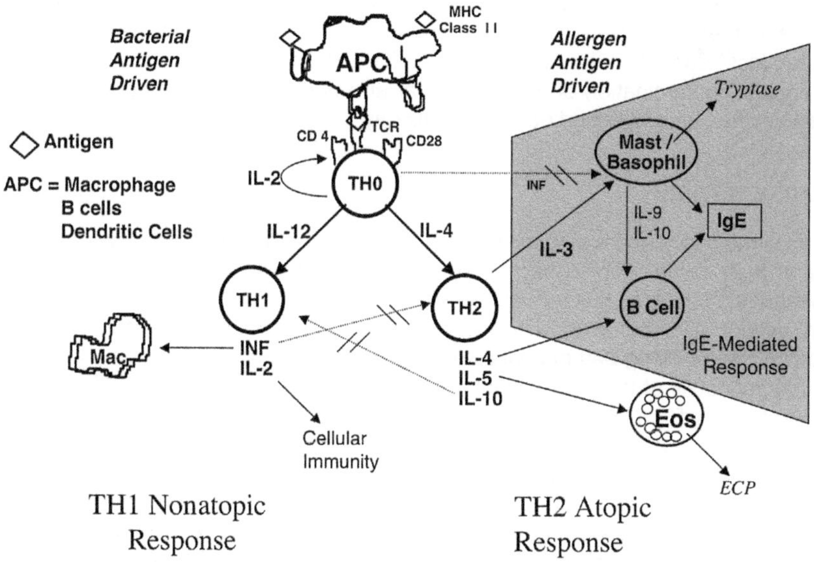

Fig. 2. A representation of current concepts of T, B, and antigen-presenting cell (APC) interrelationships. Bacterial antigen-induced (T_H1) and allergen-induced (T_H2) reactions lead to the release of cell mediators such as tryptase, eosinophil cationic protein (ECP) and MPO. APCs include macrophages (Mac), B cells, and dendritic cells. Cells in the trapezoid constitute the IgE-mediated early phase T_H2 response. Eosinophils and IL-5 are expressions of non—IgE-mediated late phase disease. Eos, eosinophils; INF, interferon; MHC, major histocompatibility complex; TCR, T cell receptor. (*Adapted from* Hurst DS, Venge P. The impact of atopy on neutrophil activity in middle ear effusion from children and adults with chronic otitis media. Arch Otolaryngol Head Neck Surg 2002;128:561; with permission.)

in ongoing disease. The presence of eosinophils does not in itself implicate IgE-mediated disease but rather reflects non—IgE-mediated hypersensitivity. Influx of eosinophils and their mediators eosinophil cationic protein (ECP) and major basic protein (MBP) are typical of some of the most refractory subtypes of asthma and rhinosinusitis and have been documented in the effusion of OME.[9]

HISTORICAL PERSPECTIVE

In 1931, Proetz[10] noted a relationship of middle ear disease with allergic rhinitis. In 1947, Koch[11] observed eosinophilia in the otorrhea from 222 children, "supporting the contention that the middle ear takes part in allergic reactions similar to those seen in the nose and sinuses." In 1965, Fernandez and McGovern[12] suggested that an allergic mechanism, although not the major cause of chronic OME, was a predisposing factor in as many as 85% of children with acute otitis. Shambaugh[13] suspected allergy as a cause of chronic draining mastoid cavities or middle ears in patients with OME and cautioned that "surgical mastoidectomy, simple or radical is not indicated. With competent allergic diagnosis and management, preferably by the otologist trained in allergic methods, the otorrhea is finally brought under control."[13]

Objective information on the allergic status of patients with OME is lacking in available otitis databases in Minnesota or Norway (Casselbrant M, personal communication, 2007), making the true incidence of allergy unknown. In studies from 1952 to 1984, Suehs,[14] Senturia and colleagues,[15] Boor,[16] Siirala,[17] Lim and Brick,[18] and Reisman and Bernstein[19] using the techniques of their day, could not find any clinical basis of allergy in the formation of OME. Suehs[14] reported an absence of eosinophils in the middle ear effusion (MEE) of 50 patients, as did Senturia[20] in 1960. Sade and colleagues[21] attributed the basic cause of OME to infection in the nasopharynx with retrograde contamination of the middle ear and edema of the eustachian tube (ET). This thinking has dominated otology to this day.

ALLERGY TESTING

Studies that find no increased allergy in subjects with OME often rely on less-objective criteria than actual skin testing to arrive at a diagnosis of allergy. Tomonaga and colleagues[22] criticized many of these methodologically flawed studies in the "Discussion" section of of their work. The study revealed that 21% of 605 patients with allergy had OME, but among 259 patients with OME, 87% were atopic by skin testing, even though only 50% of them had nasal allergy.

The study by Bernstein and colleagues[23] in 1981, although sentinel in being among the first to link allergy to otitis, probably underestimated the role of allergy in OME because it reported that less than 30% of OME was related to allergy. This low percentage results from the very narrow definition of atopy, which required both rhinitis and a total IgE level greater than 100 μg/L or positive results of prick testing. Ten years ago, the author's group showed that the mean total IgE level among atopic patients was 93.8 μg/L, with two-thirds of atopic patients with OME having a serum IgE level less than 100 μg/L.[24] Otitis is thus similar to rhinitis. It is a "low level IgE disease" having no relation to the total IgE level, unlike asthma, which does show a correlation with IgE levels.[25] Because OME is a low-level IgE disease, prick testing misses more than 80% of patients with OME whose disease actually resolves when those particular allergens that give positive results on intradermal testing are included in their immunotherapy (IT).[26] The reported prevalence of atopy of 81% to 100% by the author among the group of more than 240 patients with OME[9,24,26] may reflect the increased sensitivity of intradermal testing compared with results obtained from specific IgE in vitro testing,[27,28] and/or its equivalent skin prick testing (SPT).

There are several large literature reviews of the relationship of allergy to OME. Ojala[29] surmised that "It would seem that atopy is probably one cause of persistent therapy-resistant otitis media and it must be taken into account when considering the treatment of a chronic ear." Sprinkle and Veltri[30] found "solid evidence....to suggest that *(Gell Coombs)* Type I immune injury can be considered a major contributing factor to persistent middle ear effusion.," and that type III hypersensitivity reactions that require the presence of microorganisms were "very important," and type IV reactions may also "play a role in causing and potentiating serous otitis media in man." Doyle[31] concluded that "it has been reasonably well demonstrated that allergy is a risk factor for otitis media." Skoner and colleagues[32] in his article on OM, with more than 209 references note that "evidence that allergy contributes to the pathogenesis of OME is derived from epidemiologic, mechanistic, and therapeutic lines of investigation." Tewfik and Mazer[5] concluded "in-vitro and clinical evidence now indicates that, as in asthma and allergic rhinitis, Th2 mediated allergic inflammation is found in middle ear effusion in some patients with OME. As in asthma, this may be a result of direct allergen exposure."

EPIDEMIOLOGY

OME is a multifactorial disease, of which allergy is only 1 risk factor. Parental smoking, day care classrooms having more than 6 students, asthma, and viral upper respiratory tract infection are also known to predispose one for OME. Yet allergy adds unique comorbidity and is by far a greater risk factor than other identified factors, conferring a 2- to 4.5-fold increased incidence of OME compared with the incidence of OME in nonallergic people.[33,34] Thus a child who has an episode of acute OM is up to 3 times more likely to develop OME if that same child is also allergic.

Epidemiologic studies in Japan[22] and Sweden[35] have shown a significant relation of allergy to OME. Although only 6% to 20% of the general population is atopic and among atopic patients only 21% have OME, more than 87% of patients with OME were found to be atopic and/or have allergy symptoms.[22] Irander and colleagues[35] found that among 54 Swedish infants, 38% with OME had respiratory tract allergy. Infants with allergic symptoms were 5 times more likely to develop OME than nonatopic patients. Jero and colleagues[36] found similar results in Finland where allergy posed a risk factor of 4.4 for children failing to clear an acute otitis. Allergy certainly puts a patient at risk for recurrent sinus infections because it adds to conditions that can lead to an environment that is suitable for mucostasis, bacterial overgrowth, and chronic inflammation.[37] The author's group has found that among 97 patients with OME, 62% had documentation of additional atopic signs and symptoms, including asthma in 22%, allergic rhinitis in 48%, eczema in 4%, and chronic nasal congestion in 8%.[24]

Based on SPT, a Greek study[34] found a much higher incidence of allergy among 88 children with chronic OME than in the controls. It was concluded that allergy is an independent risk factor for developing OME. A study in Mexico found that 15% of 80 children with positive skin test result to dust, corn, and cockroach had abnormal tympanograms when compared with 50 controls all of who had normal Type A tympanograms and negative results of SPT for the same 3 allergens. Among children with rhinitis, allergy presented an increased risk for difficulty in opening their ET.[38]

Doner and colleagues[39] evaluated 22 children who required an myringotomy and tubes (M&T) and adenoidectomy. Only 8% of those with no recurrence of their middle ear disease had positive skin test result. This result compared with those of 22 children who had recurrent middle ear effusions requiring repeat M&T. Thirty-eight percent of this group had positive SPT result. The investigators concluded that allergy seemed to be a major contributing factor for recurrent disease.

Viral infections seem to be a trigger for OME. Chonmaitree and colleagues[40] found that 39% of 84 children with MEE had positive viral cultures of their effusion and/or nasal lavage at the time of their acute episode. Only 15% of the patients had no pathogen (bacteria or virus) in the effusion. Other studies showed that human rhinovirus RNA is present in 30% of the effusions of children with OME.[41] Endotoxin has been demonstrated in 52% to 87% of effusions.[42] Polymerase chain reaction has detected the presence of various bacteria in as many as 85% of the cases.[43]

Viral sensitization may contribute to the initial inflammatory process leading to OME. Respiratory syncytial virus (RSV), a common virus in the middle ear and nasopharynx, induces a state of IgE-mediated allergy in the nasopharynx[44] wherein patients with elevated number of mast cells in the adenoid bed are more prone to OME on viral exposure.[45] RSV enhances the synthesis of proinflammatory cytokines (IL-1b, tumor necrosis factor-α, IL-6) and cell adhesion molecules (ICAM-1, ELAM-1, VCAM-1)[46] in the middle ear of infected individuals. Ohashi and colleagues[47] found VCAM-1 levels to be significantly more elevated in the ears of atopic patients. It has been suggested that both a respiratory virus infection and the presence of bacteria in the nasopharynx are required for the development of acute otitis. Garofalo and colleagues[48] examined the effusion from 20 children with acute otitis. They found that tryptase levels were elevated in 79% of the patients. Samples that were negative for viral culture did not contain detectable levels of tryptase. It was suggested that viral pathogens were "an essential trigger or priming factor for mast cell degranulation." Neither virus nor bacteria alone seems to be capable of causing otitis as frequently as the 2 combined, especially in atopic patients.

HISTOLOGIC STUDIES

Inflammation is exclusively an in vivo phenomenon that only occurs in living tissues with an active microcirculation.[49] Purulence in the middle ear has previously been shown to elevate levels of both eosinophil and neutrophil mediators.[9] Perpetuation of inflammation, regardless of origin, is the crucial difference between recurrent acute OM and OME. A basic question is whether the middle ear inflammation was the result of infection, allergy, or both. Atopy seems to have a significant relationship to whatever produces a response from eosinophils and mast cells in the middle ear.[24] This is a significant observation not only in regard to the association to allergy but also because human eosinophils are much more toxic than neutrophils, making them particularly harmful to host tissues.[50]

The fact that conventional histology does not readily detect degranulated or activated neutrophils, mast cells, or eosinophils has led to various conclusions[29,51–53] and is the major reason this controversy has been perpetuated. There is also disagreement as to whether mediators in MEE come from the plasma or local tissue. In the initial stages of serous otitis, mast cells are found in the lamina propria and the pars flacida of diseased human middle ears.[54] Mast cells release inflammatory mediators producing vasodilatation and mucosal edema, as well as neutrophil chemotaxis. Using animal studies, Nakata and colleagues[55] found few eosinophils in the effusion of immunized chinchillas in the acute phase of inflammation but also concluded that "middle ear effusion is a local product of the middle ear mucosa rather than a transudate from plasma." Histopathologic examination of effusion demonstrates that eosinophils and neutrophils are integral components in these secretions.[52,56]

In addition to the cytotoxic effects of ECP, myeloperoxidase (MPO), and tryptase, these mediators are always accompanied by the other proteases, lysozomasol enzymes, and oxidizers that are released simultaneously from their respective cells. ECP attracts other inflammatory cells, including neutrophils, and also delays apoptosis. This may be why the atopic patient continues to produce additional fluid, when compared with the nonatopic patient. This condition was seen in allergic mice, which produced twice the amount of MEE as nonallergic mice on antigen challenge.[57] ECP has also been shown to decrease ciliary function and impair ET clearance.

The very high concentrations of mediators released by eosinophils and mast cells may also account for the great destruction, osteitis, and granulation tissue described on histologic examination of temporal bones from patients with chronic OME.[51] Both heparin and tryptase contribute to fibrosis and bone resorption.[58] This finding may have added significance in understanding the pathophysiology of chronic scarring in the middle ear as well as in the bone destruction observed in cholesteatoma. A prospective study of 117 patients found that "patients with cholesteatoma had a higher prevalence of IgE-mediated hypersensitivity than patients without that condition." The researchers concluded that "allergy might contribute to chronic otitis media especially in cases with a cholesteatoma."[59]

One of the unique features of the middle ear response in OME is the involvement of neutrophils. Most atopic patients have increased levels of MPO in addition to ECP in their ear effusion, even though there is no evidence of acute inflammation.[24] Paired samples confirm that in an acutely infected ear, purulent otitis is associated with a significant elevation of both mediators, but with a disproportionately greater elevation of MPO in the infected side when compared with the nonpurulent ear.[60] Yet even in the nonpurulent ear, the levels of MPO were much higher in atopic patients than in nonatopic patients. The inflammatory response to putative inciting agents such as bacterial and viral products may be amplified in atopy, perhaps via IL-8. Another explanation for the increased MPO level reported in nonpurulent MEE is that an increase in neutrophils may occur as a result of weak stimulation of these cells because bacteria are being cleared from the site of inflammation.[61] Bacterial messenger RNA (mRNA) present in otherwise sterile MEE may serve as a stimulus to T-cell activation.[62] Regardless of whether the relationship between allergy and OME is direct or indirect, marked elevation of effusion MPO levels in atopic patients, but very low levels in nonatopic patients, suggests that atopy may contribute to elevated levels of neutrophil activity in OME to a disproportionate degree among atopic patients.[60]

Neutrophils are reported in IgE-mediated late phase reactions in the nose and skin.[63] Thus the presence of neutrophils in MEE is not necessarily an argument against OME being an allergic disease. Atopy contributes to the elevated levels of MPO by causing the atopic child to respond differently to the products of acute inflammation because of its primed inflammatory cells. This is demonstrated most vividly in the classroom struck by a viral upper respiratory tract infection. Whereas most normal children only experience a cold, their atopic classmates frequently go on to trigger asthma attacks requiring nebulizer treatments.

The destructive potential of these mediators in effusion is often overlooked, as is hearing loss, yet serves as a further justification for the removal of this fluid at the time of myringotomy and for prevention of its reoccurrence by appropriate surgical and allergy management. Allergy testing is frequently recommended in children requiring a second set of tubes, in order that this common predisposing factor for OME can be addressed.

ET DYSFUNCTION

ET dysfunction (ETD), either extrinsic or intrinsic, is regarded as the underlying pathophysiologic event that leads to most cases of chronic middle ear disease. Causes of ETD include ciliary dysmotility, nasopharynx carcinoma, cleft palate, gastroesophageal reflux,[64] and adenoid hypertrophy, but these causes only account for a minority of patients. Allergy and reflux are the best explanations for the intermittent nature of ETD. Bluestone[65] outlined 4 hypothetical mechanisms by which allergy could be responsible for ETD leading to the production of OME. These mechanisms included (1) the middle ear functioning directly as a shock organ, (2) ETD due to intrinsic mechanical obstruction from inflammatory swelling of the ET itself, (3) inflammatory obstruction of the nose, or (4) aspiration of bacteria-laden allergic secretions from the nasopharynx into the middle ear. As hypothesized, these explanations have all been documented to occur at times because of allergy.

Obstruction of the ET in humans has been clearly demonstrated to result from antigen challenge.[66] The ET has been shown to be involved functionally and morphologically in type I reactions of the nose.[67] In a double-blind protocol, Friedman and colleagues[68] demonstrated that intranasal pollen challenge of atopic individuals produced allergic rhinitis followed by ET obstruction, which did not occur with the placebo. The allergic reaction inhibited even transient dilations of the ET during swallowing. Several other double-blind protocols with intranasal allergen or histamine challenge produced similar severe functional obstruction of the ET.[69] All these results confirm the hypothesis that the ET may become dysfunctional due to allergic inflammation causing intrinsic mucosal edema and obstruction. Skoner and colleagues[32] in their review state, "much of the research into OM pathophysiology has indicated that there is a pivotal role for allergen-induced dysfunction of the Eustachian tube... Allergen-induced blockage subverts the normal mechanism of gas exchange between the middle ear and the environment, thus setting the stage for development of middle ear underpressured OME."

The most frequently cited objection of past decades to the allergy hypothesis is that an allergen is unlikely to get into the middle ear itself because of the structural gatekeeper function of the ET.[70] Possible mechanisms of immune response in the ear have been proposed. Secretory immunity does not rely on the premise of direct allergen transport to the middle ear, but rather depends on the newer understanding of both humoral and cell-mediated immunology. These concepts are best explained in the section "Unified Airway."

Evidence-based medicine has dispelled previously held assumptions. It has been shown that "there are no substantial differences in ET function between ears that develop OME recurrence and ears that do not."[71] It is also a commonly held myth that the ET will grow to normal size as children mature despite evidence that there is no difference in the size of either the isthmus or the pharyngeal portion of the ET in children with OME versus normals.[72] Sade and colleagues[72] showed that the ET of patients with OM does not have an "immature morphology." Parents are also falsely told that their otitis-prone children cannot equalize the pressure in their middle ears, yet the fact is that there is no organic obstruction or stenosis of the ET in patients with OME. Only 11% of patients with active OME have abnormally high opening pressures.[73] Finally, there is the myth of antibiotics. Rosenfeld and Bluestone[74] have shown that a meta-analysis of all treatment studies demonstrate antibiotics to be no better than placebo in treating chronic OME. Chronic OME is usually not an infection.

UNIFIED AIRWAY

The middle ear is not a privileged site devoid of immune response mechanisms as was taught in the 1960s. Middle ear mucosa, which evolves from the same ectoderm as the rest of the upper respiratory tract epithelium, has been found in animal studies to have the same active intrinsic immunologic responsiveness to antigenic stimulus as do the nasal tract, sinuses, and bronchi.[62] It is now recognized that human nasal airway mucosa is the focus of absorption of allergens as well as microorganisms that activate the mucosal defense systems. Secretory immunity is the best-defined effector mechanism of antigen presentation and stimulation of the immune system in humans and is elegantly described by Jahnsen and Brandtzaeg.[75]

Since 2000, both the European Academy of Allergy and Clinical Immunology and the American Allergy Academy of Allergy Asthma and Immunology have come to view the upper respiratory tract as a unified airway system. The underlying concept is that allergy can affect different target organs at different ages. So, just as most asthmas are hyper reactive diseases of the airway mucosa, all allergic diseases, including OME, are hyper reactive mucosal diseases regardless of the location of the mucous membrane within the respiratory tract. This concept is developed in detail by Krouse.[76] Extrapolating from the landmark study by Braunstahl and colleagues[77] in which nonasthmatic patients with allergic rhinitis were administered nasal provocation with pollen, he demonstrated eosinophilic infiltration in the lungs, through bronchial washings, even though the lungs were never stimulated with antigen. He concluded that the upper respiratory tract responded as one unified airway.

Similarly, Hamid and colleague[78] simultaneously took biopsies from the middle ear mucosa and the nasopharyngeal mucosa just next to the ET orifice. He measured eosinophils, CD3 T cells, IL-4 levels, and mRNA levels for IL-5 and found them all to be elevated at both ends of the ET. He concluded that the middle ear may behave in a "similar manner to the lungs under allergic inflammatory insults" and that the "middle ear may be included in the united airways."

OM: AN ALLERGIC DISEASE

Because asthma is heterogeneous, some forms are categorized predominantly with a non–IgE-mediated eosinophilic histotype. Current medical therapy for asthma now relies on antileukotrienes and steroid inhalers as agents to downregulate the eosinophil mediators and activation. Exactly the same cells and chemical mediators found in the lung and sinuses in allergic disease are also found in the middle ear.

Proof of the hypothesis that chronic OME is an allergic disease requires the following 4 steps.

The first is to establish a relevant, associated, objective diagnosis of atopy in patients with persistent effusion or middle ear drainage. The low sensitivity of conventional prick or radioallergosorbent testing hampers the diagnosis of this low-level IgE-mediated disease.[26,79] As mentioned, investigators using objective intradermal testing demonstrate that 72% to 100% of children with OME are atopic (**Table 1**).

The second step is to establish an association of allergic T_H2 immune-mediated histochemical reactivity within the target organ itself. The concept that active immunologic processes may be a localized phenomena in the middle ear has been established in animal models[57] as well as in humans. Lymphocytes necessary for antibody production are recruited nonspecifically into the mucosa in OM. T lymphocytes are

Table 1
Studies of patients with OME with allergy confirmed by skin testing

References	Number with Positive Skin Test	% of Positive Tests	% Improved with Allergy Therapy
Dohlman,[80] 1943	178	56%	—
Mao,[81] 1942	252	29% of pathologically deaf children 2% of normal children	—
Jordan,[82] 1949	123	74%	98%
Solow,[83] 1958	50	72%	—
Lecks,[84] 1961	82	88%	—
Fernandez and McGovern,[12] 1965	113	55%	95%
Whitcomb,[85] 1965	38	100%	87%
Draper,[86] 1967	340	53%	91%
Hall and Lukat,[87] 1981	92	100%	82%
McMahan et al,[88,a] 1981	119	93%	86%
Sanz et al,[89,a] 1986	20	30%	—
Tomonaga et al,[22] 1988	259	72% of OME cases	
Hurst,[90,b] 1990	20	100%	100%
Becker et al,[91] 1991	35	34%	SPT
Nsouli et al,[92,a] 1994	104	78%	86%
Corey et al,[93,a] 1994	89	61%	—
Hurst,[9] 1996	73	87%	—
Psifidis et al,[94] 1998	148	59%	78%
Doner et al,[39] 2004	22	38%	SPT
Lasisi et al,[95] 2008	80	80%	SPT
Hurst,[26,b] 2008	89	100%	89% of OME resolve 0% of controls

[a] In vitro testing.
[b] Patients not included in previous study.

Data from Hurst DS. The middle ear: the inflammatory response in children with otitis media with effusion and the impact of atopy. Clinical and histochemical studies. In: Comprehensive Summaries of Uppsala Dissertations from the Faculty of Medicine, Dept of Immunology and Clinical Chemistry #978. Uppsala (Sweden): Uppsala University Sweden; 2000. p. 14; as modified in Hurst DS. Freedom from Chronic Ear Infections: The Role of Allergies and the Way to a Cure. Portsmouth, NH: Back Channel Press; 2011. p. 130; with permission.

common in serous or mucoid effusions.[96] IL-5 is produced predominately by stimulated T_H2 and not T_H1 cells (see **Fig. 2**),[97] and its levels are increased during the late phase reaction of chronic middle ear disease.[98] IL-5 mRNA in middle ear mucosa biopsies provides strong evidence that the middle ear is actively participating in a T_H2 response.[99]

Proof of a relation of allergy to asthma or sinus disease required researchers to demonstrate tryptase from mast cells and, more importantly, ECP or MBP from eosinophils in the lung and sinuses. Similarly, studies in China, Japan, the United States, Canada, and Sweden have demonstrated that all the mediators required for a T_H2 inflammatory response, including ECP, tryptase, and/or IL-5 mRNA cells, $CD3^+T$

cells,[99] eosinophils,[100] mast cells,[101] Rantes,[102] prostaglandins,[78] and specific IgE for foods and inhalants[103] are present in most ears with chronic effusion. Antitryptase antibody (AA1) staining[101] has shown that mast cells are present in the mucosa and submucosa in atopic patients and not in controls. Lasisi and colleagues[103] studied the secretion of IgE in the middle ear of patients with CSOM and controls. They found that "allergy appears to play a contributory role in CSOM and elevated IgE in the middle ear secretions suggests a likely mucosal response."[103] Furthermore, they found that a positive skin reaction in 80% of patients with CSOM suggested a "substantial potentiating role of allergy in SOM."

The third step needed to prove that the middle ear behaves as a target organ of allergy is to demonstrate that the inflammation within the middle ear is truly allergic in nature, and not merely coincidental. This demonstration requires an examination of the epidemiologic mechanisms and treatment studies for patients with chronic OME. These studies were reviewed earlier under the section "Etiology."

Direct demonstration of serum and middle ear immunoglobulins being associated with a T_H2 response in the middle ear itself has been provided by Hamid,[78] Lasisi and colleagues,[103] and Hurst and colleagues.[104] The evidence is conclusive enough for the 2004 guidelines published by the academies of Pediatrics, Family Practice, and Otolaryngology-Head and Neck Surgery to conclude that the middle ear epithelium of atopic patients has all the components required to behave in a manner similar to that of the rest of the upper respiratory system, and that "like other parts of respiratory mucosa, the mucosa lining the middle ear cleft is capable of an allergic response."[105] Roland's review[106] surmised that significant data supports "the concept that chronic OME in atopic patients represents a local Th2 allergy response."

The fourth and final step needed to prove the hypothesis of an allergy connection requires direct evidence of a dose-response curve and consistency of results. A call for treatment studies has been made every 4 years at the International Symposia on Middle Ear Disease as well as by the Committee on Guidelines which states, "no recommendation is made regarding allergy management...based on insufficient evidence of therapeutic efficacy or causal relationship between allergy and OME."[105]

EFFICACY OF IMMUNOTHERAPY FOR OME

Sporadic reports of therapeutic efficacy of IT for OME have lacked documented controls until recently. In a study of 89 patients aged 4 to 70 years with intractable middle ear disease who presented with chronic effusion or chronic draining perforations or tubes all proved to be atopic by intradermal skin testing. All were offered allergy IT based on the results of their intradermal testing. A total of 21 individuals self-selected to be a "control cohort" by choosing not to proceed with IT for a variety of reasons. Specific allergy IT completely resolved 85% of 127 diseased ears and significantly improved an additional 5.5%. The condition in all children younger than 15 years and most adults resolved within 4 months and they remained free of disease while on allergy IT for 2 to 8 years of follow-up. None of the controls' 39 ears resolved spontaneously ($P<.001$). The average patient with OME proved to be sensitive to 9 allergens (range 4–15). This study documented that in a select population, antiallergy therapy is efficacious in preventing or limiting the duration of OME while comparing treatment patients to a control cohort.[26] These findings are in keeping with other studies (see **Table 1**) that although lacking a control group, have demonstrated that when a patient's allergies are properly treated with IT and/or diet elimination, the effusion resolves in most patients.

Because chronic otitis has been shown to be a low-level IgE-mediated disease similar to allergic rhinitis, with two-thirds of patients with OME having a serum IgE level less than 100 μg/L (mean 93.8 μg/L),[24] intradermal testing was chosen for its greater sensitivity and reproducibility as the test for atopy. IT was chosen to treat the underlying allergy because it has been shown to have a long-lasting effect on T lymphocytes, it acts in the earliest stages of immunologic response, and it can revert an atopic patient from a T_H2 response back to being a normal T_H1 responder.[107] This has been documented in cases of asthma, allergic sinusitis, and, now, clinically in chronic OME.[78]

This cohort study demonstrated conclusively that almost all patients with OME were atopic. Eighty-seven percent of patients with chronic middle ear fluid who presented with draining tubes, draining perforations, or a history of OME showed resolution of the disease and stayed free of disease from 1 to 8 years follow-up on allergy IT, whereas none of the controls had disease resolution spontaneously. Direct proof that allergy contributes to chronic OME and/or other manifestations of chronic middle ear disease is best given by a randomized, double-blind placebo-controlled trial. None have been published.

Not all OMEs are the result of allergy. What makes the middle ear mucosa the target organ of some allergies and the lung, sinuses, or skin the target of others is unknown. Allergy seems to play a role in more than 85% of those adults or children who present with chronic OME.

Several reviewers suggest that otolaryngologists consider the possible use of allergy treatment for chronic middle ear disease. Lieberman and Blaiss[108] conclude that "in patients with OME in which allergy may be a contributing factor, appropriate allergy treatment of avoidance of particular allergens, medications, and immunotherapy may be indicated." The review by Tewfik and Mazer[5] suggests that it may be prudent to screen every child with OME for allergic rhinitis and, ultimately, to manage those with allergic inflammation differently than nonatopic individuals with OME.

SUMMARY

Current medical evidence supports the link between allergy and OME. The application of newly gained knowledge of inflammation provided by modern immunology and cellular biology gleaned from the study of chronic mucosal inflammatory diseases of the unified airway helps us to understand the pathophysiology underlying chronic middle ear disease. Histologic, epidemiologic, and clinical studies based on objective allergy testing have thus far achieved the following:

1. Established that most patients with OME (see **Table 1**) are atopic
2. Demonstrated that all the mediators necessary for a T_H2 allergic response are present in the middle ear
3. Provided medical evidence to support the conclusion that "the middle ear (mucosa) is capable of an allergic response"[105]
4. Shown using intradermal testing that patients with OME are almost universally atopic and that their chronic middle ear disease does resolve with IT in more than 85% of cases when compared with 0% of a control cohort ($P<.001$).[26]

Review of recent medical evidence supports the hypothesis that chronic OME is an allergic disease. It raises a call for further studies to confirm that treatment using immunotherapy, an established conventional modality recognized to be effective in treating and reversing allergic rhinitis and asthma, is worth considering for the treatment of the otherwise frequently intractable middle ear disease.

REFERENCES

1. Teele DW, Klein JO, Rosner B. Otitis media with effusion during the first three years of life and the development of speech and language. Pediatrics 1984; 74:282–6.
2. Shekelle P, Takata G, Chan LS, et al. Diagnosis, natural history, and late effects of otitis media with effusion. Evidence report/technology assessment no. 55. Rockville (MD): Agency for Healthcare Research and Quality; 2003. AHRQ Publication No. 03-E023.
3. Grundfast K, Schwartz R, Rodriguez W. Duration of middle ear effusion after acute otitis media. Pediatr Infect Dis 1984;3:204–7.
4. Roland P, Finitzo T, Friel-Patti S, et al. Otitis media-incidence, duration, and hearing status. Arch Otolaryngol Head Neck Surg 1989;115:1049–53.
5. Tewfik TL, Mazer B. The links between allergy and otitis media with effusion. Curr Opin Otolaryngol Head Neck Surg 2006;14(3):187–90.
6. Stool SE, Berg AO, Berman A, et al, editors. Otitis media with effusion in young children. Rockville (MD): U.S. Dpeartment of Health and Human Services; Clinical Practice Guideline No. 12; No. AHCRP Publication No. 94-0622; 1994.
7. Johansson SG, Bieber T, Dahl R, et al. Revised nomenclature for allergy for global use: report of the nomenclature review committee of the world allergy organization, October 2003. J Allergy Clin Immunol 2004;113(5):832–6.
8. Romagnani S. Type 1 T helper and type 2 T helper cells: functions, regulation and role in protection and disease. Int J Clin Lab Res 1991;21(2):152–8.
9. Hurst DS. The association of otitis media with effusion and allergy as demonstrated by intradermal skin testing and eosinophil cationic protein levels in both middle ear effusions and mucosal biopsies. Laryngoscope 1996;106:1128–37.
10. Proetz AW. Allergy in middle and internal ear. Ann Otol 1931;40:67.
11. Koch H. Allergical investigations of chronic otitis. Acta Otolaryngol 1947;(Suppl 62): 1–202.
12. Fernandez A, McGovern J. Secretory otitis media in allergic infants and children. South Med J 1965;58:581–6.
13. Shambaugh G Jr. Pathology and clinical course of inflammatory diseases of the middle ear. In: Shambaugh G, editor. Surgery of the ear. 2nd edition. Philadelphia: W.B. Saunders Co; 1967. p. 210–1, p. 271–2.
14. Suehs OW. Serous otitis media. Laryngoscope 1952;62:998–1027.
15. Senturia BH, Jessert CF, Carr CD, et al. Studies concerned with tubal tympanitis. Ann Otol Rhinol Laryngol 1958;67:440.
16. Boor SW. Management of secretory otitis media. Arch Otolaryngol 1962;75: 1305–18.
17. Siirala U. Otitis media adhesiva. Arch Otolaryngol 1964;80:287–96.
18. Lim DJ, Brick H. Ultrastructural pathology of the middle ear mucosa in serous otitis media. Ann Otol Rhinol Laryngol 1971;80:838–53.
19. Reisman RE, Bernstein J. Allergy and secretory otitis media. Pediatr Clin North Am 1975;22:251.
20. Senturia BH. Allergic manifestations in otologic disease. Laryngoscope 1960;70:287.
21. Sade J, Carr DD, Senturia BH. Middle ear effusions produced experimentally in dogs. Ann Otol Rhinol Laryngol 1959;68:1017–27.
22. Tomonaga K, Kurono Y, Moge G. The role of nasal allergy in otitis media with effusion, a clinical study. Acta Otolaryngol Suppl 1988;458:41–7.
23. Bernstein JM, Ellis E, Li P. The role of IgE-mediated hypersensitivity in otitis media with effusion. Otolaryngol Head Neck Surg 1981;89:874.

24. Hurst DS, Venge P. Evidence of eosinophil, neutrophil, and mast-cell mediators in the effusion of OME patients with and without atopy. Allergy 2000;55(5):435–41.
25. Burrows B, Martinez FD, Halonen M, et al. Association of asthma with serum IgE levels and skin-test reactivity to allergens. N Engl J Med 1989;320:271–7.
26. Hurst DS. Efficacy of allergy immunotherapy as a treatment for patients with chronic otitis media with effusion. Int J Pediatr Otorhinolaryngol 2008;72(8):1215–23.
27. Coulson CJ, Drake-Lee AB, Plant T, et al. Total serum IgE and IgE antibodies specific to house dust mite found in two aged-matched cohorts of children with and without otitis media with effusion. Clin Otolaryngol 2006;31(2):130–3.
28. Firat Y, Koc C, Olcay I, et al. The incidence of atopy in adults with recurrent secretory otitis media: screening with Phadiatop. Kulak Burun Bogaz Ihtis Derg 2006;16(1):11–7.
29. Ojala K, Sipila P, Sorri M, et al. Role of atopic allergy in chronic otitis media: evaluation based on serum IgE and nasal/aural cytologic findings in patients with operated chronic ears. Acta Otolaryngol 1982;93:55–60.
30. Sprinkle P, Veltri R. Pathophysiology of serous otitis media. Am J Otol 1986;7:113–8.
31. Doyle WJ. The link between allergic rhinitis and otitis media. Curr Opin Allergy Clin Immunol 2002;2(1):21–5.
32. Skoner D, Gentile D, Mandel E, et al. Otitis media. In: Adkinson N, Bochner BJ, Yunginger J, et al, editors. 6th edition. Middleton's allergy principles & practice, vol. 2. Philadelphia: Mosby, Inc; 2003. p. 1437–54.
33. Stenstrom C, Ingvarsson L. General illness and need of medical care in otitis prone children. Int J Pediatr Otorhinolaryngol 1994;29(1):23–32.
34. Chantzi FM, Kafetzis DA, Bairamis T, et al. IgE sensitization, respiratory allergy symptoms, and heritability independently increase the risk of otitis media with effusion. Allergy 2006;61(3):332–6.
35. Irander K, Borres MP, Björksten B. Middle ear diseases in relation to atopy and nasal metachromatic cells in infancy. Int J Pediatr Otorhinolaryngol 1993;26:1–9.
36. Jero J, Virolainen A, Virtanen M, et al. Prognosis of acute otitis media: factors associated with poor outcome. Acta Otolaryngol 1997;117(2):278–83.
37. Benninger MS, Ferguson BJ, Hadley JA, et al. Adult chronic rhinosinusitis: definitions, diagnosis, epidemiology, and pathophysiology. Otolaryngol Head Neck Surg 2003;129(Suppl 3):S1–32.
38. Lazo-Saenz JG, Galvan-Aguilera AA, Martinez-Ordaz VA, et al. Eustachian tube dysfunction in allergic rhinitis. Otolaryngol Head Neck Surg 2005;132(4):626–9.
39. Doner F, Yariktas M, Demirci M. The role of allergy in recurrent otitis media with effusion. J Investig Allergol Clin Immunol 2004;14(2):154–8.
40. Chonmaitree T, Howie VM, Truant AL. Presence of respiratory viruses in middle ear fluids and nasal wash specimens from children with acute otitis media. Pediatrics 1986;77:698–702.
41. Pitkaranta A, Jero J, Arruda E, et al. Polymerase chain reaction-based detection of rhinovirus, respiratory syncytial virus, and coronavirus in otitis media with effusion. J Pediatr 1998;133:390–4.
42. Dingman J, Rayner M, Mishra S, et al. Correlation between presence of viable bacteria and presence of endotoxin in middle-ear effusions. J Clin Microbiol 1998;36:3417–9.
43. Hendolin P, Karkkainen U, Himi T, et al. High incidence of Alloiococcus otitis in otitis media with effusion. Pediatr Infect Dis J 1999;18:860–5.

44. Bernstein JM. The role of IgE-mediated hypersensitivity in the development of otitis media with effusion. Department of Otolaryngology SUNY, ed. Otolaryngol Clin North Am 1992;25:197–211 Buffalo.
45. Ulualp SO, Sahin D, Yilmaz N, et al. Increased adenoid mast cells in patients with otitis media with effusion. Int J Pediatr Otorhinolaryngol 1999; 49:107–14.
46. Okamoto Y, Kudo K, Ishikawa K, et al. Presence of respiratory syncytial virus genomic sequences in middle ear fluid and its relationship to expression of cytokines and cell adhesion molecules. J Infect Dis 1993;168:1277–81.
47. Ohashi Y, Nakai Y, Tanaka A, et al. Soluble adhesion molecules in middle ear effusions from patients with chronic otitis media with effusion. Clin Otolaryngol 1998;23:231–4.
48. Garofalo R, Enander I, Nilsson M, et al. Mast cell degranulation in middle ear of children with acute otitis media. In: Lim D, Bluestone C, Casselbrant M, et al, editors. Proceedings of the Sixth International Symposium on Otitis Media. vol Abs. Hamilton (ON): BC Decker; 1996. p. 22.
49. Persson CG. Airway mucosal exudation of plasma as a measure of subepithelial inflammation. In: Chung F, Barnes P, editors. Pharmacology of the respiratory tract. Lung biology in health and disease. New York: Decker; 1993. p. 483–504.
50. Roberts RL, Ank BJ, Stiehm ER. Human eosinophils are more toxic than neutrophils in antibody-independent killing. J Allergy Clin Immunol 1991;87: 1105–15.
51. Meyerhoff W, Kim CS, Paparella MM. Pathology of chronic otitis media. Ann Otol Rhinol Laryngol 1978;87(6):749–61.
52. Palva T, Johnsson L. Findings in a pair of temporal bones from a patient with secretory otitis media and chronic middle ear infection. Acta Otolaryngol 1984;98:208–20.
53. Suzuki M, Kawauchi H, Moge G. Immune-mediated otitis media with effusion. Am J Otolaryngol 1988;9:199–209.
54. Hellstrom S, Salen B, Stenfors LE. The site of initial production and transport of effusion materials in otitis media serosa. Acta Otolaryngol 1982;93:435–40.
55. Nakata J, Suzuki M, Kawauchi H, et al. Experimental otitis media with effusion induced by middle ear effusion. Laryngoscope 1992;102(9):1037–42.
56. Kahonen K, Palva T, Bergroth V, et al. Immunohistochemical identification of inflammatory cells in secretory and chronic otitis media and cholesteatoma using monoclonal antibodies. Acta Otolaryngol 1984;97:431–6.
57. Labadie RF, Jewett BS, Hart CF, et al. Allergy increases susceptibility to otitis media with effusion in a rat model. Second place–Resident Clinical Science Award 1998. Otolaryngol Head Neck Surg 1999;121(6):687–92.
58. Berger G, Hawke M, Ekem JK. Bone resorption in chronic otitis media: the role of mast cells. Acta Otolaryngol 1985;100:72–80.
59. Hong SD, Cho YS, Hong SH, et al. Chronic otitis media and immunoglobulin E-mediated hypersensitivity in adults: is it a contributor of cholesteatoma? Otolaryngol Head Neck Surg 2008;138(5):637–40.
60. Hurst DS, Venge P. The impact of atopy on neutrophil activity in middle ear effusion from children and adults with chronic otitis media. Arch Otolaryngol Head Neck Surg 2002;128(5):561–6.
61. Hallett MB. The significance of stimulus-response coupling in the neutrophil for physiology and pathology. In: Hallet MB, editor. The neutrophil: cellular biochemistry and physiology. Boca Raton (FL): CRC Press; 1989. p. 1–18.

62. Takeuchi K, Tomemori T, Iriyoshi N, et al. Analysis of T cell receptor b chain repertoire in middle ear effusions. Ann Otol Rhinol Laryngol 1996;105:213–7.
63. Ott N, Gleich G, Peterson E, et al. Assessment of eosinophil and neutrophil participation in atopic dermatitis: comparison with the IgE- mediated late-phase reaction. J Allergy Clin Immunol 1994;94:120–8.
64. O'Reilly RC, He Z, Bloedon E, et al. The role of extraesophageal reflux in otitis media in infants and children. Laryngoscope 2008;118(7 Part 2 Suppl 116):1–9.
65. Bluestone CD. Eustachian tube function and allergy in otitis media. Pediatrics 1978;61(5):753–60.
66. Ackerman M, Friedman R, Doyle W, et al. Antigen-induced eustachian tube obstruction: an internasal provocative challenge test. J Allergy Clin Immunol 1984;73:604–9.
67. Skoner DP, Doyle WJ, Chamovitz AH, et al. Eustachian tube obstruction after internasal challenge with house dust mite. Arch Otolaryngol Head Neck Surg 1986;112:840–2.
68. Friedman RA, Doyle WJ, Casselbrant ML, et al. Immunologic-mediated eustachian tube obstruction: a double-blind crossover study. J Allergy Clin Immunol 1983;71:442–7.
69. Doyle WE, Takahara T, Fireman P. The role of allergy in the pathogenesis of otitis media with effusion. Arch Otolaryngol 1985;111:502–6.
70. Ichimiya I, Kawauchi H, Mogi G. Analysis of immunocompetent cells in the middle ear mucosa. Arch Otolaryngol Head Neck Surg 1990;116:324–30.
71. Straetemans M, van Heerbeek N, Schilder AG, et al. Eustachian tube function before recurrence of otitis media with effusion. Arch Otolaryngol Head Neck Surg 2005;131(2):118–23.
72. Sade J, Wolfson S, Sachs Z, et al. The infant's eustachian tube lumen: the pharyngeal part. J Laryngol Otol 1986;100:129–34.
73. Takahashi H, Hayashi M, Sato H, et al. Primary deficits in eustachian tube function in patients with otitis media with effusion. Arch Otolaryngol Head Neck Surg 1989;115:581–4.
74. Rosenfeld RM, Bluestone CD. Evidenced-based otitis media. Hamilton (Canada): B.C. Decker Inc; 1999.
75. Jahnsen FL, Brandtzaeg P. Antigen presentation and stimulation of the immune system in human airways. Allergy 1999;54(Suppl 57):37–49.
76. Krouse JH. The unified airway. Otolaryngol Clin North Am 2008;41(2):257–66, v.
77. Braunstahl GJ, Overbeek SE, Kleinjan A, et al. Nasal allergen provocation induces adhesion molecule expression and tissue eosinophilia in upper and lower airways. J Allergy Clin Immunol 2001;107(3):469–76.
78. Nguyen LH, Manoukian JJ, Sobol SE, et al. Similar allergic inflammation in the middle ear and the upper airway: evidence linking otitis media with effusion to the united airways concept. J Allergy Clin Immunol 2004;114(5):1110–5.
79. Chinoy B, Yee E, Bahna SL. Skin testing versus radioallergosorbent testing for indoor allergens. Clin Mol Allergy 2005;3(1):4.
80. Dohlman FG. Allergiska Processer i Mellanorat. Nord med tidskr 1943;20:2231 [in Swedish].
81. Mao CY. Allergy as a contributing factor to biologic deafness. Arch Otolaryngol 1942;35:582–6.
82. Jordan R. Chronic secretory otitis media. Laryngoscope 1949;59(9):1002–15.
83. Solow IA. Is serous otitis media due to allergy or infection? Ann Allergy 1958;16:297–9.
84. Lecks HL. Allergic aspects of serous otitis media in childhood. N Y State J Med 1961;61:2737–43.

85. Whitcomb NJ. Allergy therapy in serous otitis media associated with allergic rhinitis. Ann Allergy 1965;23:232–6.
86. Draper WL. Secretory otitis media in children: a study of 540 children. Laryngoscope 1967;77:636–53.
87. Hall LJ, Lukat RM. Results of allergy treatment on the Eustachian tube in chronic serous otitis media. Am J Otol 1981;3(2):116–21.
88. McMahan JT, Calenoff E, Croft DJ, et al. Chronic otitis media with effusion and allergy: modified RAST analysis of 119 cases. Otolaryngol Head Neck Surg 1981;89(3 Pt 1):427–31.
89. Sanz M, Tabar A, Manrique M, et al. Local serum IgE in patients affected by otitis media with effusion. Allergol Immunopathol (Madr) 1986;14:483–7.
90. Hurst DS. Allergy management of refractory serous otitis media. Otolaryngol Head Neck Surg 1990;102(6):664–9.
91. Becker S, Koch T, Philipp A. Allergic origin of recurrent middle ear effusion and adenoids in young children. Klinik, Medizinischen Hochschule Hannover. HNO 1991;39:122–4 [in German].
92. Nsouli TM, Nsouli SM, Linde RE, et al. The role of food allergy in serous otitis media. Ann Allergy 1994;73(3):215–9.
93. Corey J, Adham R, Abbass A, et al. The role of IgE-mediated hypersensitivity in otitis media with effusion. Am J Otolaryngol 1994;15:138–44.
94. Psifidis A, Hatzistilianou M, Samaras K, et al. Atopy and otitis media in children. Paper presented at Proceedings of the 7th International Congress of Pediatric Otorhinolaryngology. Helsinki (Finland); 1998.
95. Lasisi AO, Arinola OG, Bakare RA. Serum and middle ear immunoglobulins in suppurative otitis media. ORL J Otorhinolaryngol Relat Spec 2008;70(6): 389–92.
96. Palva T, Hayry P, Yikoski J. Lymphocyte morphology in middle ear effusions. Ann Otol Rhinol Laryngol 1980;89(Suppl 68):143–6.
97. Egan RW, Umland SP, Cuss RM, et al. Biology of interleukin-5 and its relevance to allergic disease. Allergy 1996;51:71–81.
98. Bikhazi P, Ryan AF. Expression of immunoregulatory cytokines during acute and chronic middle ear immune response. Laryngoscope 1995;105:629–34.
99. Wright ED, Hurst D, Miotto D, et al. Increased expression of major basic protein (MBP) and interleukin-5(IL-5) in middle ear biopsy specimens from atopic patients with persistent otitis media with effusion. Otolaryngol Head Neck Surg 2000;123(5):533–8.
100. Hurst DS. The middle ear: the inflammatory response in children with otitis media with effusion and the impact of atopy. Clinical and histochemical studies. [PhD]. Uppsala (Sweden): Comprehensive Summaries of Uppsala Dessertations from the Faculty of Medicine, Dept of Immunology and Clincal Chemistry #978, Uppsala University. Sweden; 2000.
101. Hurst DS, Amin K, Sevéus L, et al. Evidence of mast cell activity in the middle ear of children with otitis media with effusion. Laryngoscope 1999;109:471–7.
102. Jang CH, Kim YH. Demonstration of RANTES and eosinophilic cataionic protein in otitis media with effusion with allergy. Int J Pediatr Otorhinolaryngol 2003; 67(5):531–3.
103. Lasisi AO, Arinola OG, Olayemi O. Role of elevated immunoglobulin E levels in suppurative otitis media. Ann Trop Paediatr 2008;28(2):123–7.
104. Hurst DS, Ramanarayanan MP, Weekley M. Evidence of possible localized specific IgE production in middle ear fluid as demonstrated by ELISA testing. Otolaryngol Head Neck Surg 1999;121:224–30.

105. Rosenfeld RM, Culpepper L, Doyle KJ, et al. Clinical practice guideline: otitis media with effusion. Otolaryngol Head Neck Surg 2004;130(Suppl 5):S95–118.
106. Luong A, Roland PS. The link between allergic rhinitis and chronic otitis media with effusion in atopic patients. Otolaryngol Clin North Am 2008;41(2):311–23, vi.
107. Passalacqua G, Canonica GW. Long-lasting clinical efficacy of allergen specific immunotherapy. Allergy 2002;57(4):275–6.
108. Lieberman P, Blaiss M. Allergic diseases of the eye and ear. In: Leslie Grammer PG, editor. Patterson's allergic diseases. 6th edition. Philadelphia: Lippincott Williams & Wilkins; 2002. p. 209–23.

Allergic and Immunologic Features of Ménière's Disease

M. Jennifer Derebery, MD

KEYWORDS

• Ménière's disease • Allergy • Endolymphatic hydrops • Vertigo

Key Points: Allergic and Immunologic Features of Ménière's Disease

- The endolymphatic sac is not only capable of processing antigen, but also producing its own antibody response to immune stimulation.
- The prevalence of confirmed allergy in patients with MD is 41%, as compared with 14% to 20% of the US population as a whole.
- A large subset of patients with MD also has migraine headaches. The vast majority of these also have allergy, which may play a triggering role in both entities.
- First-generation antihistamines, although having a beneficial anticholinergic effect on the symptom of vertigo, do not change the underlying pathophysiology of the allergic immune response.
- The allergic stimulation of symptoms seen in some patients with MD is more effectively managed with allergy immunotherapy for inhalant allergies, and dietary elimination of food allergies.

In 1861, Prosper Ménière's first associated dizziness with the inner ear.[1] Later, the syndrome of fluctuating sensorineural hearing loss, episodic vertigo, and tinnitus was named for him. Since then, the pathogenesis of Ménière's disease (MD) was found to be a hydropic distension of the endolymphatic system. In its guidelines for MD diagnosis and evaluation of treatment, the American Academy of Otolaryngology–Head and Neck Surgery (AAO-HNS) describes MD as a "clinical disorder defined as the idiopathic syndrome of endolymphatic hydrops. For clinical purposes (treatment and reporting), the presence of endolymphatic hydrops can be inferred

Clinical Studies Department, House Ear Institute, 2100 West Third Street, 5th Floor, Los Angeles, CA 90057, USA
E-mail address: jderebery@hei.org

Otolaryngol Clin N Am 44 (2011) 655–666
doi:10.1016/j.otc.2011.03.004 oto.theclinics.com
0030-6665/11/$ – see front matter

during life by the presence of the syndrome of endolymphatic hydrops. This syndrome is defined as the presence of ... : recurrent, spontaneous episodic vertigo; hearing loss; aural fullness; and tinnitus."[2(pp 181–5)] AAO-HNS guidelines further define the vertigo episodes as a "spontaneous rotational vertigo lasting at least 20 minutes." **Box 1** lists the classification of MD based on the AAO-HNS criteria.

The initial vertigo attack—the feeling of intense motion when sitting or standing still—can cause the subject to fall to the ground and is accompanied by nausea and vomiting. An incidence rate of 15 per 100,000 and a prevalence rate of 218 per 100,000 have been reported for MD in the United States.[4] Although idiopathic, MD has been ascribed to various causes, including trauma, viral infections, metabolic disorders, allergies, and autoimmune factors. The author emphasizes that MD, at the time of this writing, is idiopathic. The author believes that there may be some genetic predisposition to the development of MD and/or endolymphatic hydrops, with the final "insult" resulting in disease development being either inflammatory or a dysregulation of ion channels. The author does not believe that MD, per se, is "caused" by allergies, but rather, in some patients who likely have a genetic predisposition, an allergic reaction produced by a food and/or inhalant allergen may stimulate an inflammatory reaction resulting in the development of symptoms. In this article, the author specifically looks at the evidence, both historical and current, linking some cases of MD to an underlying allergic state. Briefly addressed are other potential stimuli, such as viral antigen and autoimmune factors, in addition to the Type I Gel and Coombs reaction characterized as "allergy."

First, the immunology of the inner ear is reviewed. Then, the literature from 2002 to 2010 regarding MD, allergy, and autoimmunity is reviewed.

Box 1
Classification of Ménière's disease based on the AAO-HNS criteria

- *Certain Ménière's disease*
  - Definite Ménière's disease, plus histopathological confirmation
- *Definite Ménière's disease*
  - Two or more definite spontaneous episodes of rotational vertigo for 20 minutes or longer
  - Audiometrically documented hearing loss (unilateral or bilateral) on at least one occasion
  - Tinnitus or aural fullness in the affected ear
  - Other causes excluded, such as vestibular schwannoma
- *Probable Ménière's disease*
  - One definite episode of rotational vertigo
  - Audiometrically documented hearing loss (unilateral or bilateral) on at least one occasion
  - Tinnitus or aural fullness in the affected ear
  - Other causes excluded
- *Possible Ménière's disease*
  - Episodic vertigo of the Ménière's type without documented hearing loss, or
  - Sensorineural hearing loss (unilateral or bilateral, fluctuating or fixed, with disequilibrium but without definite episodes of vertigo)
  - Other causes excluded[3]

REVIEW OF IMMUNOLOGY

The inner ear demonstrates both cellular and humoral immunity. Most leukocytes enter the cochlea via the spiral modiolar vein.[5] The innate immunity of the cochlea has been suggested to allow an adaptive local response to antigen challenge.[6] Hashimoto and colleagues[6] have suggested that the inner ear may be "primed" by lipopolysaccharides or other viral or bacterial antigens, resulting in the upregulation of interleukin (IL)-1C in the spiral ligament fibrocytes, permitting leukocytes to enter. Subsequently, in those having lymphocytes primed to react against inner-ear antigens, an initiated immune response may result in local inflammation. Altermatt and colleagues[7] have suggested that the seat of immune activity in the inner ear appears to be the endolymphatic sac (ES) and duct. Immunoglobulin (Ig) G, IgM, IgA, and secretory components are found in the ES, and numerous plasma cells and macrophages reside in the perisaccular connective tissue.

Additionally, the labyrinth exhibits active components of allergic reactivity. Mast cells have been identified in the perisaccular connective tissue. Following sensitization, IgE-mediated degranulation of mast cells has resulted in eosinophilic infiltration of the peri connective tissue and, clinically, the production of endolymphatic hydrops.[8]

The ES is capable of both processing antigen and producing its own local antibody response.[9,10] Surgical destruction of the ES results in decreased antigen and antibody responses.[10] The highly vascular subepithelial space of the ES contains numerous fenestrated blood vessels,[11] with arterial branches of the posterior meningeal artery supplying the ES and duct.[12] Although the labyrinth is protected by the blood-labyrinthine barrier, the posterior meningeal artery is fenestrated, offering a peripheral portal of circulation. Fenestrated vessels supplying organs involved in absorption (eg, kidney, choroid) are especially susceptible to damage by immune complex deposition.

Despite evidence of immune activity, only 30% of patients with MD show a true autoantibody response on Western blot assay to specific anticochlear antibody.[13] Tests of abnormal cell-mediated immunity are either inconsistent or normal, even in patients with known causes of inner ear autoimmune dysfunction, including Cogan syndrome.[13] Despite increased understanding of labyrinthine immunoreactivity, a reliable laboratory marker to "prove" autoimmune or allergic causation in patients with suspected inflammatory hearing loss has not yet been developed.

The first published report of MD believed to be provoked by an allergic reaction was in 1923.[14] Both inhalant and food allergies have been linked with MD symptoms.[15] Many of MD's clinical characteristics suggest an underlying inflammatory, if not autoimmune, etiology, such as its propensity to wax and wane, with periods of remission. It is also bilateral in a significant number of cases.[16,17]

There are different possible mechanisms by which an allergic reaction produces MD symptoms.[18] First, the ES itself could be a target organ of the allergic reaction. The sac's peripheral and fenestrated blood vessels could allow antigen entry, stimulating mast cell degranulation in the perisaccular connective tissue. The resulting inflammatory mediator release could affect the sac's filtering capability, resulting in a toxic accumulation of metabolic products, and interfering with hair cell function. Also, the fenestrated blood vessels to the ES could be pharmacologically vulnerable to the effects of vasoactive mediators such as histamine, which are released in a distal allergic reaction. The unique blood supply of the interosseus ES would serve as a portal for these mediators to exert a direct pharmacologic effect. The potent vasodilating effects of histamine or other mediators could affect the resorptive capacity of the ES. Yan and colleagues[19] have shown that Waldeyer ring in the nasopharynx is the anatomic site of T-cell homing to the ES. In systemically sensitized rodents, intranasal antigen stimulation with keyhole limpet hemocyanin (KLH) in Waldeyer ring resulted in an antigen-specific reaction in the ES and perilymphatic vessels, suggesting that viral or allergic antigen could be processed in the nasopharynx, with the resulting specific immune reaction occurring at the ES.

A second possible mechanism involves the production of a circulating immune complex, such as a food antigen, which is then deposited through the fenestrated blood vessels of the ES, producing inflammation. An increased incidence of circulating immune complexes in the serum has been described in both MD and allergic rhinitis.[20,21] The inflammatory response resulting from the deposition of immune complexes along vascular basement membranes is the hallmark of an immune complex disease. Although the binding of the complexes to the cell membranes facilitates their phagocytosis, it also results in the release of tissue-damaging enzymes. This is believed to be the mechanism of unexplained sensorineural hearing loss in patients with Wegener granulomatosis, a prototype immune-complex–mediated disease. Upon examining the temporal bones of patients with Wegener granulomatosis and unexplained sensorineural hearing loss, the cochlea is found to be normal; the pathology occurs in the ES.[22]

Alternatively, circulating immune complexes may be deposited in the stria, causing the normally intact blood-labyrinthine barrier to leak as a result of increased vascular permeability. In addition to disrupting normal ionic and fluid balance in the extracapillary spaces, this could facilitate the entry of autoantibodies into the inner ear.

A third possible mechanism is a viral antigen-allergic interaction. A predisposing viral upper respiratory infection in childhood (eg, mumps, herpes) antigenically stimulates Waldeyer ring, with subsequent T-cell homing to the ES,[23] resulting in a chronic low-grade inflammation. This is not enough initially to result in hearing loss or vertigo, but it does produce mild impairment of ES absorption. Later in adult life, "something" in the system then stimulates excess fluid production. Several investigators have assumed that viral infections play a direct or indirect role in the etiology of MD. Gacek[24] recently published temporal bone evidence of viral particles enclosed in transport vesicles in a patient with a history of MD. He also noted that antiviral treatment controlled vertigo in most patients with both MD and viral neuronitis.

Viruses are also capable of exacerbating allergic symptoms by several mechanisms. Both live and ultraviolet light–inactivated viruses have been shown to enhance histamine release, an effect believed to be mediated by interferon. Viruses can also damage epithelial surfaces, thereby enhancing antigen entry and increasing the responsiveness of target organs to histamine. It has long been noted that patients with poorly controlled allergy are more likely than nonallergic persons to develop upper and lower respiratory viral infections.

The herpes virus family would appear to be the most likely candidate for a viral stimulus. Patients with MD have elevations in serum antibody against herpes simplex and enterovirus.[25] Additionally, Heat Shock Protein 70, an antibody frequently seen elevated in both MD and autoimmune inner ear disease (AIED), is often upregulated in viral infections.

EPIDEMIOLOGY OF MD

In a survey performed of 734 patients with Ménière's syndrome, the prevalence of skin test–confirmed concurrent allergic disease was 41%.[23] Although the prevalence of allergic rhinitis is often quoted as 20% or more, the recent Allergies in America report,[26] the largest survey to date regarding prevalence and disease burden of allergic rhinitis, found that physician-diagnosed allergic rhinitis in patients with rhinitic symptoms is 14%. Hence, the prevalence of physician-diagnosed allergy in American patients diagnosed with MD is almost 3 times that of the general population.[23] In a more recent survey of patients with MD, Derebery and Berliner found that patients reported a 58% rate of allergy history and, again, a 41% rate of positive skin or in vitro test.[17]

In his original description, Prosper Ménière's suggested an association between migraine and MD.[1] Since then, many investigators have noted paroxysmal headache independently occurring in many patients with MD.[27–29] Radtke and colleagues[30] published a well-designed prospective trial based on strict diagnostic criteria, which clearly established an increased lifetime prevalence of migraine in patients diagnosed with MD.

A recent study reported both an increased incidence of self-reported migraine and allergic rhinitis in patients with MD as compared with a control group of age- and sex-matched patients without MD attending an otolaryngology clinic.[31] Sen and colleagues[31] used a Web-based questionnaire to recruit 108 patients with MD, and a control group of 100 patients attending the otolaryngology clinic for other problems. The migraine prevalence in MD sufferers was 39.0% compared with 18.0% in the control group, whereas the prevalence of allergy in those with MD was 51.9%, compared with 23.0% in the control group. In the MD group, a history of allergy was significantly more prevalent in patients with migraine (71%) than in those without migraine (39%). There was no such link between allergy and migraine in the control group, with the combination of allergy and migraine 9 times more prevalent in the MD group.

The Sen and colleagues' study[31] is interesting because it suggests that in that large subset of patients with MD who also have migraine, the vast majority report an additional diagnosis of allergy. In reviewing their Web-based questionnaire, one weakness would be that the allergy history is obtained by simply asking the subjects whether they or family members suffer from any allergy, without confirmatory skin or in vitro testing. However, the fact that all patients—control group and patients with MD—were asked the same question and gave such differing responses adds credence to the supposition that there is a much higher incidence of allergy and migraine in patients with MD.

Although the list of "causes" for migraine is quite extensive, it has long been noted that allergic reactions were a common trigger in many sufferers. There are striking similarities among MD, allergy, and migraines concerning both symptom presentation and vascular changes. All 3 tend to recur cyclically, and sufferers are often able to note a cause and effect between a particular suspected "exposure" or event and the subsequent development of symptoms. The entities all show similar vascular changes as well: vasoconstriction, vasodilatation, and plasma extravasations, during the course of symptom production. Ibekwe and colleagues[32] reported that there is an elevation in IgG containing immune complexes in the meningeal vessels of patients with migraine, as well as in the subepithelial layer of the endolymphatic sac in patients with MD. They hypothesized that there may be a common defective ion channel in both disease states, with the predominant expression in the inner ear and brain, resulting in a local increase in extracellular potassium and the production of symptoms.

PATHOPHYSIOLOGY OF MD

Paparella and Djalilian[33] provide an excellent review for the practitioner of the temporal bone correlates of the clinical symptoms of MD. They review various theorized "causes" of MD symptoms, including allergy. They conclude that the fundamental etiology of MD is likely a multifactorial inheritance, suggesting that the most likely predisposing factors are hypoplasia of the mastoid air cell system, vestibular aqueduct, and ES, and the other physical abnormalities that have been frequently reported in patients with MD.

The author also believes that MD is likely multifactorial in etiology. It is not the author's contention that MD is "caused" by allergy. However, if we accept that most patients with MD do have an anatomic abnormality, including a smaller than average ES size, factors that may affect either excessive endolymph production or reduction of endolymph absorption may promote MD symptoms. Inflammatory stimulation by an inhaled or ingested allergen in a genetically predisposed individual should be considered as one possible trigger.

IMMUNOPATHOLOGY OF MD

Many investigators have looked at serologic evidence of immunopathology or changes in patients with MD. Savastano and colleagues[34] found more than half of 200 patients with MD had increased circulating immune complexes, as well as an increase in the number of IL-2 receptors and autoantibodies, compared with healthy controls. There were no elevations of IgG, IgM, IgA, erythrocyte sedimentation rate, C-reactive protein, complement factors, and cryoglobulins in most patients.

Of interest, Savastano and colleagues[34] also attempted to relate immunologic findings to disease severity, using the 1985 AAO-HNS Pearson and Brackmann classification of disability for reporting results in MD treatment. (It is unclear why they did not use the currently accepted AAO-HNS functional disability scale from the 1995 guidelines.) In the 1985 system, grade I exhibits no or mild disability with intermittent or continuous dizziness precluding work in a hazardous environment; grade II exhibits moderate disability with intermittent or continuous dizziness/unsteadiness requiring employment in a sedentary occupation; and grade III exhibits severe disability/disabling symptoms precluding gainful employment. There was a significant relationship between disease severity and test abnormalities for circulating immune complexes, CD4, and CD4 to CD8 ratio, with the highest rate of serologic abnormalities found in group III with disabling symptoms and the lowest rate in group I. A trend was also found for differences in C-reactive protein, C3 complement, and early T-activation.

Elevated circulating immune complexes in patients with MD have been reported by Brookes[20] and by Derebery and Berliner.[23] It would have been interesting for Savastano and colleagues[34] to have done a subanalysis of patients with bilateral MD (not identified in the text). Derebery and Berliner[23] found a direct relationship between larger elevations in circulating immune complexes and disease bilaterality.

Keles and colleagues[35] performed another study of MD immunopathology. They attempted to evaluate the possible role of allergy in producing Ménière's symptoms by examining the cytokine profiles, allergic parameters, and lymphocyte subgroups of patients with MD versus controls.

Forty-six adult patients with classic MD were compared with an identical number of healthy volunteers in the same age group and socioeconomic class, living in the same region of Turkey. These researchers measured lymphocyte subtypes, including CD4, CD8,CD23 antibodies, interferon (IFN)-H, IL-4, total serum IgE, and antigen-specific IgE to regionally important tree pollens, molds, and common foods in the local diet.

Significant differences were found between the patients with MD and the controls in CD4, CD4/CD8, CD23, IFN-H, and IL-4 levels. Keles and colleagues[35] also found significant positive correlations between levels of CD23 and total serum IgE, CD8 and total serum IgE, CD4/CD8 and IgE, and CD23 and CD8, although correlation coefficients were not provided for the reader to determine strength of the relationships. Elevation of total serum IgE was found in 43.3% of the MD group compared with only 19.5% of the control group. Additionally, 67.3% of the patients with MD gave a positive history of allergy, whereas the same was found in only 34.7% of the control group, leading Keles and colleagues[35] to suggest that potentially beneficial future therapies would be suppression of production of IL-4 and IL-1, or stimulation of a helper T1 (Th1) cell predominance with the application of Bacillus Calmette-Guérin (BCG) vaccination.

This interesting study does not change the current treatment parameters for MD[35]; however, it documents that unselected patients with MD have serologic findings that correlate strongly with atopy.

Oral steroids have commonly been used for treatment of patients with MD as a "rescue" and are the only treatment shown to offer efficacy in the treatment of AIED, many of whom present with a rapidly progressive form of bilateral MD.[36] However, long-term use of steroids are fraught with potential side effects, including osteoporosis, cataracts, and hyperglycemia. Intratympanic (IT) dexamethasone is used increasingly in an attempt to obtain the anti-inflammatory benefits of steroids without the systemic side effects. Herraiz and colleagues[37] recently reported that IT dexamethasone gave excellent improvement in tinnitus and decreased vertigo, as well as good preservation in hearing in a group of 34 patients with MD treated with IT dexamethasone in an open-label study, with improvement persisting for up to 24 months. The reader is also encouraged to read a review by McCall and colleagues[38] regarding other potential forms of drug delivery that may be applicable to treating patients with MD.

TREATMENT OF MD

The standard therapy in the United States and many other areas in the world for treatment of MD are sodium restriction, diuretics, and rescue vestibular suppressants for vertigo attacks. Many if not most patients get good results with this treatment, which, although not curative, can offer acceptable relief from vertigo most of the time. There is no treatment for MD that has been shown to be effective at hearing stabilization, at the time of this writing. The patient with MD should never be told "nothing can be done for it." Should medications not work, progressively more aggressive management, including endolymphatic shunt surgery, intratympanic gentamicin, or ablative procedures, such as vestibular nerve section or labyrinthectomy in the case of nonserviceable hearing, can be effective. Some patients will benefit by the use of the Meniett pressure-regulating device.

In addition to these, the author reviews several studies related to treatment of MD on immunologic and allergic aspects of the disease. Jeck-Thole and Wagner[39] published a review of safety data on betahistine, which is often sold under the trade name Serc (Solvay Pharmaceuticals, Marietta, GA, USA). Betahistine contains a structural analog of histamine, and is prescribed in the treatment of vestibular disorders, such as MD, for symptomatic treatment of vertigo. Betahistine is said to be the most commonly prescribed medication for MD in the world. Although not currently available in the United States, it can be obtained by compounding pharmacies or through sources in Canada or Europe. The typical adult dose is 16 mg 3 times daily. The reader may see a patient with MD using betahistine and reporting good clinical results.

In the United States, the most commonly prescribed medications for treating symptoms of MD are antihistamines (eg, meclizine, diphenhydramine, and dimenhydrinate). These medications are felt to be effective by exerting an anticholinergic central suppressive effect on the symptom of vertigo. Therefore, it might appear to be counterintuitive to prescribe a histamine analog to treat these same symptoms. In tissue, histamine is primarily stored in mast cells and may be released by various drugs, venoms, or allergens, resulting in hypersensitivity reactions, gastric acid secretion, and increased capillary permeability. In association with the peripheral actions of histamine, its function as a central neurotransmitter was postulated. Subsequently, various receptor subtypes were described, including histamine H_1, H_2, H_3, and, eventually, H_4.[40,41]

Betahistine acts as a neurotransmitter modulator of the complex histaminergic receptor system with no known affinity for any other receptors.[42] Betahistine is a weak partial H_1 receptor agonist with a distinctly lower affinity than histamine. It has almost no affinity for the H_2 receptor, having extremely weak effects on gastric secretion.[43] In contrast, betahistine shows a potent antagonistic effect on the H_3 receptor. The H_3 heteroreceptor, belonging to a class of presynaptic receptors, is involved in the synthesis and release of histamine and other neurotransmitters, including dopamine, H-aminobutyric acid (GABA), acetylcholine, norepinephrine, and serotonin.[44] Actions that are mediated by the H_1 receptor are blocked by negative H_3 receptor feedback. Betahistine has an antagonistic effect on the H_3 receptor, followed by an increased histamine release. Betahistine's H_3 receptor antagonistic action is believed to be responsible for improvement in the inner ear microcirculation and subsequent reduction of endolymphatic pressure.[45,46] Betahistine has also been shown to inhibit the basal spike generation of the vestibular neurons in the lateral and medial vestibular nuclei, both crucial for controlling posture. A recent meta-analysis of treatment with betahistine in treating vertigo in non-Ménière's patients has shown it to be efficacious.[47]

In terms of side effects or drug interaction, betahistine is nonsedating and free from psychomotor impairment. Theoretically, because betahistine and histamine are similar, betahistine could interact with an antihistaminic agent such as diphenhydramine or cetirizine, or even induce or support hypersensitivity reactions with regard to the H_1-agonistic quality. However, betahistine affinity at the receptor site has been shown to be significantly weaker than histamine affinity. In addition, betahistine-induced histamine release from mast cells has not been described.[48]

INDICATIONS FOR TESTING

How does one select which patient with MD should undergo diagnostic testing? Classically, Powers[15] described suggestive history, including a seasonal relationship of symptoms (eg, hearing loss, vertigo attacks), as well as the presence of "other symptoms" suggesting allergy, such as rhinitis, as indicators. These are actually a useful guide. The author also feels other details of history are useful guides, including bilateral symptoms, strong family history of allergy, a history of childhood allergy that one has "outgrown," as well as obvious factors such as the production of MD symptoms within a short time after exposure to a food or inhaled antigen.

As for testing modalities, there are varying thoughts regarding the relative sensitivity versus specificity of various tests, including prick testing, intradermal, intradermal titration, intradermal dilutional provocative food testing, as well as in vitro. The reader is encouraged to perform his or her own review of the subject. The author suggests that, whatever testing type is selected, the patient be tested with both inhalants as well as food antigens, despite the acknowledged lesser sensitivity of food testing when compared with inhalant.

Our preferred method of testing is intradermal titration, or, less so, prick testing with single-dilution intradermal testing in the case of negative results with a prick test. The author has observed that the reactivity of patients with suspected inhalant allergic triggers to their MD symptoms are often relatively low, typically in the range of

1/500 wt/vol of antigen.[49] Likewise, Topuz and colleagues[50] also noted that there was a large increase of abnormal electrocochleography results before and/or after prick testing in patients with MD (29% of diseased ears vs 78% after testing), as well as that the inner ear did not appear to require a strong antigen dose to be objectively stimulated. Similar electrocochleography changes have also been noted in patients with MD who have been tested with dietary antigen stimulation by provocative food testing, nasal provocation with inhalant antigens, and prick testing.[51] The reader is advised to recall that the purpose of testing for allergy is to establish objectively whether a patient is allergic to a particular allergen or not, rather than to infer that the amount of antigen that produces a positive skin test directly relates to what type or how severe those induced symptoms will be.

TREATMENT OUTCOME STUDIES

We evaluated the effect of specific allergy immunotherapy and food elimination of suspected food allergens on patients with MD for whom allergy treatment had been recommended[20] via a questionnaire regarding their symptoms. The 113 patients treated by desensitization and diet showed a significant improvement after treatment, both in allergy symptoms and in Ménière's symptoms. The patient ratings of frequency, severity, and interference with daily activities of their Ménière's symptoms also appeared better after allergy treatment, compared with ratings from the control group of 24 untreated patients. Results indicated that patients with MD can show improvement in tinnitus and vertigo symptoms when receiving specific allergy therapy, suggesting the inner ear may also be a direct or indirect target of an allergic reaction.

Because the first study asked patients to retrospectively rate their pretreatment symptoms, a prospective study was undertaken in which 68 patients completed the questionnaire before allergy treatment and at an average of 23 months after treatment.[52] Severity of vertigo, tinnitus, and unsteadiness improved significantly, as did frequency of vertigo, frequency and interference of unsteadiness, and ratings on the AAO-HNS disability scale. Quality of life improved significantly on 4 of 8 SF-36 Health Survey scales. Initial SF-36 scores indicated that patients with both MD and allergy score more poorly than the general US adult population on several quality-of-life aspects. Paired comparisons between SF-36 scale scores at initial and follow-up intervals identified significant improvements in subtests that were below normal initially. Statistical analyses strongly suggested that these improvements were independent of natural history and of other medical treatment for MD that the patients may have received during the immunotherapy period.

A weakness of these and other studies is that there are no control groups receiving saline injections or given diets eliminating foods that were negative on testing. It has been observed that patients with MD are reluctant to commit to months or a year of possible placebo injections to "prove" that immunotherapy may help improve symptoms of vertigo, hearing loss, and/or tinnitus. Presently, we rely on using statistical control as well as research that clearly demonstrates the ability of allergy immunotherapy to downregulate Th2 cell–driven inflammatory responses in patients with allergic rhinitis and asthma.[53] If MD is believed to be a chronic condition with an inflammatory component, it is logical that downregulating the production and release of both proinflammatory and vasoactive mediators promoting fluid extravasation and/or retention could help lessen symptoms. This is the rationale for using steroids and restricting dietary salt in patients with MD.

The classic first-generation antihistamines commonly used for their desired anticholinergic effects to lessen vertigo severity do not change the underlying pathology of hydropic distention of the endolymphatic space. Pharmacologically, these agents have limited effect, and do not block the effects of other inflammatory mediators, such as leukotrienes, released with mast cell degranulation. In the author's experience, nonsedating antihistamines have limited benefit in treating vertigo and/or dizziness. Effective immunotherapy, with its induced immunologic changes, can prevent mast cell degranulation. Additionally, an appropriate elimination diet for documented food allergies can prevent an immune-mediated reaction. In the author's clinical experience, the symptoms of MD are generally better controlled, with fewer vertigo attacks and more stable hearing, in those patients with allergy and MD whose underlying allergic disorder is downregulated with immunotherapy and/or dietary avoidance of reactive food allergens. The ideal "proof" of the role of allergy in a large subset of patients who develop MD would be a double-blind, placebo-controlled trial of immunotherapy, for the minimum of 2 years as required by AAO-HNS for evaluating the effects of surgical procedures for MD; however, realistically, recruiting patients for such a study would be a challenge because of the potentially disabling symptoms of MD.

SUMMARY

The prevalence of both migraine and atopy is much higher in patients with MD than in the healthy population. Unselected patients with MD have serologic findings that correlate both with underlying atopy and inflammation. Indications for testing for allergy in a patient with MD should include symptoms associated with a seasonal relationship or food ingestion to symptom production, a known history of allergy or clear allergic symptoms in a patient with MD, or a known past childhood history or a strong family history of allergy. Additional consideration should be given for testing in those patients with bilateral MD. Although there are no double-blind, placebo-controlled trials comparing outcomes of patients with MD treated with specific allergy immunotherapy, clinical case reports strongly suggest that such treatment lessens severity and frequency of vertigo and results in more stable hearing. Objective outcomes of successful medical and surgical treatment of MD symptoms have been established and published, and may be used as a reference for assessing treatment response by specific allergy immunotherapy, or dietary elimination of food allergy.

REFERENCES

1. Ménière's P. Pathologieauriculaire: mémoire sur des lésions de l'oreille interne donnant lieu a des symptômes de congestion cerebrale apoplectiform. Gaz Med Paris 1861;16:597–601 [in French].
2. American Academy of Otolaryngology—Head and Neck Foundation. Committee on hearing and equilibrium guidelines for the diagnosis and evaluation of therapy in Ménière's disease. Otolaryngol Head Neck Surg 1995;113:181–5.
3. Hamid MA. Ménière's disease. Pract Neurol 2009;9:157–62.
4. Wladislavosky-Wasserman P, Facer GW, Mokri B, et al. Ménière's disease: a 30-year epidemiologic and clinical study in Rochester, MN, 1951–1980. Laryngoscope 1984;94:1098–102.
5. Stearns GS, Keithley EM, Harris JP. Development of high endothelial venule-like characteristics in the spiral modiolar vein induced by viral labyrinthitis. Laryngoscope 1993;103:890–8.
6. Hashimoto S, Billings P, Harris JP, et al. Innate immunity contributes to cochlear adaptive immune responses. Audiol Neurootol 2005;10:35–43.

7. Altermatt HJ, Gebbers JO, Muller C, et al. Human endolymphatic sac: evidence for a role in inner ear immune defence. ORL J Otorhinolaryngol Relat Spec 1990; 52:143–8.
8. Uno K, Miyamura K, Kanzaki Y, et al. Type I allergy in the inner ear of the guinea pig. Ann Otol Rhinol Laryngol 1992;101(Suppl 157):78–81.
9. Harris JP. Immunology of the inner ear: evidence of local antibody production. Ann Otol Rhinol Laryngol 1984;93:157–62.
10. Tomiyama S, Harris JP. The role of the endolymphatic sac in inner ear immunity. Acta Otolaryngol 1987;103:182–8.
11. Wackym PA, Friberg U, Linthicum FH Jr, et al. Human endolymphatic sac: morphologic evidence of immunologic function. Ann Otol Rhinol Laryngol 1987; 96:276–81.
12. Gadre AK, Fayad JN, O'Leary MJ, et al. Arterial supply of the human endolymphatic duct and sac. Otolaryngol Head Neck Surg 1993;108:141–8.
13. Harris JP, Ryan AF. Fundamental immune mechanisms of the brain and inner ear. Otolaryngol Head Neck Surg 1995;112:639–53.
14. Duke W. Ménière's syndrome caused by allergy. JAMA 1923;81:2179–82.
15. Powers WH. Allergic factors in Ménière's disease. Trans Am Acad Ophthalmol Otolaryngol 1973;77:22.
16. House JW, Doherty JK, Fisher LM, et al. Ménière's disease: prevalence of contralateral ear involvement. Otol Neurotol 2006;27:355–61.
17. Derebery MJ, Berliner KI. Characteristics, onset and progression in Ménière's disease. In: Lim DJ, editor. Proceedings of the 5th International Symposium on Ménière's's Disease and Inner Ear Homeostasis Disorders. Los Angeles (CA): House Ear Institute; 2005. p. 128–130.
18. Derebery MJ. Allergic management of Ménière's disease: an outcome study. Otolaryngol Head Neck Surg 2000;122:174–82.
19. Yan Z, Wang JB, Gong SS, et al. Cell proliferation in the endolymphatic sac in situ after the rat Waldeyer ring equivalent immunostimulation. Laryngoscope 2003; 113:1609–14.
20. Brookes GB. Circulating immune complexes in Ménière's disease. Arch Otolaryngol Head Neck Surg 1986;112:536–40.
21. Derebery MJ, Rao VS, Siglock TJ, et al. Ménière's disease: an immune complex-mediated illness? Laryngoscope 1991;101:225–9.
22. Leone CA, Feghali JG, Linthicum FH Jr. Endolymphatic sac: possible role in autoimmune sensorineural hearing loss. Ann Otol Rhinol Laryngol 1984;93:208–9.
23. Derebery MJ, Berliner KI. Prevalence of allergy in Ménière's disease. Otolaryngol Head Neck Surg 2000;123:69–75.
24. Gacek RR. Ménière's disease is a viral neuropathy. ORL J Otorhinolaryngol Relat Spec 2009;71(2):78–86.
25. Ruckenstein MJ. Immunologic aspects of Meniere's disease. Am J Otolaryngol 1999;20:161–5.
26. Allergies in America. A landmark survey of nasal allergy sufferers. Available at: http://www.myallergiesinamerica.com/. Accessed November 20, 2009.
27. Atkinson M. Migraine and Ménière's disease. Arch Otolaryngol 1962;75:48–51.
28. Hinchcliffe R. Headache and Ménière's disease. Acta Otolaryngol 1967;63:384–90.
29. Dolowitz DA. Ménière's—an inner ear seizure. Laryngoscope 1979;89:67–77.
30. Radtke A, Lempert T, Gresty MA, et al. Migraine and Ménière's disease: is there a link? Neurology 2002;5:1700–4.
31. Sen P, Georgalas C, Papesch M. Co-morbidity of migraine and Ménière's disease: is allergy the link? J Laryngol Otol 2005;119:455–60.

32. Ibekwe TS, Fasunla JA, Ibekwe PU, et al. Migraine and Ménière's disease: two different phenomena with frequently observed concomitant occurrences. J Natl Med Assoc 2008;100:334–8.
33. Paparella MM, Djalilian HR. Etiology, pathophysiology of symptoms, and pathogenesis of Ménière's disease. Otolaryngol Clin North Am 2002;35:529–45.
34. Savastano M, Giacomelli L, Marioni G. Non-specific immunological determinations in Ménière's disease: any role in clinical practice? Eur Arch Otorhinolaryngol 2007;264:15–9.
35. Keles E, Godekmerdan A, Kalidag T, et al. Ménière's disease and allergy: allergens and cytokines. J Laryngol Otol 2004;118:688–93.
36. Harris J, Weisman MH, Derebery JM, et al. Treatment of corticosteroid-responsive autoimmune inner ear disease with methotrexate: a randomized controlled trial. JAMA 2003;290:1875–83.
37. Herraiz C, Plaza G, Aparicio JM, et al. Transtympanic steroids for Ménière's disease. Otol Neurotol 2010;31(1):162–7.
38. McCall AA, Swan EE, Borenstein JT, et al. Drug delivery for treatment of inner ear disease: current state of knowledge. Ear Hear 2010;31(2):156–65.
39. Jeck-Thole S, Wagner W. Betahistine: a retrospective synopsis of safety data. Drug Saf 2006;29:1049–59.
40. Hill SJ, Ganellin CR, Timmerman H, et al. International union of pharmacology, XIII. Classification of histamine receptors. Pharmacol Rev 1997;49:253–77.
41. Liu C, Ma XJ, Jiang X, et al. Cloning and pharmacological characterization of a fourth histamine receptor (H4) expressed in bone marrow. Mol Pharmacol 2001;5:420–6.
42. Arrang JM, Garbarg M, Quach TT, et al. Actions of betahistine at histamine receptors in the brain. Eur J Pharmacol 1985;111:73–84.
43. Curwain BP, Holton P, Spencer J. The effect of betahistine on gastric acid secretion and mucosal blood flow in conscious dogs. Br J Pharmacol 1972;46:351–4.
44. West RE, Zweig A, Shih NY, et al. Identification of two H3-histamine receptor subtypes. Mol Pharmacol 1990;38:610–3.
45. Laurikainen EL, Miller JM, Nutall AL. The vascular mechanism of action of betahistine in the inner ear of the guinea pig. Eur Arch Otorhinolaryngol 1998;255:119–23.
46. Dziadziola JK, Laurikian EL, Rachel JD. Betahistine increases vestibular blood flow. Otolaryngol Head Neck Surg 1999;120:400–5.
47. Della PC, Guidetti G, Eandi M. Betahistine in the treatment of vertiginous syndromes: a meta-analysis. Acta Otorhinolaryngol Ital 2006;26:208–15.
48. Kohno S, Nakao S, Ogawa K, et al. Possible participation of histamine H3-receptors in the regulation of anaphylactic histamine release from isolated rat peritoneal mast cells. Jpn J Pharmacol 1994;66:173–80.
49. Derebery J, Valenzuela S. Ménière's syndrome and allergy. Otolaryngol Clin North Am 1992;25(1):213–24.
50. Topuz B, Ogmen G, Ardiç FN, et al. Provocation of endolymphatic hydrops with a prick test in Meniere's disease. Adv Ther 2007;24(4):819–25.
51. Gibbs SR, Mabry RL, Roland PS, et al. ECOG changes after intranasal allergen challenge: a possible diagnostic tool in patients with Ménière's disease. Otolaryngol Head Neck Surg 1999;121:283–4.
52. Derebery MJ, Berliner KI. Allergic management in Ménière's disease: a prospective study. Presented at the American Academy of Otolaryngic Allergy Annual Meeting. Orlando (FL); September 19, 2003.
53. Yang X. Does allergen immunotherapy alter the natural course of allergic disorders? Drugs 2001;61:365–74.

Asthma

Michael J. Parker, MD

KEYWORDS

• Asthma • Airway inflammation • Allergens • Genetic risk
• Asthma symptoms • Asthma diagnosis • Asthma management
• Hyperresponsiveness

Asthma is a common, chronic disorder of the airways, but it is a complex disorder. Asthma is characterized by:

1. Variable and recurring symptoms
2. Airflow obstruction
3. Bronchial hyperresponsiveness
4. Underlying inflammation.

The comorbid conditions of allergic rhinitis and asthma have been well documented, are frequently observed, and may represent a spectrum of the same disease entity (1-airway hypothesis).[1,2] Health care providers managing allergic rhinitis need to be comfortable with their ability to recognize and treat asthma and inflammation of the lower airway.

The clinical presentation of asthma can be highly variable over time and is often dependent on several factors:

- The inflammation of asthma in the airway of susceptible individuals causes recurrent episodes of wheezing, breathlessness, chest tightness, and coughing, which often worsen at night and in the early morning
- Episodes of inflammation are usually associated with widespread, but often variable, airflow obstruction that is frequently reversible
- This inflammation can also cause an increase in the existing bronchial hyperresponsiveness typical of asthma.

The interaction of these features of asthma determines the clinical manifestations and severity of asthma and the response to treatment.

The relationship between the upper and lower airway inflammation should not be underestimated. Rhinitis occurs in 75% to 90% of adult subjects with allergic asthma and 80% of those with nonallergic asthma.[3] The incidence of asthma is high in developed nations, constituting the most common chronic disease of childhood, affecting more than 7 million children in the United States.[4] Allergic disease is associated with the development, severity, and persistence of asthma. As an example, up to 80% of

Department of Otolaryngology and Communication Sciences, SUNY Upstate Medical University, Syracuse, NY, USA
E-mail address: mjparker.md@gmail.com

Otolaryngol Clin N Am 44 (2011) 667–684
doi:10.1016/j.otc.2011.04.001

children with atopic dermatitis develop asthma and/or allergic rhinitis later in childhood.[5] Conversely, asthma occurs in 25% to 50% of individuals with rhinitis. Adults with perennial rhinitis are more likely to have asthma than those without rhinitis.[6] The odds of developing asthma are eightfold higher in patients with allergic rhinitis and almost 12-fold higher in patients with nonallergic rhinitis.

PATHOPHYSIOLOGY OF ASTHMA

The immunohistopathologic features of asthma include an inflammatory cell infiltration into the respiratory tract. Neutrophils, eosinophils, lymphocytes, mast cell activation, and epithelial cell injury are common cellular findings. In some patients with progression of disease, persistent changes in airway structure occur, including subbasement fibrosis, mucus hypersecretion, injury to epithelial cells, smooth muscle hypertrophy, and angiogenesis. Numerous inflammatory mediators have also been implicated in the inflammatory process, and management of these mediators has held some promise in the progression and management of the reactive process of asthma. Chemokines, cytokines, cysteinyl-leukotrienes, nitric oxide, and immunoglobulin E (IgE) all play a role in the development of airway inflammation.[7–10]

Central to the variable clinical presentations of asthma is the presence of underlying airway inflammation, which is also varied over time within the same individual and among individuals. This inflammatory variability has distinct, but overlapping, patterns that reflect different aspects of the clinical presentation of the disease, such as intermittent versus persistent asthma or acute versus chronic manifestations.

Acute symptoms of asthma usually arise from bronchospasm and require and respond to bronchodilator therapy. Acute and chronic inflammation can affect not only the airway caliber and airflow but also underlying bronchial hyperresponsiveness, which enhances susceptibility to bronchospasm.[11]

RISK FACTORS FOR ASTHMA

The variables that result in the initiation of the inflammatory process in some individuals are being investigated. Although no definitive pattern exists, there is evidence that the origin of the airway inflammation occurs early. The expression of the clinical presentation of asthma is complex and involves interaction between genetic host factors and environmental exposures occurring at a critical time in the development of the immune system. The development of asthma likely results from complex interactions between multiple genetic and environmental influences (**Box 1**).[12] The onset of asthma for most patients begins early in life, with the pattern of disease persistence determined by early, recognizable risk factors including atopic disease, recurrent wheezing, and a parental history of asthma.

Box 1
Variables influencing the development of asthma

- Innate Immunity
- Genetics
- Sex
- Allergens/type and timing of exposure
- Respiratory infections
- Environmental exposures

The genetic predisposition for the development of an IgE-mediated response to common aeroallergens is the strongest identifiable predisposing factor for developing asthma. The Third National Health and Nutrition Examination Survey (NHANES) found that one-half of asthma cases were attributable to atopy.[13]

Additional precipitating events may be important variables for exacerbation of asthma and may also contribute to the development of asthma. These events include viral respiratory infections, exposure to environmental tobacco smoke, and obesity (**Fig. 1**).[14–16]

NATURAL HISTORY OF ASTHMA

Persistence and severity of asthma seems to involve a progression of airway inflammation resulting in airway remodeling and eventual irreversible airway obstruction. An important question is whether antiinflammatory medication (ie, inhaled corticosteroids [ICS]) given early in the course of disease might interrupt this process and prevent permanent declines in lung function, or whether the progression to more persistent and severe disease is predetermined by other variables.

Early studies have indicated that, although current treatments are effective in controlling symptoms, reducing airflow limitations, and preventing exacerbations, present treatments for persistent disease (eg, ICS) do not seem to prevent the underlying severity of asthma from progressing,[17] which suggests that currently available therapy controls, but does not modify, the underlying disease process.

In the pediatric population, age 3 years or younger, patients most at risk for developing progressive disease were most likely to have had 4 or more episodes of

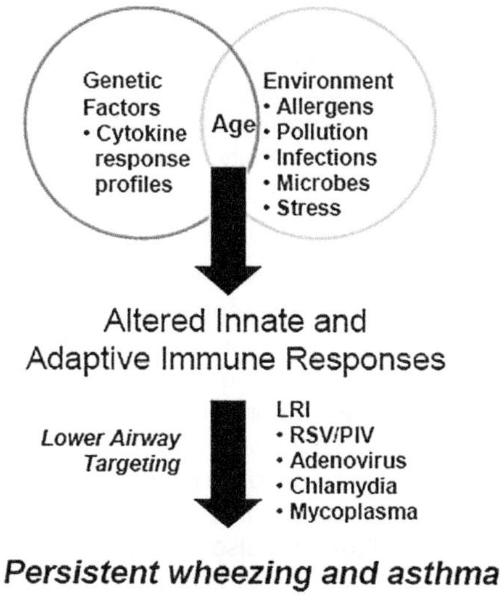

Fig. 1. Host factors and environmental exposures. Guideline for the diagnosis and management of asthma. (*From* National Asthma Education and Prevention Program: Expert Panel Report III: guidelines for the diagnosis and management of asthma. Bethesda (MD): National Heart, Lung, and Blood Institute; 2007. [NIH publication no. 08-4051]. Available at: www.nhlbi.nih.gov/guidelines/asthma/asthgdln.htm. Accessed on September 01, 2007.)

wheezing during the previous year, and either a parental history of asthma, a diagnosis of atopic dermatitis, or evidence of sensitization to aeroallergens.[17]

Data on adult onset asthma are inconclusive on the ability of ICS to alter progression of disease, but seem promising. In 2 long-term observational studies, an association was noted between ICS therapy and reduced decline in forced expiratory volume in 1 second (FEV_1) in adults who had asthma.[18,19]

If ICS can change the natural course of asthma, some continued improvement in lung function might be expected once ICS are discontinued. The best available evidence in children aged 5 to 12 years[20] and aged 2 to 3 years[17] showed that, although ICS provide superior control and prevention of symptoms and exacerbations during treatment, symptoms and airway hyperresponsiveness worsen when treatment is withdrawn. This evidence suggests that currently available therapy controls, but does not modify, the underlying disease process.

Asthma Management: Assessment and Monitoring

Key elements of assessment and monitoring include evaluation of severity of symptoms, control of symptoms, and responsiveness to therapy. Severity, defined as the intrinsic intensity of the disease process, can often be easily measured and should be assessed when the patient is not receiving long-term control therapy. Controls of symptoms are defined as the degree to which the clinical manifestations of asthma can be minimized. Assessment of symptoms, functional impairment, and risks of future events should be minimized. Responsiveness is defined as the ease with which asthma control is achieved.

The diagnosis of asthma is the initial step in reducing the symptoms, functional limitations, impairment in quality of life, and risk of adverse future events that accompany the disease. The ultimate goal of treatment is to enable patients to live with none of the manifestations of asthma.

The initial assessment of the severity of the disease allows for an estimate of the type and intensity of treatment needed. Responsiveness to asthma treatment is variable; therefore, to achieve the goals of therapy, follow-up assessment must be made and treatment should be adjusted accordingly. Patients who have asthma that is well controlled at the time of a clinical assessment should be monitored over time, as the processes of asthma can vary in intensity, and treatment should be adjusted accordingly.

HISTORICAL INFORMATION

Some patients with asthma report or present with the classic triad of symptoms: wheeze, cough (typically worsening at night), and shortness of breath or difficulty breathing. Wheezing does not have a standard meaning for patients and may be used by those without a medical background to describe a variety of sounds. Cough may be dry or productive. Other patients have only 1 or 2 of these symptoms. Some patients describe chest tightness or a bandlike constriction. In contrast, chest pain is uncommonly used to describe the sensation of asthma.

Because the symptoms of asthma are also seen in a myriad of other respiratory diseases, it may be difficult to be certain of the diagnosis of asthma based on history alone.[21–23] However, certain historical features heighten the prior probability of asthma:

- Episodic symptoms: asthmatic symptoms characteristically come and go, resolving spontaneously with removal from the triggering stimulus or in response to antiasthmatic medications. Patients with asthma also may remain asymptomatic for long periods of time

- Characteristic triggers of asthma include exercise, cold air, and exposure to allergens. Similarly, viral infections are common triggers for asthma, although they can trigger exacerbations in other chronic respiratory conditions as well. A strong family history of asthma and allergies or a personal history of atopic diseases (specifically, atopic dermatitis, seasonal allergic rhinitis and conjunctivitis, or hives) favors a diagnosis of asthma in a patient with suggestive symptoms.

Physical Findings

Widespread, high-pitched, musical wheezes are characteristic of asthma, although these findings are not specific and are often absent between exacerbations of the disease. Wheezes are heard most commonly on expiration, but can also occur during inspiration. The presence or absence of wheezing on physical examination is a poor predictor of the severity of airflow obstruction in asthma. Wheezing may be heard in patients with mild, moderate, or severe airway narrowing, whereas widespread airway narrowing may be present in individuals without wheezing. Thus, the presence of wheezing suggests the likely presence of airway narrowing, but not its severity.

PULMONARY FUNCTION TESTING

Variability of patient symptoms and disease exacerbations has resulted in pulmonary function testing becoming a critical tool in the diagnosis and management of asthma. Measurement of peak expiratory flow rate and spirometry are used most frequently.

Peak Expiratory Flow Rate

The peak expiratory flow rate (PEFR) is the measure of airflow during a brief, forceful exhalation. The measurement of peak flow rates can be taught to the patient and routinely used at home to monitor disease severity. As with most pulmonary function testing, the resulting measurements are highly dependent on the patient's expiratory effort and technique. Thus, it is important that the clinician assesses and monitors the patient's technique and effort level and corrects any mistakes. The PEFR maneuver can be performed sitting or standing. Proper technique involves taking a maximally large breath in, putting the peak flow meter quickly to the mouth and sealing the lips around the mouthpiece, and blowing as hard and fast as possible into the meter. For PEFR, the effort does not need to be sustained beyond 1 to 2 seconds. The patient should perform the maneuver 3 times and record the highest of the 3 measurements. Patients should perform the test routinely 2 to 3 times per day and keep a log, establishing a personal-best PEFR. PEFRs may be misleading and mild airflow obstruction may be present when the peak flow remains within the normal range. Reduced peak flow measurements do not differentiate between obstructive and restrictive diseases; spirometry and sometimes measurement of lung volumes are necessary to distinguish the two. Peak flow measurements are not sufficient to distinguish upper airway obstruction (eg, vocal cord dysfunction) from asthma. The validity of PEFR measurements depends on patient effort and technique. There is also no standardization among peak flow measurements. Despite the shortcomings, many patients use PEFR to successfully follow the progression of their asthmatic disease.

Spirometry

Spirometry, which includes measurement of FEV_1 and forced vital capacity (FVC), provides valuable information that is useful in the diagnosis of asthma. Spirometry is a simple office procedure that can be completed in 10 to 15 minutes with virtually no risk to the patient. The test is dependent on patient effort, although standard protocols and normative values have been established.

Spirometry can be used to determine normal from abnormal lung function and can categorize the abnormalities into obstructive or restrictive patterns. Spirometry can also be used to characterize the severity of the asthma and can be used to assess the reversibility of the obstructive abnormality if the testing is repeated after administration of a bronchodilator.

Variable airflow obstruction is the hallmark of asthma. An atopic patient with a cough, shortness of breath, and/or wheezing who has expiratory airflow obstruction pattern on spirometry that reverses to normal with treatment almost certainly has asthma. In contrast, the person with cough and chest congestion who has consistently normal spirometry probably does not have asthma, and alternative explanations (eg, recurrent bronchitis) should be sought.

An obstructive pattern on spirometry is identified numerically by a reduction in the ratio of FEV_1 to the FVC. When FEV_1/FVC is reduced to less than normal (best defined by 95% confidence intervals around the normal values, information that is provided electronically by modern computerized spirometers), airflow obstruction is present. When the FEV_1/FVC ratio is normal or increased, there is no expiratory airflow obstruction.

Having identified the presence of airflow obstruction by a reduction in FEV_1/FVC, the severity of airflow obstruction is then categorized by the degree of reduction of the FEV_1 less than normal. By convention, the severity of airflow obstruction based on spirometry is graded as mild, moderate, severe, and very severe based on the reduction in FEV_1. These categories are used for pulmonary function interpretation and are not the same as categories used to stage asthma severity.

Bronchodilator Response

The ability to acutely reverse airflow obstruction is tested by administering 2 to 4 puffs of a quick-acting bronchodilator (albuterol) and repeating spirometry 10 to 15 minutes later. The variability of the measurement is such that an increase of less than 12% may occur simply because of making repeated measurements. However, an increase in FEV_1 of 12% or more, accompanied by an absolute increase in FEV_1 of at least 200 mL, can be attributed to bronchodilator responsiveness with 95% certainty (**Fig. 2**).

Occasionally, patients with asthma have airflow obstruction on spirometry, but fail to exhibit a 12% or greater increase in FEV_1 following bronchodilator (a false-negative response). There are several reasons for false-negative response to a bronchodilator:

- Incomplete inhalation of the bronchodilator caused by using the metered-dose inhaler incorrectly
- Recent use of a bronchodilator resulting in near-maximal bronchodilation before testing
- Minimal airflow obstruction at the time of testing (FEV_1 already close to 100%)
- In some patients with asthma, the presence of irreversible airways obstruction caused by chronic airways inflammation or scarring (so-called airway remodeling).

Bronchoprovocation Testing

Bronchoprovocation testing is another tool for diagnosing asthma. Bronchoprovocation is used to attempt to provoke airflow obstruction using a stimulus known to elicit airway narrowing. Patients with asthma are more sensitive to such stimuli than are

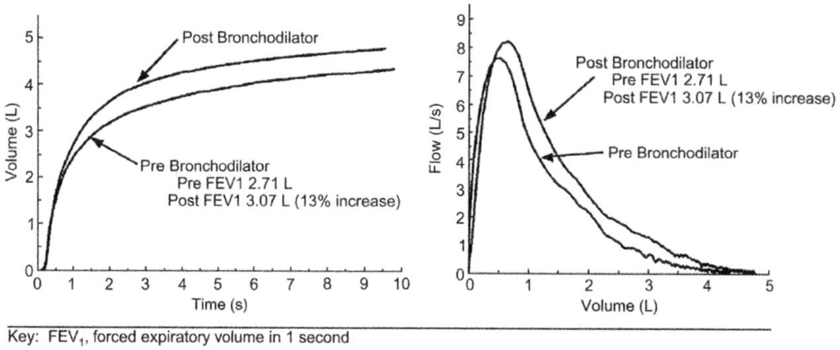

Fig. 2. Sample spirometry: volume time and flow volume curves. (*From* National Asthma Education and Prevention Program: Expert Panel Report III: guidelines for the diagnosis and management of asthma. Bethesda (MD): National Heart, Lung, and Blood Institute; 2007. [NIH publication no. 08-4051]. Available at: www.nhlbi.nih.gov/guidelines/asthma/asthgdln.htm. Accessed on September 01, 2007.)

patients without asthma. Methacholine, exercise, hyperventilation of cold dry air, and inhaled histamine have all been used to provoke bronchoconstriction.

PATIENT MONITORING/PATIENT EDUCATION

Effective asthma management requires a proactive, preventive approach. Routine follow-up visits for patients with asthma are recommended, at a frequency of every 1 to 6 months, depending on the severity of symptoms and patients' responsiveness to therapy. Signs and symptoms of active disease and pulmonary function testing should be reviewed regularly. Quality-of-life questions, number of exacerbations, adherence with treatment, medication side effects, satisfaction with care, and expectations of therapy should all be discussed.

Symptom Assessment

Symptoms over the past 2 to 4 weeks should be assessed at each visit. Assessment should address daytime symptoms, nighttime symptoms, use of short-acting inhaled β-agonists to relieve symptoms, and difficulty in performing normal activities and exercise. There are several validated questionnaires that are easy for patients to complete.[24–30] An example is the Asthma Control Test (http://www.asthmacontrol.com).

The following questions are representative:

Assessment of impairment

- Has your asthma awakened you at night or in the early morning?
- Have you needed your quick-acting relief medication more than usual?
- Have you needed any unscheduled care for your asthma, including calling in, an office visit, or going to the emergency room?
- Have you been able to participate in school/work and recreational activities as desired?
- If you are measuring your peak flow, has it been lower than your personal best?
- Have you had any side effects from your asthma medications?

Assessment of risk

- Have you needed any unscheduled care for your asthma, including calling in, an office visit, or going to the emergency room?
- Have you taken any oral glucocorticoids for your asthma?

Well-controlled asthma is characterized by daytime symptoms no more than twice per week and nighttime symptoms no more than twice per month. Short-acting β-agonists for relief of asthma symptoms should be needed less often than twice weekly, and there should be no interference with normal activity (preventive use of a short-acting β-agonist, such as before exercise, is acceptable even if used in this way on a daily basis). Peak flow should remain normal or near normal. Oral glucocorticoid courses and/or urgent-care visits should be needed no more than once per year.[31]

Environmental Controls/Controlling Triggers

The identification and avoidance of asthma triggers is a critical component of successful asthma management, and successful avoidance or remediation may reduce the patient's need for medications. Directed questions can identify specific triggers and contributing conditions.

Adults should be questioned about symptoms not only in the home but also in the workplace, because asthma can be exacerbated by both irritant and allergen exposures in occupational settings. Some triggers are unavoidable, such as upper respiratory tract illnesses, exercise, hormonal fluctuations, and extreme emotion, and patients should be taught to adjust their management accordingly.

Allergen provocation of asthma is common and the patient should be questioned about symptoms triggered by common inhaled allergens. Indoor allergens, such as dust mites, animal dander, molds, and cockroaches, are of particular importance as triggers of asthma. If the history suggests that the patient has allergic triggers, basic avoidance measures should be advised, and further evaluation, including specific allergen testing via in vitro or skin testing techniques, is warranted.

Inhaled irritants as a trigger of asthma are also common and include tobacco smoke, wood smoke from stoves or fireplaces, strong perfumes and odors, chlorine-based cleaning products, and air pollutants. These exposures should always be considered when discussing environmental controls.

Patients should be cognizant of avoiding irritants, and avoid exertion outdoors on days when levels of air pollution are increased.

Clinicians should be vigilant for comorbid conditions in patients with poorly controlled asthma. In adults, these conditions include chronic obstructive pulmonary disease (COPD)/emphysema, allergic bronchopulmonary aspergillosis, gastroesophageal reflux, obesity, obstructive sleep apnea, rhinitis/sinusitis, vocal cord dysfunction, and depression/chronic stress. In young children, contributing conditions include respiratory syncytial virus infection, foreign body aspiration, bronchopulmonary dysplasia, cystic fibrosis, and obesity.[32]

Medication reactions also need to be considered when discussing the control of asthma triggers. Nonselective β-blockers can trigger severe asthmatic attacks, even in the small amounts absorbed systemically from topical ophthalmic solutions. Selective β-1 blockers have also been shown to aggravate asthma in some patients, especially at higher doses.

Aspirin and nonsteroidal antiinflammatory drugs can trigger asthma symptoms in approximately 3% to 5% of adult asthmatic patients. The incidence of aspirin-exacerbated respiratory disease is higher among asthmatic patients with nasal polyposis (constituting triad asthma or Samter triad). Aspirin-sensitive asthma is uncommon in children.

Annual administration of influenza vaccine is recommended for patients with asthma because they are at risk for complications of infection. However, vaccination does not reduce the number or severity of asthma exacerbations during the influenza season, and providers should ensure that patients understand this distinction.

Administration of pneumococcal vaccination is recommended for adults whose asthma is severe enough to require controller medication and for children with asthma who require chronic oral glucocorticoid therapy.[33]

Dietary sulfites (used in foods to prevent discoloration) have been shown to provoke asthma. As many as 5% of patients with asthma may note significant and reproducible exacerbations following ingestion of sulfite-treated foods and beverages, such as beer, wine, processed potatoes, dried fruit, sauerkraut, or shrimp.

PHARMACOLOGIC TREATMENT

Pharmacologic treatment is the mainstay of management in most patients with asthma. The 2007 National Asthma Education and Prevention Program (NAEPP) Expert Panel Report presented a stepwise approach to pharmacologic therapy, which is reflected in this review.[32]

These guidelines are well written and are intended to support, as opposed to dictate, care. Allowing for treatment is based on the clinician's clinical judgment.

The stepwise approach to pharmacotherapy is based on increasing medications until asthma is controlled, and decreasing medications, when possible, to minimize side effects. Decisions regarding the patient's management should be discussed at every visit. The initial step in determining appropriate therapy for patients who have not been treated with a controller medication is classifying the severity of the patient's asthma.

Categories of Asthma Severity

Asthma severity is determined by considering the following 3 factors[32]:

1. Reported symptoms over the previous 2 to 4 weeks
2. Current level of lung function (FEV_1 and FEV_1/FVC values)
3. Number of exacerbations requiring oral glucocorticoids per year

The use of these 3 elements to determine severity in adolescents more than 12 years of age and in adults is presented in **Table 1**.

The classification of severity in children aged 5 to 11 years is similar to that in adults (**Table 2**).

However, severity in children less than 4 years of age is classified differently (**Table 3**).

The classification for children older than 12 years of age to adults divides asthma severity into intermittent or persistent based on frequency of symptoms. Persistent asthma is further classified into mild, moderate, or severe depending on symptom severity and objective testing.

Intermittent Asthma

The criteria for adolescents and adults diagnosed with intermittent asthma are:

- Daytime asthma symptoms occurring 2 or fewer days per week
- Two or fewer nocturnal awakenings per month
- Use of short-acting β-agonists to relieve symptoms fewer than 2 times a week
- No interference with normal activities between exacerbations
- FEV_1 measurements between exacerbations are consistently within the normal range (ie, equal to 80% of predicted normal)
- Only 1 or no exacerbations of symptoms requiring oral glucocorticoids per year.

Table 1
The 3 elements used to determine asthma severity in adolescents older than 12 years and in adults

Components of Severity		Classification of Asthma Severity (Youths ≥12 y of Age and Adults)			
			Persistent		
		Intermittent	Mild	Moderate	Severe
Impairment	Symptoms	≤2 d/wk	>2 d/wk but not daily	Daily	Throughout the day
Normal FEV_1/FVC:	Nighttime awakenings	≤2x/mo	3–4/mo	>1/wk but not nightly	Often 7/wk
8–19 y 85% 20–39 y 80% 40–59 y 75%	Short-acting β_2-agonist use for symptom control (not prevention of EIB)	≤2 d/wk	>2 d/wk but not >1/d	Daily	Several times per day
60–80 y 70%	Interference with normal activity	None	Minor limitation	Some limitation	Extremely limit
	Lung function	Normal FEV_1 between exacerbations FEV_1 >80% predicted FEV_1/FVC normal	FEV_1 ≥80% predicted FEV_1/FVC normal	FEV_1 >60% but <80% predicted FEV_1/FVC reduced 5%	• FEV_1 <60% predicted • FEV_1/FVC reduced >5%
Risk	Exacerbations requiring oral systemic corticosteroids	0–1/y (see note)	≥2/y (see note) →		
		← Consider severity and interval since last exacerbation. Frequency and severity may fluctuate over time for patients in any severity category. →			
		Relative annual risk of exacerbations may be related to FEV_1			

Abbreviation: EIB, exercise-induced bronchospasm.

From National Asthma Education and Prevention Program: Expert Panel Report III: guidelines for the diagnosis and management of asthma. Bethesda (MD): National Heart, Lung, and Blood Institute; 2007. [NIH publication no. 08-4051]. Available at: www.nhlbi.nih.gov/guidelines/asthma/asthgdln.htm. Accessed on September 01, 2007.

Table 2
The classification of severity in children aged 5 to 11 years

Components of Control		Classification of Asthma Control (Children 5–11 y of Age) Well Controlled	Not Well Controlled	Very Poorly Controlled
Impairment	Symptoms	≤2 d/wk but not more than once on each day	>2 d/wk or multiple times on ≤2 d/wk	Throughout the day
	Nighttime awakenings	≤1/mo	≥2/mo	≥2/wk
	Interference with normal activity	None	Some limitation	Extremely limited
	Short-acting β_2-agonist use for symptom control (not prevention of EIB)	≤2 d/wk	>2 d/wk	Several times per day
	Lung function			
	• FEV_1 or peak flow	>80% predicted/personal best	60%–80% predicted/personal best	<60% predicted/personal best
	• FEV_1/FVC	>80%	75%–80%	<75%
Risk	Exacerbations requiring oral systemic corticosteroids	0–1/y	≥2/y (see note)	
		Consider severity and interval since last exacerbation		
	Reduction in lung growth	Evaluation requires long-term follow-up		
	Treatment-related adverse effects	Medication side effects can vary in intensity from none to very troublesome and worrisome. The level of intensity does not correlate to specific levels of control but should be considered in the overall assessment of risk		

Abbreviation: EIB, exercise-induced bronchospasm.

From National Asthma Education and Prevention Program: Expert Panel Report III: guidelines for the diagnosis and management of asthma. Bethesda (MD): National Heart, Lung, and Blood Institute; 2007. [NIH publication no. 08-4051]. Available at: www.nhlbi.nih.gov/guidelines/asthma/asthgdln.htm. Accessed on September 01, 2007.

Table 3
Severity in children less than 4 years of age

	Components of Control	Classification of Asthma Control (Children 0–4 y of Age)		
		Well Controlled	Not Well Controlled	Very Poorly Controlled
Impairment	Symptoms	≤2 d/wk	>2 d/wk	Throughout the day
	Nighttime awakenings	≤1/mo	>1/mo	>1/wk
	Interference with normal activity	None	Some limitation	Extremely limited
	Short-acting β_2-agonist use for symptom control (not prevention of EIB)	≤2 d/wk	>2 d/wk	Several times per day
Risk	Exacerbations requiring oral systemic corticosteroids	0–1/y	2–3/y	>3/y
	Treatment-related adverse effects	Medication side effects can vary in intensity from none to very troublesome and worrisome. The level of intensity does not correlate to specific levels of control but should be considered in the overall assessment of risk		

From National Asthma Education and Prevention Program: Expert Panel Report III: guidelines for the diagnosis and management of asthma. Bethesda (MD): National Heart, Lung, and Blood Institute; 2007. [NIH publication no. 08-4051]. Available at: www.nhlbi.nih.gov/guidelines/asthma/asthgdln.htm. Accessed on September 01, 2007.

If these various elements are discordant, the patient's asthma should be categorized at the level of the most severe.

In addition, a person using a short-acting β-agonist to prevent exercise-induced asthmatic symptoms might fit into this category even if exercising more than twice per week. Others in whom asthmatic symptoms arise only in certain infrequently occurring circumstances (eg, on encountering a cat or during viral respiratory tract infections) are also considered to have intermittent asthma.

Mild Persistent Asthma

Mild persistent asthma is characterized by:

- Symptoms occurring more than twice weekly (although < daily)
- Between 3 and 4 nocturnal awakenings per month caused by asthma
- Need to use short-acting β-agonists to relieve symptoms more than 2 times a week (but not daily)
- Minor interference with normal activities
- FEV_1measurements within normal range (equal to 80% of predicted normal) and the FEV_1/FVC ratio is normal (based on age-adjusted values)
- Two or more exacerbations requiring oral glucocorticoids per year.

If the various elements are discordant, the patient's asthma should be categorized at the level of the most severe.

Moderate Persistent Asthma

The presence of any of the following is considered an indication of moderate disease severity classified as moderate persistent asthma:

- Daily symptoms of asthma
- Nocturnal awakenings more than once per week
- Daily need for short-acting β-agonists for symptom relief
- Some limitation in normal activity
- Spirometry in mild persistent asthmatics shows an FEV_1between 60% and 80% of predicted and the FEV_1/FVC ratio is reduced to less than normal (based on age-adjusted values)
- Two or more exacerbations annually requiring oral glucocorticoids.

Severe Persistent Asthma

Patients with severe persistent asthma experience 1 or more of the following symptoms of asthma:

- Symptoms of asthma throughout the day
- Nocturnal awakenings nightly
- Need for short-acting β-agonists for symptom relief several times per day
- Extreme limitation in normal activity
- Objective pulmonary function testing reveals FEV_1 less than 60% of predicted and an FEV_1/FVC reduced to less than normal (based on age-adjusted values).

These patients require oral glucocorticoids 2 or more times per year.

PHARMACOTHERAPY FOR ASTHMA

Initiating Therapy in Previously Untreated Patients

The initiation of asthma therapy in a stable patient who is not already receiving medications is based on the severity of the individual's asthma. A stepwise treatment approach has been developed in children younger than 15 years of age to adults (**Fig. 3**), children aged 5 to 15 years (**Fig. 4**), and in children younger than 4 years of age. These guidelines are offered in an attempt to facilitate rapid control of symptoms with the least amount of medications required. Increasing or reducing therapy, as symptoms dictate, reflects the variable nature of asthma.[32]

Intermittent (Step 1)

Patients with mild intermittent asthma are best treated with a quick-acting inhaled β2-selective adrenergic agonist, taken as needed for relief of symptoms (see **Fig. 3**).[34] Patients for whom triggering of asthmatic symptoms can be predicted (eg, exercise-induced bronchoconstriction) are encouraged to use their inhaled β-agonist approximately 10 minutes before exposure to prevent the onset of symptoms.

Mild Persistent (Step 2)

The distinction between intermittent and mild persistent asthma is important, because current guidelines for mild persistent asthma call for initiation of daily long-term controller medication. For mild persistent asthma, the preferred long-term controller is a low-dose inhaled glucocorticoid (see **Fig. 3**). Regular use of inhaled glucocorticoids reduces the frequency of symptoms (and the need for short-acting β-agonists

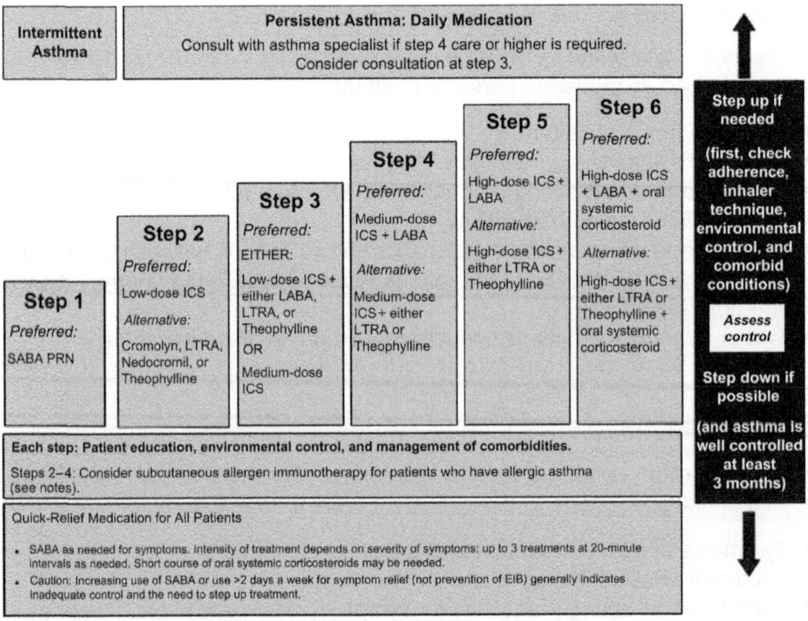

Fig. 3. Stepwise approach for managing asthma in children 5 to 11 years of age. (*From* National Asthma Education and Prevention Program: Expert Panel Report III: guidelines for the diagnosis and management of asthma. Bethesda (MD): National Heart, Lung, and Blood Institute; 2007. [NIH publication no. 08-4051]. Available at: www.nhlbi.nih.gov/guidelines/asthma/asthgdln.htm. Accessed on September 01, 2007.)

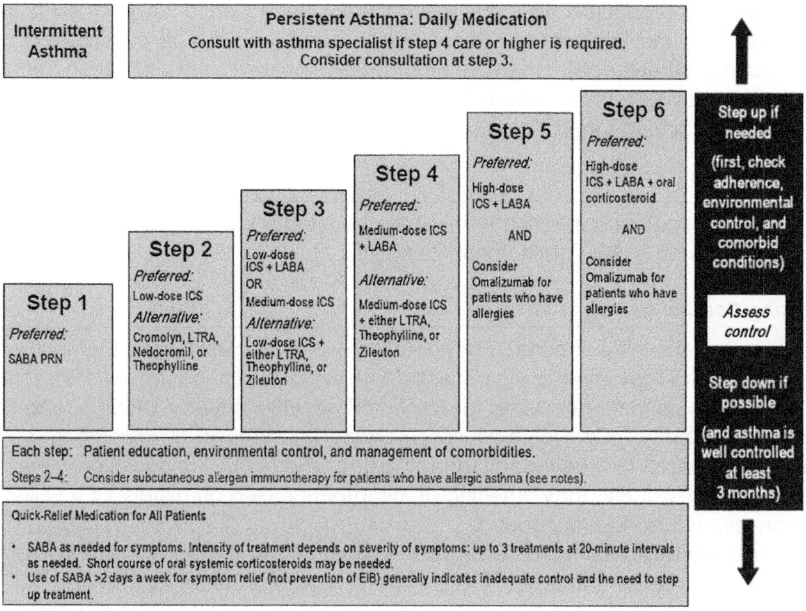

Fig. 4. Stepwise approach for managing asthma in youths more than 12 years of age and adults. (*From* National Asthma Education and Prevention Program: Expert Panel Report III: guidelines for the diagnosis and management of asthma. Bethesda (MD): National Heart, Lung, and Blood Institute; 2007. [NIH publication no. 08-4051]. Available at: www.nhlbi.nih.gov/guidelines/asthma/asthgdln.htm. Accessed on September 01, 2007.)

for symptom relief), improves the overall quality of life, and decreases the risk of serious exacerbations.[35–37] Regular use of inhaled glucocorticoids has not been shown to definitively prevent progressive loss of lung function over time.

Alternative strategies for treatment of mild persistent asthma include leukotriene receptor antagonists, theophylline, and cromoglycates (see **Fig. 3**). Patients receiving long-term controller therapy should continue to use their short-acting β-agonist as needed for relief of symptoms and before exposure to known triggers of their symptoms.

Moderate Persistent (Step 3)

For moderate persistent asthma, the preferred therapies are either low doses of an inhaled glucocorticoid plus a long-acting inhaled β-agonist, or medium doses of an inhaled glucocorticoid (see **Fig. 3**). The former combination has proved more effective in controlling asthmatic symptoms than increasing the dose of inhaled glucocorticoids, although it entails the potential risk of adverse outcomes that have been reported in association with long-acting inhaled β-agonists.[38,39]

Alternative strategies include adding a leukotriene modifier (leukotriene receptor antagonist or lipoxygenase inhibitor) or theophylline to low-dose inhaled glucocorticoids.

Severe Persistent (Step 4 or 5)

For severe persistent asthma, the preferred treatments are medium (step 4) or high (step 5) doses of an inhaled glucocorticoid, in combination with a long-acting inhaled β-agonist (see **Fig. 3**).

In addition, for patients who are inadequately controlled on high-dose inhaled glucocorticoids and long-acting β-agonists, the anti-IgE therapy omalizumab may be considered if there is objective evidence (allergy skin tests or in vitro measurements of allergen-specific IgE) of sensitivity to a perennial allergen and if the serum IgE level is within the established target range.

Step 6 Therapy

For severe asthma not controlled through step 5, step 6 involves the addition of oral glucocorticoids on a daily or alternate-day basis.

Assessing Control to Adjust Therapy

Assessment of the level of control, rather than severity of classification, of disease is used to adjust therapy in returning patients. Assessing level of control also is useful to alter therapy in patients evaluated for the first time while already taking a long-term controller medication. Control is assessed based on the level of impairment/symptoms over the past 2 to 4 weeks and through using current FEV_1 or peak flow measurements. Estimates of risk for worsening of symptoms based on history or a validated questionnaire is also a useful tool.[32]

The clinician should determine whether the patient's asthma is well controlled or not using the information gathered. If the asthma is well controlled, therapy can be continued or possibly reduced to minimize medication side effects. If the asthma is not well controlled, therapy should be increased. Therapy should be readjusted at each visit, because of the inherent variability of asthma. The management of asthma is a dynamic process that changes in accordance with the patient's needs over time. Educating the patient with respect to the nature of the disease and the control process facilitates management.

Efficacy of Asthma Management

A prospective, randomized trial applied the management recommendations of previous NAEPP guidelines to approximately 1500 patients with a variety of severities of asthma for a period of 12 months.[40] The use of guideline-based management resulted in significant improvement in health-related quality of life in most patients, regardless of disease severity. In this study, subjects who required inhaled glucocorticoids were randomly assigned to receive either fluticasone propionate (FP) alone or the combination of FP and salmeterol (S). Subjects were evaluated every 3 months and medications were stepped up as needed. With both treatments, more than one-half of patients achieved well-controlled or totally controlled asthma, although control was slightly better with FP plus S. The greatest improvements occurred in the first few months of therapy. Thus, the stepwise approach to asthma management is effective in reducing symptoms and improving health-related quality of life. The current guidelines have expanded on this same basic approach.[32]

REFERENCES

1. Slavin RG. The upper and lower airways: the epidemiological and pathophysiological connection. Allergy Asthma Proc 2008;29:553.
2. Greenberger PA. Allergic rhinitis and asthma connection: treatment implications. Allergy Asthma Proc 2008;29:557.
3. Sibbald B, Rink E. Epidemiology of seasonal and perennial rhinitis: clinical presentation and medical history. Thorax 1991;46:895.

4. National Health Interview Survey (NHIS 2005). Hyattsville (MD): National Center for Health Statistics (NCHS), Centers for Disease Control and Prevention; 2005. Available at: www.cdc.gov/nchs/fastats/asthma.htm. Accessed August 28, 2010 and September 27, 2010.
5. Eichenfield LF, Hanifin JM, Beck LA, et al. Atopic dermatitis and asthma: parallels in the evolution of treatment. Pediatrics 2003;111(3):608–16.
6. Leynaert B, Bousquet J, Neukirch C, et al. Perennial rhinitis: an independent risk factor for asthma in nonatopic subjects: results from the European Community Respiratory Health Survey. J Allergy Clin Immunol 1999;104:301.
7. Zimmermann N, Hershey GK, Foster PS, et al. Chemokines in asthma: cooperative interaction between chemokines and IL-13. J Allergy Clin Immunol 2003; 111(2):227–42.
8. Busse WW. The role of leukotrienes in asthma and allergic rhinitis [review]. Clin Exp Allergy 1996;26(8):868–79.
9. Deykin A, Massaro AF, Drazen JM, et al. Exhaled nitric oxide as a diagnostic test for asthma: online versus offline techniques and effect of flow rate. Am J Respir Crit Care Med 2002;165(12):1597–601.
10. Boyce JA. Mast cells: beyond IgE. J Allergy Clin Immunol 2003;111(1):24–32 [quiz: 33].
11. Cohn L, Elias JA, Chupp GL. Asthma: mechanisms of disease [review]. Annu Rev Immunol 2004;22:789–815.
12. Allen M, Heinzmann A, Noguchi E, et al. Positional cloning of a novel gene influencing asthma from chromosome 2q14. Nat Genet 2003;35:258.
13. Arbes SJ Jr, Gergen PJ, Vaughn B, et al. Asthma cases attributable to atopy: results from the Third National Health and Nutrition Examination Survey. J Allergy Clin Immunol 2007;120:1139.
14. Johnston SL, Pattemore PK, Sanderson G, et al. Community study of role of viral infections in exacerbations of asthma in 9–11 year old children. BMJ 1995;310:1225.
15. Cunningham J, O'Connor GT, Dockery DW, et al. Environmental tobacco smoke, wheezing, and asthma in children in 24 communities. Am J Respir Crit Care Med 1996;153:218.
16. Beuther DA, Sutherland ER. Overweight, obesity, and incident asthma: a meta-analysis of prospective epidemiologic studies. Am J Respir Crit Care Med 2007;175:661.
17. Guilbert TW, Morgan WJ, Zeiger RS, et al. Long-term inhaled corticosteroids in preschool children at high risk for asthma. N Engl J Med 2006;354(19): 1985–97.
18. Dijkstra A, Vonk JM, Jongepier H, et al. Lung function decline in asthma: association with inhaled corticosteroids, smoking and sex. Thorax 2006;61(2):105–10.
19. Lange P, Scharling H, Ulrik CS, et al. Inhaled corticosteroids and decline of lung function in community residents with asthma. Thorax 2006;61(2):100–4.
20. Childhood Asthma Management Program Research Group (CAMP). Long-term effects of budesonide or nedocromil in children with asthma. N Engl J Med 2000;343(15):1054–63.
21. Pratter MR, Hingston DM, Irwin RS. Diagnosis of bronchial asthma by clinical evaluation. An unreliable method. Chest 1983;84:42.
22. Irwin RS, Curley FJ, French CL. Chronic cough. The spectrum and frequency of causes, key components of the diagnostic evaluation, and outcome of specific therapy. Am Rev Respir Dis 1990;141:640.
23. Pratter MR, Curley FJ, Dubois J, et al. Cause and evaluation of chronic dyspnea in a pulmonary disease clinic. Arch Intern Med 1989;149:2277.

24. Juniper EF, O'Byrne PM, Guyatt GH, et al. Development and validation of a questionnaire to measure asthma control. Eur Respir J 1999;14:902.
25. Vollmer WM, Markson LE, O'Connor E, et al. Association of asthma control with health care utilization and quality of life. Am J Respir Crit Care Med 1999; 160:1647.
26. Boulet LP, Boulet V, Milot J. How should we quantify asthma control? A proposal. Chest 2002;122:2217.
27. Nathan RA, Sorkness CA, Kosinski M, et al. Development of the Asthma Control Test: a survey for assessing asthma control. J Allergy Clin Immunol 2004;113:59.
28. Patino CM, Okelo SO, Rand CS, et al. The asthma control and communication instrument: a clinical tool developed for ethnically diverse populations. J Allergy Clin Immunol 2008;122:936.
29. Schatz M, Kosinski M, Yarlas AS, et al. The minimally important difference of the Asthma Control Test. J Allergy Clin Immunol 2009;124:719.
30. Liu AH, Zeiger RS, Sorkness CA, et al. The Childhood Asthma Control Test: retrospective determination and clinical validation of a cut point to identify children with very poorly controlled asthma. J Allergy Clin Immunol 2010;126:267.
31. Bateman ED, Reddel HK, Eriksson G, et al. Overall asthma control: the relationship between current control and future risk. J Allergy Clin Immunol 2010;125:600.
32. National Asthma Education and Prevention Program: Expert Panel Report III: guidelines for the diagnosis and management of asthma. Bethesda (MD): National Heart, Lung, and Blood Institute; 2007. (NIH publication no. 08-4051). Available at: www.nhlbi.nih.gov/guidelines/asthma/asthgdln.htm. Accessed September 27, 2010.
33. Klemets P, Lyytikäinen O, Ruutu P, et al. Risk of invasive pneumococcal infections among working age adults with asthma. Thorax 2010;65:698.
34. Nelson HS. Beta-adrenergic bronchodilators. N Engl J Med 1995;333:499.
35. Haahtela T, Järvinen M, Kava T, et al. Comparison of a beta 2-agonist, terbutaline, with an inhaled corticosteroid, budesonide, in newly detected asthma. N Engl J Med 1991;325:388.
36. Dutoit JI, Salome CM, Woolcock AJ. Inhaled corticosteroids reduce the severity of bronchial hyperresponsiveness in asthma but oral theophylline does not. Am Rev Respir Dis 1987;136:1174.
37. Juniper EF, Kline PA, Vanzieleghem MA, et al. Effect of long-term treatment with an inhaled corticosteroid (budesonide) on airway hyperresponsiveness and clinical asthma in nonsteroid-dependent asthmatics. Am Rev Respir Dis 1990; 142:832.
38. Chowdhury BA, Dal Pan G. The FDA and safe use of long-acting beta-agonists in the treatment of asthma. N Engl J Med 2010;362:1169.
39. FDA drug safety communication: new safety requirements for long-acting inhaled medications called long-acting beta-agonists (LABAs). Available at: www.fda.gov/Drugs/DrugSafety/PostmarketDrugSafetyInformationforPatientsandProviders/ucm200776.htm. Accessed September 05, 2010.
40. Bateman ED, Bousquet J, Keech ML, et al. The correlation between asthma control and health status: the GOAL study. Eur Respir J 2007;29:56.

Nasal Polyps: Pathogenesis and Treatment Implications

Michael A. DeMarcantonio, MD, Joseph K. Han, MD*

KEYWORDS

- Sinusitis • Asthma • Unified airway
- Allergy • Rhinosinusitis • Polyp

Key Points: Nasal Polyps: Pathogenesis and Treatment Implications

- Nasal polyp (NP) is the end product of chronic rhinosinusitis (CRS).
- NPs are created through multiple inflammatory or infectious pathways.
- All types of CRS have the potential to develop NPs, given enough time and insult.
- Medical treatment depends on the pathogenesis of NPs.
- Surgical removal of inflammatory cell and mediators followed by medical treatment is likely to have the best success in patients with severe nasal polyposis.
- Evaluation of allergy, whether it is negative or positive, is important in the management of patients with nasal polyposis.

NPs represent a common clinical end point for a myriad of inflammatory disease processes involving the paranasal sinuses. NP is common, with 1% to 4% of the general population having evidence of an NP on autopsy.[1] However, not everyone with NP develops clinical symptoms because only a portion of population becomes symptomatic, with a yearly incidence of 0.627 per 1000 people.[1] Men seem to outnumber women (2:1), with the overall incidence increasing in both sexes with age. Even though these numbers of individuals with NP are small compared with that of other more common chronic illnesses, such as hypertension, the overall effect of NP should not be underestimated. In fact, NPs have been shown to have a significant detrimental effect on the quality of life, which is similar in severity to chronic obstructive pulmonary disease.[2]

The authors have nothing to declare.
Department of Otolaryngology–Head and Neck Surgery, Eastern Virginia Medical School, 600 Gresham Drive, Suite 1100, Norfolk, VA 23507, USA
* Corresponding author.
E-mail address: hanjk@evms.edu

Otolaryngol Clin N Am 44 (2011) 685–695
doi:10.1016/j.otc.2011.03.005
oto.theclinics.com

CLINICAL PRESENTATION AND DIAGNOSIS

When discussing trends in clinical presentation, the diversity of patients with NPs must always be respected, and broad generalizations should be avoided. Nevertheless, trends in clinical complaints have been shown when comparing patients with CRS with polyps with those without evidence of polyps. Patients with NPs are more likely to complain of a constellation of symptoms, including diminished olfaction, headache, and postnasal drip.[3] In addition, symptoms are more likely to be described as bilateral in 80% to 90% of patients.[4] Although a thorough clinical history taking is invaluable, the gold standard for diagnosis of NPs remains endoscopy.[5] In an effort to quantify endoscopic findings, multiple staging systems have been proposed. The utility of these systems lie primarily in their ability to allow for preinterventional and postinterventional comparison. Lund and Mackay[6] used a 3-tier system with scoring as follows: 0, no polyps; 1, confined to middle meatus; and 2, beyond middle meatus. Lildholdt and colleagues[7] used a slightly varied system to assess the effect of multiple treatment methods. The 4-point system developed used the upper and lower edges of the inferior turbinate as a landmark to describe polyp extension. The highest score available extended to the inferior edge of the inferior turbinate, essentially contacting the floor and filling the nasal cavity. To assess these systems and several new methods, Johansson and colleagues[5] evaluated interobserver and intraobserver variability in a well-designed clinical study. The Lildholdt system was found to provide good repeatability and less interexaminer variability in comparison with the Lund-Mackay scoring system. Of note, researchers have shown poor reliability or correlation between patients' recorded visual analog scores for nasal obstruction and the objective polyp burden regardless of the scoring system. Although objective measures are needed for treatment studies, this lack of correlation with symptoms highlights the weakness of using staging systems in clinical practice.

IMAGING FOR NASAL POLYPS

It is undeniable that computed tomographic (CT) imaging has become an essential tool for the diagnosis and surgical management of sinusitis. Classically, CT scans of sinuses in patients with NP are described as possessing polypoid masses associated with partial or complete opacification of paranasal sinuses with infundibulum widening.[8] With respect to its use as a diagnostic tool, CT imaging's major weakness lies in its inability to differentiate polyps from mucous and other soft tissue masses. However, many patients with CRS eventually require operative intervention, and therefore, a major benefit of CT imaging remains in its ability to provide a road map for surgical planning. For patients with nasal polyposis, this information can be invaluable because the deforming nature of the disease can lead to intraoperative disorientation, making knowledge of anatomic variations crucial.

CHRONIC RHINOSINUSITIS AND NASAL POLYP

The largest proportion of patients with NP has a diagnosis of CRS. CRS affects about 30 million Americans, imparting an annual medical cost of $2.4 billion. Societal effects are further compounded by sick days, lost work hours, and other indirect costs.[9] To standardize a formerly amorphous clinical diagnosis, CRS criteria have been set forth. A diagnosis of CRS requires a symptom duration longer than 12 weeks with 2 of the following symptoms: facial pain/pressure, hyposmia/anosmia, nasal obstruction, or anterior/posterior nasal drip.[10] Even though all types of CRS have the potential to develop NPs, given enough time and insult, the presence of NPs has been used as a way to subdivide CRS into 2 groups: CRS with NPs (CRSwNP) and CRS without NPs (CRSsNP). CRSwNP represents 20% to 33% of overall CRS cases,[11] although this can vary depending on the geographic location. Although only a portion of patients with CRS have nasal polyposis, these patients likely represent a disproportionate number of recalcitrant patients.

A diverse collection of chronic sinusitis can present with NPs, which include allergic fungal sinusitis, aspirin-exacerbated respiratory disease (AERD), and cystic fibrosis (CF). Despite having similar macroscopic findings, each of these disorders represents a complex pathology and varying treatment strategy. This article outlines the current understanding of pathogenesis in nasal polyposis and discusses the implications on therapy.

PATHOGENESIS

In attempting to understand pathogenesis in nasal polyposis, it must be remembered that this subject represents a topic in flux. To date, there exists no delineated pathway that can clearly explain the journey from insult to tissue change. The current understanding is instead limited to comprehending and elucidating differing inflammatory promoters and pathways. Much as in the mastery of any sport, it is essential to understand the roles of the key players before tackling overall strategy. It is hoped that by understanding the various inflammatory pathways and their effects eventually, detailed classification will allow for prediction of clinical course and tailoring of intervention.

Cytokines

The division of CRSwNP and CRSsNP has long centered on the separation of the inflammatory pathways that drive them. Classically, CRSsNP is a helper T cell (T_H) subtype 1–dominant and neutrophil-dominant process, whereas CRSwNP represents an eosinophilic T_H2 process.[12] This paradigm has been supported by the finding that 60% to 90% of the cell population in NPs is composed of eosinophils.[13,14] It is presumed that through degranulation and release of cytotoxic compounds, such as eosinophilic cationic protein (ECP), these invading cells propagate inflammation and cell damage.[15] High levels of the T_H2 cytokines interleukin (IL)-5 and IL-4 have long been confirmed in NP tissues.[4] Research in reactive airway diseases has also demonstrated a clear link between these cytokines and both tissue and blood eosinophilia.[16] IL-4 in particular seems to promote not only eosinophil migration and activation but also T-cell differentiation from T_H0 to T_H2. The resultant cyclical T_H2 upregulation further spurs on eosinophilic inflammation.[17] IL-5 arguably plays the most important role in eosinophilic-driven processes. Like IL-4, this cytokine has a dual action and influence, prompting propagation and activation while simultaneously preventing apoptosis.[18]

CRSsNP can be characterized by the presence of the T_H1 cytokine interferon γ (INF-γ). INF-γ plays an essential role in both innate immunity and acute inflammation.[19] In contrast to IL-4 and IL-5, INF-γ has been shown to prevent airway eosinophilia and allergic response.[17] As would be expected, the INF-γ level is found to be decreased in NPs.[3] The role of another T_H1 cytokine, IL-8, is not completely discerned. IL-8 represents a neutrophil chemoattractant that is frequently associated with acute sinus infections. In patients with CRSwNP, Chen and colleagues[20] demonstrated that IL-8 was diffusely upregulated throughout mucosa but without specific association with polyp tissue.

The real goal of delineating the cytokine profile is to allow for the differentiation of CRS subtypes. Van Zele and colleagues,[3] in an attempt to realize this goal, evaluated inflammatory cells and mediators in those with CRSsNP, CRSwNP, and CF and in controls. This group confirmed statistically significant IL-5 and eosinophil levels in individuals with CRSwNP compared with abundant INF-γ in those with CRSsNP. In contrast, individuals with CF nasal polyps (CF-NP) displayed neutrophil-dominant markers with increases in IL-8 and myeloperoxidase (MPO) levels. The inflammatory process responsible for CF-NP formation is not driven by the T_H2 process or eosinophils as most typical CRSwNP but rather by the T_H1 process. In addition, using receiver operating characteristic analysis, the best cytokine profiles to differentiate each group were identified. Of note, a sensitivity and specificity rate of 75% was observed using IL-5, ECP, and IgE levels to differentiate CRSwNP from CRSsNP. INF-γ was found to offer a similar rate of successful differentiation. IL-8 and MPO were found to provide a sensitivity and specificity of 75% for differentiation between other forms of CRS. Such research offers a window into the future of CRS management in which inflammatory cells and mediators may be used in combination with history taking and examination to classify patients with CRS.

T-cell Regulation and Transforming Growth Factor β1

Once the primary cytokines involved in NPs have been described, it becomes essential to examine the intracellular processes upstream that lead to T-cell differentiation and propagation. An interesting avenue of research in this field examines the interplay of forkhead box P3 (FoxP3) and T regulatory (T_{reg}) cells. T_{reg} cells, also described as suppressor T cells, function to maintain self-tolerance and immune hemostasis.[21] The lack of adequate function can result in rampant and uncontrolled immune activation seen in fatal autoimmune disease. The FoxP3 gene exerts control over immune hemostasis by regulating T_{reg} production.[21] The characterization of this pathway has provided insight into a wide array of allergic and inflammatory pathways. In the realm of CRS, Van Bruaene and colleagues[22] have demonstrated diminished FoxP3 expression and T_{reg} production in those with CRSwNP compared with both those with CRSsNP and controls. It can be suggested that such an environment of diminished immune control may act as the priming pump for excessive inflammation. Levels of transforming growth factor β1 (TGF-β1) were also proportionally decreased in NPs for the CRSwNP group. This association offers a possible link between the upregulation of inflammation and TGF-β1–associated tissue damage. TGF-β1 is a cytokine produced by lymphocytes, macrophages, eosinophils, and fibroblasts and is associated with local deposition of extracellular matrix and eventual cellular damage.[19,23] TGF-β1 seems to exert an influence on fibroblasts, resulting in the production of fibrous stroma and hypertrophic scar tissue.[24,25] This propensity for thick fibrous tissue formation offers an additional point of differentiation between CRSwNP and CRSsNP. A cellular disparity could explain the obvious differences in the gross pathology between the edematous polypoid mucosa of CRSwNP and the thickened scarred sinuses of CRSsNP.

The function of TGF-β1, however, does not seem to be 1-dimensional. In in vitro studies of fibroblast activity, TGF-β1 has been shown to be increased 3-fold in patients with NPs when exposed to IL-4.[25] In a follow-up study, Little and colleagues[26] examined the influence of increased TGF-β1 levels on NP-derived fibroblasts. Although proliferation and fibrotic potential were clearly increased, TGF-β1 was also associated with decreased levels of eotaxin and other eosinophilic inflammation promoters. The investigators propose these findings to help define a dual role for TGF-β1 as both an antiinflammatory agent and a promoter of fibrosis. Such a system could explain the transition from acute/chronic inflammation to fibrotic changes.[26]

EOSINOPHILIC AND NONEOSINOPHILIC NASAL POLYPOSIS

It has been well accepted that not all patients with CRS that form NPs demonstrate T_H2 eosinophilic-dominant pathology.[27,28] New emphasis on noneosinophilic nasal polyposis has emerged primarily from Asian research groups. It is notable that 80% of Western patients with CRSwNP demonstrate tissue eosinophilia compared with less than 35% of Korean patients.[29] To examine the possible differences in Western and Eastern nasal polyposis, Zhang and colleagues[30] compared Chinese patients with CRSwNP with their Belgian counterparts. These groups were found to have similar symptoms, CT findings, and endoscopic examination results compared with controls. In addition, both groups expressed upregulation of IL-2 levels and downregulation of FoxP3 T_{reg} cells and TGF-β1 levels, confirming previous findings.[22,30] Differences were, however, noted with regard to inflammatory cells and T-cell dominance. The Belgian contingent confirmed previous findings of T_H2-dominant eosinophilic inflammation. In comparison, the Chinese group displayed a neutrophilic pattern with T_H1/T_H17 T-cell upregulation.

The role of T_H17 in immunology has only recently been elucidated. Over the past 5 years, the basic CD4 differentiation pathway into T_H1 and T_H2 cells has been challenged by the discovery of T_H17 as an alternative end point. The discovery of T_H17 and its associated cytokines IL-23 and IL-17 was prompted by the inability of T_H1/T_H2 subtypes to explain murine autoimmune models.[31] Instead of IL-4 (T_H2) or IL-12 (T_H1), induction of T_H17 differentiation is promoted by IL-1 and IL-6.[31] Such a profile was confirmed by Zhang and colleagues[30] when patients with noneosinophilia displayed an upregulation in IL-1, IL-6, IL-17, and T_H17 levels. This production eventually results in the production of proinflammatory mediators, fibroblasts, and tissue change.[20]

STAPHYLOCOCCUS AUREUS ENTEROTOXIN

S aureus enterotoxin (SAE) has been suggested as a possible instigating and/or modifying factor in nasal polyposis. As in other superantigen reactions, SAE acts to nonspecifically activate T cells by binding the major histocompatibility II complex.[32] The unregulated upregulation results in an increase of T_H2-biased proinflammatory cytokine levels.[33] This outcome is enhanced by *S aureus* colonization, with 60% of patients with CRSwNP demonstrating colonization compared with 33% in controls.[34] The effect of this colonization as shown by SAE IgE is not universal among patients with CRSwNP. Instead, asthmatic patients are more likely to have colonization of *S aureus* and detectable IgE levels, therefore resulting in elevated IL-5, eotaxin, and ECP levels.[4,34] Despite their different clinical and inflammatory phenotypes, Chinese patients with asthma were also more likely to have detectable SAE levels.[35] Although these results are interesting, further work is needed to correlate SAE effects with clinical symptoms and course. Further research should focus on defining the effect that SAE plays, particularly in asthmatic eosinophilic CRSwNP.

ASPIRIN-EXACERBATED RESPIRATORY DISEASE

A small portion of patients with NPs and CRS are classified as having AERD, also known as Samter triad or aspirin triad. These patients present with the classic Samter triad with aspirin sensitivity, polyposis, and asthma. An additional near-universal feature of these patients is hyperplastic eosinophilic sinusitis.[36] The increased tissue eosinophilia, infiltrating mast cells producing histamine, and increased levels of cysteinyl leukotrienes secondary to overexpression of leukotriene C_4 synthase contribute to systemic inflammation of this disease.[37] Also for AERD, symptoms are worsened by the introduction of cyclooxygenase (COX) 2 inhibitors with a metabolic shift of arachidonic acid toward lipoxygenase pathways with resultant increased leukotriene products.[36] Nasal mucosa of these patients has also been found to have diminished COX-1 and COX-2 productions. Therefore, even before insult, these patients produce less of the protective prostaglandin E_2 (PGE_2).[38] Validation of this baseline deficiency has been addressed by Sestini and colleagues.[39] These researchers were able to prevent aspirin-induced bronchospasm by using inhaled PGE_2. Their findings were confirmed objectively by forced expiratory volume in the first second of expiration (FEV_1) and urinary leukotriene E_4 level measures. Also, when compared with other patients with severe nasal polyposis and asthma, the incidence of allergy in these patients with AERD are likely to be lower. Therefore, the examination of allergy is especially important in the evaluation and diagnosis of patients with severe nasal polyposis and adult-onset asthma.

CYSTIC FIBROSIS

CF is a rare autosomal recessive genetic disorder affecting approximately 1 in every 2500 people. All patients with CF develop chronic sinusitis, but of these patients, 7% to 48% demonstrate NPs (CF-NP).[40] CF-NP stands out from other NP groups by way of its obvious phenotype and diagnosis. Defects of ciliary clearance in these patients create an environment in which bacterial colonization, particularly with *Pseudomonas aeruginosa*, is a virtual constant.[41] The resultant neutrophilic response to these pathogens may explain the dominance of IL-8 and MPO in the inflammatory cascade.[3] The role of bacterial pathogens is further supported by the role of toll-like receptors (TLRs) and lack of clear benefit of corticosteroids in CF-NP.[40,42]

IL-8 and MPO levels have been previously shown to be increased in patients with CF-NP compared with both those with CRS and bronchitis.[3,43] Claeys and colleagues[42] evaluated the differentiation of CF-NP from non–CF-NP by comparison of inflammatory cytokines, innate antimicrobial peptides, and innate pattern recognition receptors (PRRs). IL-8 and MPO were confirmed to dominate CF-NP compared with ECP, eotaxin, and IgE in non–CF-NP. The innate antimicrobial peptide human defensin β2 (HBD2) and PRR TLR-2 levels were found to be significantly higher in CF-NP as well. These findings suggest an inflammatory pathway instigated by bacterial exposure. In such a system, TLRs recognize pathogen-associated molecular patterns with resultant production of antimicrobial peptides and stimulation of an inflammatory cascade.[44,45] A system of excessive inflammatory response is supported by the findings that children with CF display disproportionate neutrophil and IL-8 responses to bacteria compared with controls.[46] More research is required to assess the feasibility that in CF, bacterial colonization may upregulate TLR-2, HBD2, and subsequently IL-8 levels, leading to inflammation and polyp formation.

TREATMENT

Medical Therapy

Corticosteroids

For decades, corticosteroids have been the mainstay of therapy for nasal polyposis. The mechanism of action involves the downregulating of inflammatory protein-encoding genes by the activation of intracellular glucocorticoid receptors.[47,48] Nasal topical steroids have been shown to both decrease polyp size and improve nasal symptoms.[47] The use of these steroids postoperatively has also proved to reduce recurrence and the need for systemic therapy.[49] The undeniable benefits of nasal steroids have made them the first line of therapy in nasal polyposis. The benefit of oral steroids, however, remains less definitive with little randomized data available and the risk of systemic effect from oral steroids. Nevertheless, their use remains near universal as a means to abate NP symptoms. Regardless of documented effect, the use of oral steroids will continue to be limited by their extensive and well-documented long-term side effects.

Antileukotrienes

Cysteinyl leukotriene receptor (LTR) antagonists, such as montelukast, function by blocking LTR sites. Multiple studies have shown clinical improvement in those with CRSwNP, demonstrating reduction in polyps, decreased steroid use, and improved overall symptoms.[50–52] However, there remains a dearth of well-designed randomized studies at this time. In patients with excessively high leukotriene levels, such as those with AERD, simply blocking LTRs may be insufficient to meaningfully affect symptoms. To increase effectiveness, the leukotriene pathway must be interrupted during production. The 5-lipoxygenase inhibitor zileuton functions in this manner and has been advocated in the treatment of AERD. As with LTR antagonists, further research is needed to quantify the effects and use of this medication.

Immunomodulators

The development of immunomodulators represents a crucial step in the individualized treatment of nasal polyposis. No other treatment modality offers such an obvious link to inflammatory pathogenic cytokines. The role of IL-5 in inflammation has made it a natural target for suppression. Use in CRS has been spurred on by success in patients with eosinophilic asthma, otherwise known as patients with unified airway disease.[53] In these patients, treatment with anti–IL-5 results in improved serum eosinophil levels, asthma control, and FEV_1 levels.[54] Gevaert and colleagues[55] sought to apply this therapy to patients with CRS and follow up the effect by measuring serum and nasal ECP levels. Although no statistically significant differences were noted, it was shown that responders were more likely to have higher pretreatment IL-5 levels. The treatment of all patients with anti–IL-5 would be misguided because only those with T_H2-dominant eosinophilic disease are likely to benefit. Although the cost of immunomodulators likely limits their overall use, their effect on the landscape of CRS therapy may be the greatest as a model of individualized/tailored therapy.

The future for the medical management of CRS is defined by research that accounts for and adjusts therapy with respect to pathogenesis. In a recent example of such a model, Huvenne and colleagues[56] compared in a randomized fashion doxycycline and steroid therapy in patients with NP. The results of this study are perhaps less important than the fact that the effect of each therapy was measured with respect to inflammatory cytokines. Such a strategy in combination with further classification of CRS subtypes makes targeted therapy a reality.

Surgical Therapy

CRSwNP

Endoscopic sinus surgery (ESS) has long been implemented with success in the treatment of CRS. Overall success rates have been reported at 85%, with failure rates ranging from 2% to 24%.[57] However, success has been difficult to achieve in the setting of nasal polyposis because surgical management does not rid the individual of the inflammatory sinonasal mucosa. In 65 patients with NP, Dufour and colleagues[57] examined symptom improvement with respect to nasal obstruction and anosmia. Less than 50% of patients demonstrated major improvement of nasal obstruction, with even less reporting improvement in olfaction. This failure of subjective improvement can frustrate both the patient and surgeon. Although the polyp burden can be reduced by surgical resection of the inflammatory mediators and cells, the correlation with symptoms may be lacking. In certain patient subsets, the benefit of surgery may be more or less profound. In particular, patients with asthma or unified airway have experienced significant subjective improvements after ESS,[58,59] which is not surprising because of the direct decrease of inflammatory load of these patients. Improvements of objective measures, however, have been inconsistent.[58,59] In contrast, patients with AERD seem to be particularly difficult to treat with surgery. In a study of olfaction status after ESS, AERD was found to be an independent risk factor for poor recovery.[60] It is important to remember that surgical management or resection of NPs does not prevent the recurrence of NPs, especially in individuals with inherent inflammatory mucosa. However, surgical management can be used to decrease the amount of inflammation so that the medical treatment becomes more effective and thus prevents the recurrence of NPs.

Cystic Fibrosis

In the setting of CF, ESS has been shown to be safe with a major complication rate within the range of normal.[61] Given the precarious pulmonary status of patients with CF, it is important also to note that these patients experienced no increased anesthesia risk.[61] Although ESS can safely be performed in patients with CF, the presence of NPs should not alone be considered a reason for surgery[62] because the recurrence of the sinus disease is likely to return despite surgical management. It is important to remember that less than 10% of patients with CF report sinonasal symptoms.[63] Given that surgical intervention has had mixed results demonstrating improvement in pulmonary function, especially in the long term, symptom status should be used to determine need for functional endoscopic sinus surgery.[64] In general, patients with CF are considered good surgical candidates when imaging confirms that disease burden and symptoms are persistent.[40] In this setting, surgical intervention can improve upper respiratory status, whereas the lower respiratory status remains in question.

SUMMARY POINTS: NASAL POLYPS

1. CRS is the most common cause for NPs, but not all NPs are created equally.
2. Patients with asthma and CRS represent clinical examples of the unified airway. As such, these patients benefit from treatment aimed at control of T_H2-driven eosinophilic inflammation.
3. NPs are not a uniquely T_H2-driven process. Recent research has demonstrated a clear pathogenic role for T_H1- and T_H17-driven processes.
4. Future research in understanding the development of NPs will dictate the proper medical management of NPs.

REFERENCES

1. Larsen K, Tos M. The estimated incidence of symptomatic nasal polyps. Acta Otolaryngol 2002;122(2):179–82.
2. Videler WJ, Van Drunen CM, Van Der Meulen FW, et al. Radical surgery: effect on quality of life and pain in chronic rhinosinusitis. Otolaryngol Head Neck Surg 2007;136:261–7.
3. Van Zele T, Claeys S, Gevaert P, et al. Differentiation of chronic sinus diseases by measurement of inflammatory mediators. Allergy 2006;61(11):1280–9.
4. Bachert C, Wagenmann M, Hauser U, et al. IL-5 synthesis is upregulated in human nasal polyp tissue. J Allergy Clin Immunol 1997;99(6 Pt 1):837–42.

5. Johansson L, Akerlund A, Holmberg K, et al. Evaluation of methods for endoscopic staging of nasal polyposis. Acta Otolaryngol 2000;120(1):72–6.
6. Lund VJ, Mackay IS. Staging in rhinosinusitis. Rhinology 1993;31:183–4.
7. Lildholdt T, Rundcrantz H, Bende M, et al. Glucocorticoid treatment for nasal polyps. The use of topical budesonide powder, intramuscular betamethasone, and surgical treatment. Arch Otolaryngol Head Neck Surg 1997;123(6): 595–600.
8. Drutman J, Harnsberger HR, Babbel RW, et al. Sinonasal polyposis: investigation by direct coronal CT. Neuroradiology 1994;36(6):469–72.
9. Kaliner MA, Osguthorpe JD, Fireman P, et al. Sinusitis: bench to bedside. Current findings, future directions. Otolaryngol Head Neck Surg 1997;116:S1–5.
10. Fokkens W, Lund V, Mullol J. European position paper on rhinosinusitis and nasal polyps 2007;20:1–136.
11. Chan Y, Kuhn FA. An update on the classifications, diagnosis, and treatment of rhinosinusitis. Curr Opin Otolaryngol Head Neck Surg 2009;17(3):204–8.
12. Dykewicz MS, Hamilos DL. Rhinitis and sinusitis. J Allergy Clin Immunol 2010; 125(2 Suppl 2):S103–15.
13. Pawanker R. Nasal polyposis: an update. Curr Opin Allergy Immunol 2003;3:1–6.
14. Hellquist HB. Nasal polyps update. Histopathology. Allergy Asthma Proc 1996; 17:237–42.
15. Venge P, Bystrom J, Carlson M, et al. Eosinophil cationic protein (ECP): molecular and biological properties and the use of ECP as a marker of eosinophil activation in disease. Clin Exp Allergy 1999;29:1172–86.
16. Sanderson CJ. Interleukin-5, eosinophils and disease. Blood 1992;19:3101–9.
17. Nakajima H, Takatsu K. Role of cytokines in allergic airway inflammation. Int Arch Allergy Immunol 2007;142(4):265–73.
18. Ochiai K, Kagami M, Matsumura R, et al. IL-5 but not interferon-gamma (IFN-gamma) inhibits eosinophil apoptosis by up-regulation of bcl-2 expression. Clin Exp Immunol 1997;107(1):198–204.
19. Otto BA, Wenzel SE. The role of cytokines in chronic rhinosinusitis with nasal polyps. Curr Opin Otolaryngol Head Neck Surg 2008;16(3):270–4.
20. Chen YS, Arab SF, Westhofen M, et al. Expression of interleukin-5, interleukin-8, and interleukin-10 mRNA in the osteomeatal complex in nasal polyposis. Am J Rhinol 2005;19(2):117–23.
21. Sakaguchi S, Miyara M, Costantino CM, et al. FOXP3+ regulatory T cells in the human immune system. Nat Rev Immunol 2010;10(7):490–500.
22. Van Bruaene N, Pérez-Novo CA, Basinski TM, et al. T-cell regulation in chronic paranasal sinus disease. J Allergy Clin Immunol 2008;121(6):1435–41, 1441.e1–3.
23. Wang QP. Myofibroblasts accumulation induced by transforming growth factor-beta is involved in pathogenesis of nasal polyps. Laryngoscope 1997;107: 926–31.
24. Early SB, Hise K, Han JK, et al. Hypoxic induction stimulates inflammatory and fibrotic response from nasal-polyp derived fibroblasts. Laryngoscope 2007; 117(3):511–5.
25. Bradley DT, Kountakis SE. Role of interleukins and transforming growth factor-beta in chronic rhinosinusitis and nasal polyposis. Laryngoscope 2005;115(4): 684–6.
26. Little SC, Early SB, Woodard CR, et al. Dual action of TGF-beta1 on nasal-polyp derived fibroblasts. Laryngoscope 2008;118(2):320–4.
27. Early SB, Han JK, Borish L, et al. Histologic examination reveals distinct disease subsets of chronic sinusitis. J Allergy Clin Immunol 2007;119(1):S243.

28. Payne S, Han JK, Borish L, et al. Microarray analysis of distinct gene transcription profiles in non-eosinophilic chronic sinusitis with polyps. Am J Rhinol 2008;22(6): 568–81.
29. Kim JW, Hong SL, Kim YK, et al. Histological and immunological features of non-eosinophilic nasal polyps. Otolaryngol Head Neck Surg 2007;137(6): 925–30.
30. Zhang N, Van Zele T, Perez-Novo C, et al. Different types of T-effector cells orchestrate mucosal inflammation in chronic sinus disease. J Allergy Clin Immunol 2008; 122(5):961–8.
31. Chen Z, O'Shea JJ. Th17 cells: a new fate for differentiating helper T cells. Immunol Res 2008;41(2):87–102.
32. Balaban N, Rasooly A. Staphylococcal enterotoxins. Int J Food Microbiol 2000; 61:1–103.
33. Patou J, Van Zel T, Fevaert P, et al. Staphylococcus aureus enterotoxin B, protein A, and lipoteichoic acid stimulations in nasal polyps. J Allergy Clin Immunol 2008; 121(1):110–5.
34. Van Zele T, Gevaert P, Watelet JB, et al. Staphylococcus aureus colonization and IgE antibody formation to enterotoxins is increased in nasal polyposis. J Allergy Clin Immunol 2004;114(4):981–3.
35. Bachert C, Zhang N, Holtappels G, et al. Presence of IL-5 protein and IgE antibodies to staphylococcal enterotoxins in nasal polyps is associated with comorbid asthma. J Allergy Clin Immunol 2010;126(5):962–8, e1–6.
36. Stevenson DD. Aspirin sensitivity and desensitization for asthma and sinusitis. Curr Allergy Asthma Rep 2009;9(2):155–63.
37. de Alarcon A, Caughey R, Steinke JW, et al. Overexpression of leukotriene c4 synthase and plasminogen activator inhibitor 1 gene promoter polymorphisms in sinusitis. Am J Rhinol 2006;16(10):545–9.
38. Mullol J, Fernàndez-Morata JC, Roca-Ferrer J, et al. Cyclooxygenase 1 and cyclooxygenase 2 expression is abnormally regulated in human nasal polyps. J Allergy Clin Immunol 2002;109(5):824–30.
39. Sestini P, Armetti L, Gambaro G, et al. Inhaled PGE2 prevents aspirin-induced bronchoconstriction and urinary LTE4 excretion in aspirin-sensitive asthma. Am J Respir Crit Care Med 1996;153(2):572–5.
40. Robertson JM, Friedman EM, Rubin BK. Nasal and sinus disease in cystic fibrosis. Paediatr Respir Rev 2008;9(3):213–9.
41. Laurans M, Arion A, Fines-Guyon M, et al. Pseudomonas aeruginosa and cystic fibrosis: first colonization to chronic infection. Arch Pediatr 2006;13(Suppl 1): S22–9 [in French].
42. Claeys S, Van Hoecke H, Holtappels G, et al. Nasal polyps in patients with and without cystic fibrosis: a differentiation by innate markers and inflammatory mediators. Clin Exp Allergy 2005;35(4):467–72.
43. Kim JS, Hackley GH, Okamoto K. Sputum processing for evaluation of inflammatory mediators. Pediatr Pulmonol 2001;32:152–8.
44. Raoust E, Balloy V, Garcia-Verdugo I, et al. Pseudomonas aeruginosa LPS or flagellin are sufficient to activate TLR-dependent signaling in murine alveolar macrophages and airway epithelial cells. PLoS One 2009;4(10):e7259.
45. Laube DM, Yim S, Ryan LK, et al. Antimicrobial peptides in the airway. Curr Top Microbiol Immunol 2006;306:153–82.
46. Muhlebach MS, Stewart PW, Leigh MW, et al. Quantification of inflammatory responses to bacteria in young cystic fibrosis and control patients. Am J Respir Crit Care Med 1999;160(1):186–91.

47. Mullol J, Obando A, Pujols L, et al. Corticosteroid treatment in chronic rhinosinusitis: the possibilities and the limits. Immunol Allergy Clin North Am 2009;29(4): 657–68.
48. Pujols L, Mullol J, Torrego A, et al. Glucocorticoid receptors in human airways. Allergy 2004;59(10):1042–52.
49. Rowe-Jones JM, Medcalf M, Durham SR, et al. Functional endoscopic sinus surgery: 5 year follow up and results of a prospective, randomised, stratified, double-blind, placebo controlled study of postoperative fluticasone propionate aqueous nasal spray. Rhinology 2005;43(1):2–10.
50. Parnes SM. The role of leukotriene inhibitors in patients with paranasal sinus disease. Curr Opin Otolaryngol Head Neck Surg 2003;11:184–91.
51. Ragab S, Parikh A, Darby YC, et al. An open audit of montelukast, a leukotriene receptor antagonist, in nasal polyposis associated with asthma. Clin Exp Allergy 2001;31(9):1385–91.
52. Ulualp SO, Sterman BM, Toohill RJ. Antileukotriene therapy for the relief of sinus symptoms in aspirin triad disease. Ear Nose Throat J 1999;78(8):604–6, 608, 613, passim.
53. Krouse JH, Brown RW, Fineman SJ, et al. Executive summary: asthma and the unified airway. Otolaryngol Head Neck Surg 2007;136(Suppl 5):669–706.
54. Parameswaran N, Pizzichini M, Kjarsgaard M, et al. Mepolizumab for prednisone-dependent asthma with sputum eosinophilia. N Engl J Med 2009;360(10): 985–93.
55. Gevaert P, Lang-Loidolt D, Lackner A, et al. Nasal IL-5 levels determine the response to anti-IL-5 treatment in patients with nasal polyps. J Allergy Clin Immunol 2006;118:1133–41.
56. Huvenne W, van Bruaene N, Zhang N, et al. Chronic rhinosinusitis with and without nasal polyps: what is the difference? Curr Allergy Asthma Rep 2009; 9(3):213–20.
57. Dufour X, Bedier A, Ferrie JC, et al. Diffuse nasal polyposis and endonasal endoscopic surgery: long-term results, a 65-case study. Laryngoscope 2004;114(11): 1982–7.
58. Proimos E, Papadakis CE, Chimona TS, et al. The effect of functional endoscopic sinus surgery on patients with asthma and CRS with nasal polyps. Rhinology 2010;48(3):331–8.
59. Katotomichelakis M, Riga M, Davris S, et al. Allergic rhinitis and aspirin-exacerbated respiratory disease as predictors of the olfactory outcome after endoscopic sinus surgery. Am J Rhinol Allergy 2009;23(3):348–53.
60. Albritton FD, Kingdom TT. Endoscopic sinus surgery in patients with cystic fibrosis: an analysis of complications. Am J Rhinol 2000;14(6):379–85.
61. Schulte DL, Kasperbauer JL. Safety of paranasal sinus surgery in patients with cystic fibrosis. Laryngoscope 1998;108(12):1813–5.
62. Becker SS, Han JK, Gross CW. Risk factors for recurrent sinus surgery in cystic fibrosis: review of a decade of experience. Am J Rhinol 2007;21(4):478–82.
63. King VV. Upper respiratory disease, sinusitis, and polyposis. Clin Rev Allergy 1991;9:143–57.
64. Jarrett W, Militsakh O, Anstad M, et al. Endoscopic sinus surgery in cystic fibrosis: effects on pulmonary function and ideal body weight. Ear Nose Throat J 2004;83: 118–21.

Allergic Fungal Rhinosinusitis

Matthew W. Ryan, MD

KEYWORDS

- Allergic mucin • Eosinophilic mucin • Nasal polyps
- Eosinophilic mucin rhinosinusitis • Allergic fungal sinusitis
- Immunotherapy

Key Points: Allergic Fungal Rhinosinusitis

- AFRS is a distinct form of chronic polypoid rhinosinusitis characterized by accumulation of eosinophilic mucin with fungal hyphae in the sinuses, type 1 hypersensitivity to fungi, and a propensity for mucocele formation and bone erosion
- Endoscopic sinus surgery is required for most cases and is an important component of overall management
- The best substantiated medical management options are systemic and topical corticosteroids
- Leukotriene modifiers, antibiotics, topical and systemic antifungal agents are rational medical treatment options with minimal evidence to support their use
- Allergen specific immunotherapy may be considered as an additional treatment option to address concomitant allergic disease in patients with AFRS

Does allergen-specific immunotherapy have a beneficial effect in the treatment of allergic fungal rhinosinusitis (AFRS)?

IMPLICATIONS FOR CLINICAL OUTCOMES

Type 1 hypersensitivity is believed to be one pathophysiologic component of the inflammation in AFRS. Multiple randomized, placebo-controlled trials have demonstrated the efficacy of allergen-specific immunotherapy to reduce symptoms and medication requirements in allergic rhinitis and asthma. However, there is a lack of randomized, controlled trials for the treatment of AFRS with immunotherapy. The peer reviewed literature contains low-level evidence that suggests immunotherapy may reduce inflammation and reduce steroid requirements in AFRS patients. This

Disclosures: The author is on the speaker's bureau for Merck, Inc.

Department of Otolaryngology, The University of Texas Southwestern Medical Center, 5323 Harry Hines Boulevard, Dallas, TX 75390-9035, USA
E-mail address: Matthew.Ryan@utsouthwestern.edu

Otolaryngol Clin N Am 44 (2011) 697–710
doi:10.1016/j.otc.2011.03.015
oto.theclinics.com

evidence derives from case reports, small cohort studies without comparator groups, and a single cohort study with an external control group. Immunotherapy should be considered for AFRS patients with significant allergic symptomatology, steroid dependence, or multiple polyp recurrences.

ALLERGIC FUNGAL RHINOSINUSITIS

AFRS is a well recognized label for a form of polypoid chronic rhinosinusitis (CRS) that is characterized by type 1 hypersensitivity, the accumulation of dense inspissated "eosinophilic mucin," and trapped fungi within the sinuses. AFRS was described as a distinct pathologic entity that resembled allergic bronchopulmonary aspergillosis (ABPA) with thick, dark, inspissated mucus filling the paranasal sinuses similar, grossly and microscopically, to that seen in the bronchial passages.[1–3] The nature of this condition, its diagnosis and appropriate treatment continue to generate controversy despite 30 years of investigation.

The previously accepted hallmark for the diagnosis of AFRS was the characteristic sinus contents first responsible for the description of the disease. Grossly, this "allergic mucin" or eosinophilic mucin is thick, tenacious, and darkly colored. Viewed histologically, this mucus consists of onion-skin laminations of necrotic and degranulating eosinophils in a background of mucin, occasional small hexagonal crystals of lysophospholipase (Charcot-Leyden crystals), as well as fungal hyphae. *Aspergillus* and the dematiaceous fungi are most commonly found in AFRS mucus.[4–6] Although once called "allergic" *Aspergillus* sinusitis, the preferred terminology for this condition is now "allergic fungal rhinosinusitis" or AFRS. However, investigators have noted that in some cases, the eosinophilic mucin evacuated from the sinuses does not have identifiable fungal elements.[6,7] Additionally, Ferguson[8] described an AFRS-like condition with slightly different clinical features and proposed the term "eosinophilic mucin rhinosinusitis" (EMRS) to describe cases in which fungus was not identified histologically. Some patients with clinical features of AFRS may have demonstrable fungus within their eosinophilic mucin, yet do not have allergy.[9] Others have eosinophilic mucin yet no allergy and no evidence of fungi within the mucin. The report of Ponikau and colleagues[10] suggesting that most, if not all, CRS was a hypersensitivity response to fungi and that fungi could be universally cultured from nasal secretions also further clouded the distinction between AFRS and AFRS-like CRS. AFRS is probably overdiagnosed because of clinical similarity to other forms of "eosinophilic mucin chronic rhinosinusitis" (EMCRS). The overlapping clinicopathologic features of chronic polypoid rhinosinusitis with eosinophilic mucin have led to questions about the underlying pathophysiology of AFRS. If patients with the clinical features of AFRS do not have allergy and/or do not have fungus in their eosinophilic mucin, how should these patients be classified? Is fungus the extrinsic trigger for inflammation? Is allergy an important component of the pathogenesis of AFRS? Currently it is safe to state that the clinicopathologic distinction of AFRS from other forms of EMRS requires further investigation. Questions regarding the proper diagnosis, classification, and pathogenesis of AFRS have yet to be resolved and have important implications for treatment.

PATHOPHYSIOLOGY

A hypersensitivity to fungus is believed to underlie the pathogenesis of AFRS, but the nature of this hypersensitivity is still debated. The dominant theory to explain the pathogenesis of AFRS was adopted from the model of ABPA pathogenesis[11]: in short, a combination of Gell and Coombs type 1 and type 3 hypersensitivity to fungal allergens causes sinonasal inflammation.[12] This inflammation leads to polyp formation and mucus accumulation in the sinuses, thus explaining the clinical findings in the disease. This paradigm was reinforced by the clinical association of AFRS with allergy and the detection of elevated serum levels of total and fungal antigen-specific IgE and IgG in AFRS patients. Work by Manning and Holman[13] and Stewart and Hunsaker[14] lent early support to the theory that connected AFRS pathogenesis to ABPA. Manning and Holman analyzed serum from patients with culture-confirmed AFRS (*Bipolaris*) and nonsinusitis controls and found that 82% of AFRS cases had *Bipolaris*-specific IgE by radioallergosorbent test inhibition and 94% had *Bipolaris*-specific IgG by ELISA inhibition. Stewart and Hunsaker analyzed fungal-specific serum IgE and IgG levels in nonatopic controls, allergic rhinitis patients, non-AFRS polyp patients, AFRS-like patients, and AFRS patients. Patients in the AFRS and AFRS-like group had elevated serum levels of IgE and IgG to multiple fungi. Compared with those patients with only nasal polyps, the AFRS and AFRS-like groups had significantly elevated levels of fungus-specific IgG and IgE.[14] More recent studies have also examined humoral immune responses in patients with EMCRS including AFRS cases.[15] Pant and colleagues[15] found that serum fungal-specific IgG was increased in these patients regardless of the presence of allergy or fungal elements in their eosinophilic mucin. Patients with AFRS had increases in fungal-specific IgE and total IgE but these were no different from a control group with allergic rhinitis. Pant and colleagues found a poor correlation between fungal species present in the eosinophilic mucin of AFRS patients and the specific fungal allergy (42%). However, elevated fungal-specific IgG3 appeared to be a distinguishing serologic feature that separated EMCRS and AFRS patients from those with fungal allergic rhinitis and other forms of CRS. Serum IgE levels *could* be used to distinguish EMCRS from AFRS. Finally, Luong and colleagues[16] found that peripheral blood mononuclear cells from AFRS patients are stimulated by fungal antigens to secrete TH2-type cytokines. These more recent studies continue to support a role for humoral immune factors in AFRS and EMCRS, but do not resolve the controversy about AFRS pathogenesis.

Type 1 hypersensitivity and/or dysregulation of IgE metabolism is evident locally within AFRS tissue. Most patients with AFRS have detectable fungal specific IgE in their eosinophilic mucin, whereas most patients with other forms of EMCRS do not.[17] Compared with non-AFRS sinus tissue (from nonallergic subjects) there is a local mucosal elevation in total and specific IgE to fungal and nonfungal antigens.[18] These findings again suggest a role for IgE and type 1 hypersensitivity in the pathophysiology of the disease.

However, some argue that, because EMCRS and AFRS are so similar, allergy to fungus cannot be the primary pathophysiologic force driving the inflammation in AFRS.[19] Studies comparing AFRS to other forms of EMCRS have found similar polyp histopathology, inflammatory cell infiltrate, tissue eosinophilia, and fungal-specific PBMC proliferation.[20] However, circumstantial evidence suggests that both allergic and nonallergic fungal hypersensitivity may be important components of the underlying pathophysiology of both AFRS and EMCRS.

Immunologic mechanisms alone may not account for the development of the clinical features of AFRS. It has been suggested that AFRS develops in susceptible patients with a convergence of local anatomic as well as environmental factors.[11] This may explain the propensity of AFRS to cause unilateral disease. The working theory has been that fungi entering the nose and sinuses and triggers an inflammatory response. This inflammation induces polyp formation and the accumulation of allergic mucin. Trapped fungi continue to stimulate the immune system in a vicious cycle. Over time, massive polyposis develops and mucoceles distort the sinonasal anatomy.

This model is likely an oversimplification that does not take into account many possible pathophysiologic mechanisms that are poorly understood and likely to be complex.[21]

In summary, although AFRS and EMCRS are phenotypically quite similar, a clinically important distinguishing feature of AFRS is type 1 hypersensitivity. Therefore, type 1 hypersensitivity to fungal antigens, as assessed by specific allergy tests, helps to distinguish AFRS from other forms of EMCRS and has implications for treatment.

EPIDEMIOLOGY AND MICROBIOLOGY

Allergic fungal sinusitis may be the most common form of fungal sinusitis. Allergic fungal sinusitis accounts for about 7% to 12% of cases of CRS taken to surgery in the United States, though this may be an overestimation.[22,23] Climactic factors that determine fungal growth and exposures may be responsible for the varied incidence in certain regions. In the United States, the highest incidence is in the south and along the Mississippi basin.[24] In a large pathology series of CRS cases from India, AFRS accounted for 24% of cases.[25] So clearly, the disease has a worldwide distribution, though there may be differences in the microbiology of the disease across continents.

AFRS develops primarily in young adults and adolescents.[11] Older patients with the clinical features of AFRS may be more likely have some other EMCRS syndrome. Besides being younger than other CRS patients, AFRS patients may be more likely to come from disadvantaged groups with lower socioeconomic status.[26] Affected patients are immunocompetent and have a history of atopy.[12,22] By definition, AFRS patients have allergy that should be evident by skin or in vitro testing, but only about two-thirds of patients give a history of allergic rhinitis.[13]

Aspergillus was initially believed to be the causative organism in AFRS, but further experience with cases in the United States showed that the dematiaceous fungi were most commonly found in AFRS mucus,[22,27] The terminology for this condition subsequently changed from "allergic *Aspergillus* sinusitis" to "allergic fungal sinusitis." In series of AFRS and nonallergic eosinophilic fungal sinusitis from other parts of the world, *Aspergillus* is still found to be a common isolate.[25,28–30] The specific fungal organism has not been shown to be an important or predictive clinical characteristic, but the identification of fungus in eosinophilic mucin either via histopathology or culture is still considered to be important to make the diagnosis of AFRS.

CLINICAL PRESENTATION

Symptoms of AFRS are similar to other forms of polypoid CRS. Patients with AFRS usually present with rhinosinusitis symptoms lasting months or years and they may not seek medical attention until complete nasal obstruction, headaches, visual disturbances, or facial distortion develop. Symptoms are frequently unilateral. Patients may report dark, thick nasal mucus drainage. A history of previous allergic rhinitis symptoms is common, but is not always present.

The physical examination findings in AFRS often reflect the advanced nature of disease at presentation. Proptosis or telecanthus are frequently seen at presentation, especially in younger patients.[11,28,31,32] Intranasal examination will reveal polyps that are unilateral or bilateral, and it is common for the bulk of polyp disease to be asymmetric. On nasal endoscopy, inspissated yellowish or brown mucus may be visualized among the polyps.

Testing is important to establish evidence of atopy, as demonstration of type 1 hypersensitivity is required for diagnosis. This may be accomplished with skin testing or in vitro testing for antigen-specific IgE. In addition to fungal antigens, patients should be tested against a region-specific panel of seasonal and perennial allergens. Possible laboratory abnormalities in AFRS patients include peripheral eosinophilia and dramatically elevated total IgE levels. Skin testing or in vitro IgE testing will usually demonstrate IgE-mediated hypersensitivity to multiple fungal and nonfungal antigens.[11]

DIAGNOSTIC CRITERIA

The diagnosis of AFRS requires a combination of clinical, radiographic, microbiologic, and histopathologic information. Therefore, the diagnosis of AFRS cannot be made reliably until after surgical intervention. There is still no universally recognized set of diagnostic criteria for AFRS.

A variety of diagnostic criteria for AFRS have been proposed by various investigators and these criteria have been further refined by a recent consensus conference on definitions of rhinosinusitis.[33] The classic and still widely accepted diagnostic criteria for AFRS were described by Bent and Kuhn,[34] who proposed the following: type 1 hypersensitivity, nasal polyposis, characteristic CT scan findings, eosinophilic mucus without fungal invasion into sinus tissue, and a positive fungal stain of sinus contents removed at surgery. In the absence of better defined immunologic parameters to distinguish AFRS from other forms of EMCRS, the Bent and Kuhn criteria are still important.

An important criterion is the presence of eosinophilic mucin. Grossly, eosinophilic mucin is thick, tenacious, and darkly colored; it may appear similar to a fungus ball but microscopically the two are quite different. Microscopically, eosinophilic mucin consists of onion-skin laminations of necrotic and degranulating eosinophils in a background of mucin with occasional Charcot-Leyden crystals. Fungal hyphae are present but scarce, and special fungal stains may be needed for identification. Fungal hyphae do not invade tissue: the presence of fungal tissue invasion has been considered incompatible with a diagnosis if AFRS. However, there are reports of cases with clinicopathologic features of both AFRS and chronic invasive fungal sinusitis.[25] Such cases highlight the difficulty of creating rigid diagnostic categories for fungal sinusitis, and suggest that there is a spectrum of overlapping disease features in fungal sinusitis.[25,35] In AFRS, adjacent mucosa and polyps demonstrate a prominent eosinophilic inflammatory infiltrate. Many patients with polypoid CRS and eosinophilic mucin lack other important clinical characteristics of AFRS: demonstrable fungi and fungal allergy. These patients should not be classified as having AFRS.

As discussed above, there is significant phenotypic similarity between AFRS and EMCRS. Saravanan and colleagues[29] found considerable clinical overlap in AFRS and EMCRS groups, but AFRS subjects were more likely to have bony erosion, heterogeneous opacity, and sinus expansion on CT scan. These findings are similar to those of Dhiwakar and colleagues[36] who point out that the combination of nasal polyps, CT scan hyperattenuation, and elevated titers of anti-*Aspergillus* IgE have high predictive value for AFRS, though considered in isolation they are not specific. Clearly, considerable overlap exists between AFRS, EMCRS, and CRS from other causes, and the Bent and Kuhn[34] criteria are still helpful to distinguish between these.

RADIOLOGIC FEATURES

AFRS has characteristic features on CT scan or MRI. The characteristic imaging findings of AFRS cases are still considered extremely important for diagnosis. CT scan is the initial study of choice for evaluating these patients. CT scan imaging shows multiple opacified sinuses with central hyperattenuation, sinus mucocele formation, and erosion of the lamina papyracea or skull base with a pushing border (**Fig. 1**). AFRS causes more

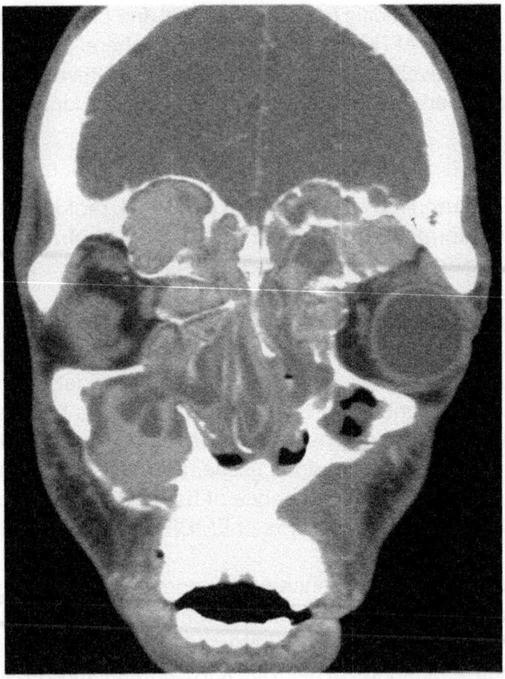

Fig. 1. Coronal contrasted CT scan image with soft tissue windowing from a patient with AFRS. There is extensive skull base distortion and orbital erosion. Low density within the sinuses represents nasal polyps; high density material is eosinophilic mucin.

bone erosion than other forms of CRS. Ghegan and colleagues[37] showed that 56% of AFRS cases presented with radiographic evidence of skull base erosion or intraorbital extension, whereas similar findings were only noticed in 5% of other cases of chronic sinusitis. African-Americans and males may have more significant bone erosion, for unclear reasons.[38] Campbell and colleagues[39] reported that 50% of children with AFRS had proptosis with orbital erosion, consistent with previous reports.[31]

The imaging features of AFRS are clearly distinguishable from other forms of chronic fungal sinusitis. In particular, chronic invasive fungal sinusitis usually involves only a few sinuses and does not cause sinus expansion.[40] Bony erosion with mucocele formation in the setting of polypoid sinusitis clearly is an important feature that should raise suspicions of AFRS.

MRI is not usually clinically necessary in the management of AFRS, but may be appropriate in cases with central nervous system or orbital complications. Nevertheless, AFRS has characteristic MRI findings. On MRI, the sinuses have a central low signal on T1 and T2 imaging that correspond with areas of eosinophilic mucin (**Fig. 2**). Peripheral high-signal intensity corresponds with inflamed mucosa.[41–43] Sometimes the sinus contents have an isointense or hypointense T1 signal (**Fig. 3**). Although the CT scan and MRI findings in AFRS are considered important in diagnosis, definitive diagnosis requires histologic verification and other clinical information.

TREATMENT

The medical and surgical treatment of AFRS improved significantly after widespread recognition that AFRS is not a form of invasive fungal sinusitis. Aggressive surgery

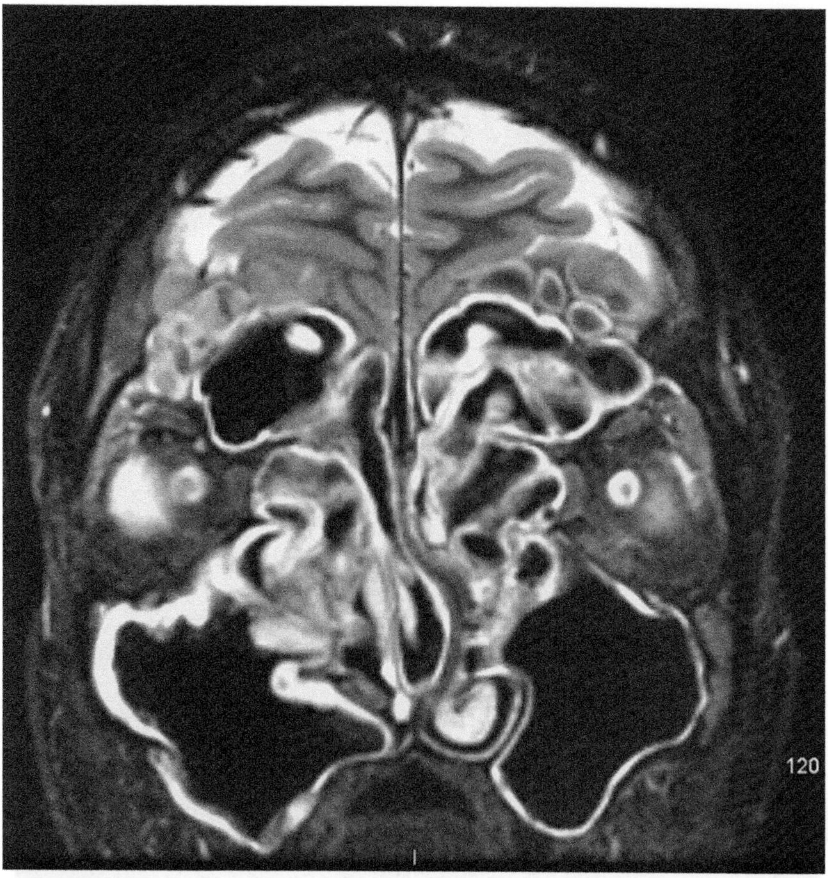

Fig. 2. T2-weighted coronal MRI from the same patient with AFRS in **Fig. 1**. Signal void in the right maxillary sinus and ethmoids corresponds with pockets of eosinophilic mucin. The left maxillary sinus is aerated; the right maxillary sinus appears aerated because of signal void.

and toxic antifungal medications have been replaced by endoscopic surgery and medical therapy directed at suppressing inflammation and reducing the burden of fungal antigen in the nose. AFRS is now considered an inflammatory disease and treatment approaches have been altered accordingly.

Surgery is required in almost all cases of AFRS. External approaches with stripping of sinus mucosa[44,45] have given way to endoscopic tissue preserving approaches that remove obstructing polyps, evacuate sinus contents, and facilitate sinus drainage.[11] External surgeries are not necessary except in rare circumstances, and obliterative procedures should be avoided. The sinonasal expansion from massive polyposis and fungal mucoceles usually facilitates surgery by widening the ethmoid cavity and frontal recess. However, the extensive polyp disease and resulting mucoceles often distort the normal intranasal landmarks and erode the important bony barriers to the orbit or brain, potentially increasing the risk of surgery. Bony lamellae can be significantly distorted such that they are not readily visible along the sinus walls. Image guidance is very helpful for orientation and to facilitate surgery that is more complete. Incomplete surgery, with retention of cells filled with eosinophilic mucin appears to

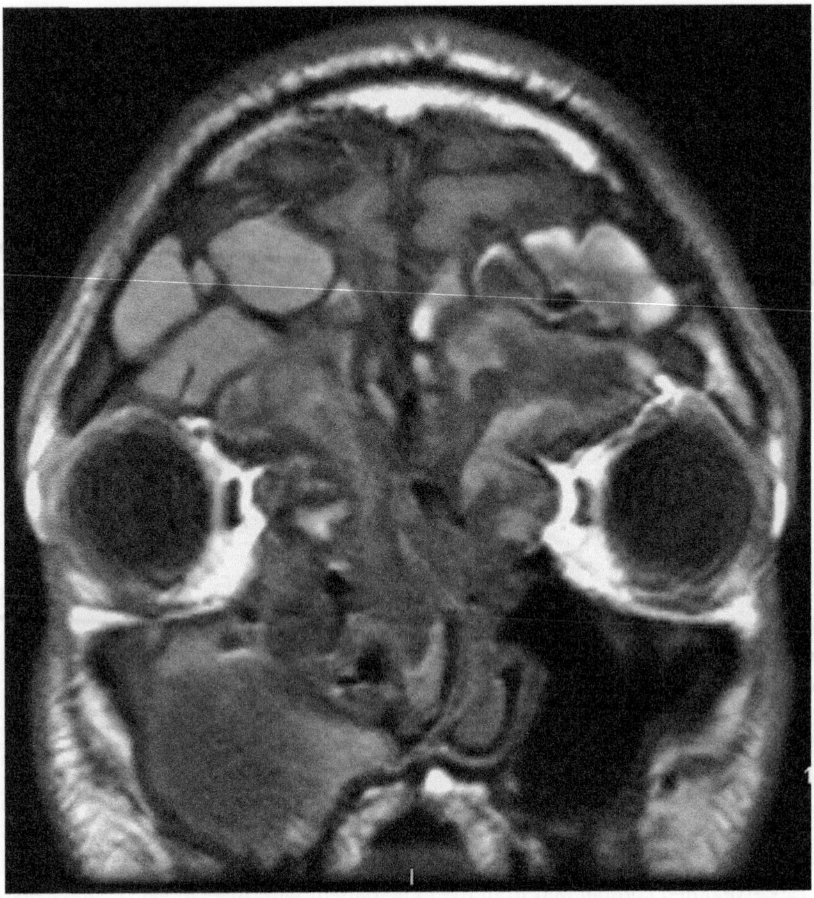

Fig. 3. T1 coronal MR image from the same patient as **Figs. 1** and **2**, in approximately the same plane, shows expanded sinuses with isointense and hyperintense (relative to brain) contents.

be a risk factor for early recurrence[46] and may limit the effectiveness of topical medical treatments. Surgical treatment for recurrences is indicated when intense medical management fails to clear an exacerbation, there is a large polyp burden, or eosinophilic mucin accumulation persists despite medical management. Intense medical therapy can reduce polyp volume, but massive polyposis and outflow tract obstruction may not respond to medical management if there is a significant polyp burden or eosinophilic mucin within the sinuses.

The goals of surgical treatment for recurrence are the same as for primary surgery, and should include the removal of remaining ethmoid lamellae and wide sinusotomies. In patients with multiply recurrent frontal disease, an endoscopic modified-Lothrop procedure may be appropriate. Despite the importance of surgery in managing AFRS, optimal outcomes depend on the combination of surgery with prolonged, comprehensive medical treatment.

Medical treatment for AFRS is essential to obtain long-term symptom control, retard polyp regrowth, and delay or prevent revision surgery. The medical treatment approach for AFRS is similar to other forms of CRS with nasal polyps or EMCRS.

A variety of medical therapies may be employed to accomplish these goals, though high level evidence from appropriately designed clinical trials that focus on AFRS is lacking.

Systemic antiinflammatory agents are usually required in the treatment of AFRS and appear to be the most effective medical therapy. Clinical experience has long shown that systemic steroids are at least transiently effective for the treatment of polypoid rhinosinusitis. This conventional wisdom has now been corroborated with placebo-controlled, randomized trials.[47,48] Among the antiinflammatory agents for AFRS, systemic steroids have the best substantiation in the literature.[49,50] As a general rule, systemic steroids are not able to completely clear polyps or eosinophilic mucin from the sinuses of patients who have not undergone surgery. However, systemic steroids may be useful in a variety of scenarios. A brief course of preoperative systemic corticosteroids will shrink polyps and decrease bleeding during surgery.[11] Systemic corticosteroids in the immediate postoperative period will prevent early recurrence of polypoid inflammation.[51] Prolonged treatment with systemic steroids may be necessary in some severe cases to maintain control of polypoid inflammation. However, long-term treatment with systemic corticosteroids increases the risk of both acute and long-term toxicities; therefore, as a general rule, systemic steroids are best confined to the perioperative period and for use in short bursts to suppress recurrent polyps and address acute exacerbations of disease.

Topical intranasal steroids play an important role in the long-term medical management of AFRS. Topical delivery avoids or minimizes most of the acute and chronic long-term toxicities of corticosteroids, yet is successful in maintaining control of inflammation for prolonged periods. Although not systematically studied in AFRS, topical steroids have been shown to be effective in the treatment of nasal polyp disease.[52] In the treatment of nasal polyp disease there does appear to be a dose-response effect, with higher doses conferring greater benefit.[53] For AFRS, some investigators have recommended that nasal steroid sprays be used at up to three times the usual dosage to boost their efficacy.[49] One emerging topical therapy is the use of budesonide respules, delivered as a drop, atomized spray, or low-volume irrigant. Topical budesonide treatment delivers a larger total dose of steroid compared with conventional steroid nasal sprays. Additionally, the mode of delivery can improve distribution to the sinus mucosa in postsurgical patients.[54] Topical budesonide therapy has not been systematically studied in AFRS. Unfortunately, although topical intranasal steroids appear to be effective, they are often not sufficient to completely eliminate the use of systemic steroids.

The recognized toxicity of repeated courses of systemic steroids has led to a search for nonsteroid treatment alternatives. Leukotriene receptor antagonists or synthesis inhibitors are sometimes employed in polypoid CRS and, although strong evidence for efficacy is lacking, these leukotriene modifiers are attractive because of their safety and possible steroid-sparing effect.[55] Other antiinflammatory agents, such as macrolide antibiotics, may have a role, though data are lacking.[50]

Antifungal treatments are sometimes employed for AFRS with the aim of decreasing the fungal exposure within the sinonasal cavities.[4,49] As with other medical treatment approaches, convincing data of their effectiveness in AFRS are still lacking. Antifungal therapy has not been widely adopted for a variety of reasons. There is little evidence that antifungals decrease reliance on systemic steroids. The fungi in AFRS are not invasive and are often present in scant numbers. Antifungal drugs have many serious toxicities and prolonged treatment may be expensive. Uncontrolled, cohort studies suggest possible efficacy with the use of itraconazole therapy.[56] Interestingly, the efficacy of agents such as itraconazole may not be due to a reduced fungal burden in the nose, but rather due to the antiinflammatory properties of the molecule or its inhibition of prednisone metabolism.

Given the toxicities of many systemic antifungals, it is rational to consider topical delivery of antifungal agents. Even agents such as amphotericin B, which have excellent activity against the usual fungi, may be administered without the significant toxicities associated with systemic administration. Like systemic antifungals, there have been no trials of topical antifungals specifically for AFRS. Randomized, controlled trials have failed to show a significant therapeutic benefit of topical antifungal (amphotericin) for the treatment of chronic polypoid rhionsinusitis.[57] Despite the purported fungal cause of AFRS, antifungal therapies need further investigation to establish their efficacy before their use is widely adopted.

Immunotherapy is another treatment modality that holds potential as an effective treatment option for AFRS. The antiinflammatory effect of specific allergen immunotherapy has the potential to decrease reliance on systemic steroids in the treatment of AFRS or may reduce the need for revision surgery. The rationale for immunotherapy is that AFRS is at least partially a result of allergen-specific IgE-mediated inflammation. Although the relative importance of type 1 hypersensitivity in AFRS continues to be debated, by definition AFRS patients have fungal allergy (and often many other aeroallergen hypersensitivities). Given that AFRS is often a severe and refractory condition that requires multiple sinus surgeries and repeated or prolonged courses of systemic steroids, it is rational to attempt to control concomitant allergic inflammation via immunotherapy. Although subcutaneous immunotherapy has clearly demonstrated efficacy in allergic rhinitis and asthma,[58,59] randomized, controlled trials that examine the efficacy of immunotherapy specifically for AFRS are lacking. Initial evidence to support the use of immunotherapy was primarily anectdotal.[60,61] However, a few cohort studies, as well as a single, controlled, comparison study suggest that allergen-specific immunotherapy is well tolerated and may result in clinical improvement in AFRS.[62] In the most rigorous study to date Folker and colleagues[5] compared AFRS patients treated with and without immunotherapy. Patients underwent comprehensive allergy testing and immunotherapy was begun approximately 1 month after endoscopic sinus surgery. Dosing consisted of weekly injections escalated to a maximally tolerated dose and continued for 3 to 5 years. After an average 33 months of follow-up, they showed that the immunotherapy-treated patients had better endoscopic mucosal appearance, lower CRS survey scores, required fewer courses of oral steroids (0 vs 2), and showed less reliance on nasal steroids (27% vs 73%). Although this was not a randomized, double-blind study, these results suggest an important role for immunotherapy in the overall management of AFRS

Currently, the recommended medical management of AFRS is based upon rational principles, reports of successful treatment approaches in the literature, and the clinical experiences of physicians who deal with the disease. Therapy is directed toward reducing inflammation and reducing fungal antigen exposure. Immunotherapy is recommended as an additional approach that holds the potential to suppress the type 1 hypersensitivity that appears to be a component of the disease process. Significant uncertainty about the ideal treatment approach will persist as long as high-level evidence from randomized, controlled trials is lacking.

NATURAL COURSE

Clinical experience has shown that, similar to other forms of polypoid CRS, recurrence of polypoid disease is common in AFRS. Kupferberg and colleagues[63] reported universal recurrence in patients treated surgically without vigorous postoperative medical treatment. The reported recurrence rates for AFRS range from 10% to 100%, and there is clearly a range of severity in these patients.[11] There are few longitudinal studies that examine the natural history of AFRS over time, but one longitudinal study showed that over a 7-year follow-up period, patients required an average of two surgical procedures and three courses of systemic steroids per year. After many years, even asymptomatic patients had persistent polypoid mucosal edema and elevated total serum IgE.[64] It appears the disease may become quiescent over a period of years, but a significant number of patients will have persistent sinonasal inflammation and require ongoing medical management. Close follow-up of these patients is warranted because recurrent disease may silently progress until intranasal polyposis again creates significant nasal obstruction. If discovered at this point, revision surgery may be required. Nasal endoscopy at regular intervals is the best way to monitor the activity of disease, and patients should be encouraged to return early for any symptom exacerbation.

SUMMARY

Since its description almost 30 years ago, the understanding of AFRS has continued to evolve. Although clinically similar to other forms of EMRS, current definitions require the demonstration of type 1 hypersensitivity to fungi to make a diagnosis of AFRS. The relative importance of type 1 hypersensitivity in the pathogenesis of the disease continues to be debated. However, given the tendency of AFRS for recurrence, the frequent need for revision endoscopic sinus surgery, and the dependence of some patients on systemic steroid treatment, it is reasonable to consider immunotherapy as one component in the overall management of these patients.

REFERENCES

1. Katzenstein AL, Sale SR, Greenberger PA. Allergic *Aspergillus* sinusitis: a newly recognized form of sinusitis. J Allergy Clin Immunol 1983;72:89–93.
2. Millar JW, Johnston A, Lamb D. Allergic *Aspergillosis* of the maxillary sinus [abstract]. Thorax 1981;36:710.
3. Safirstein B. Allergic bronchopulmonary aspergillosis with obstruction of the upper respiratory tract. Chest 1976;70:788–90.
4. Erwin GE, Fitzgerald JE. Case report: allergic bronchopulmonary aspergillosis and allergic fungal sinusitis successfully treated with voriconazole. J Asthma 2007;44:891–5.
5. Folker RJ, Marple BF, Mabry RL, et al. Treatment of allergic fungal sinusitis: a comparison trial of postoperative immunotherapy with specific fungal antigens. Laryngoscope 1998;108:1623–7.
6. Allphin AL, Strauss M, Addul-Karin FW, et al. Allergic fungal sinusitis: problems in diagnosis and treatment. Laryngoscope 1991;101:815–20.
7. Cody DT, Neel HB, Ferreiro JA, et al. Allergic fungal sinusitis: the Mayo Clinic experience. Laryngoscope 1994;104:1074–9.
8. Ferguson BJ. Eosinophilic mucin rhinosinusitis: a distinct clinicopathologic entity. Laryngoscope 2000;110:799–813.
9. Pant H, Kette FE, Smith WB, et al. Eosinophilic mucus chronic rhinosinusitis: clinical subgroups or a homogeneous pathogenic entity? Laryngoscope 2006;116:1241–7.
10. Ponikau JU, Sherris DA, Kern EB, et al. The diagnosis and incidence of allergic fungal sinusitis. Mayo Clin Proc 1999;74(9):877–84.

11. Marple BF. Allergic fungal rhinosinusitis: current theories and management strategies. Laryngoscope 2001;111:1006–19.
12. Schubert MS, Goetz DW. Evaluation and treatment of allergic fungal sinusitis. I. Demographics and diagnosis. J Allergy Clin Immunol 1998;102(3):387–94.
13. Manning SC, Holman M. Further evidence for allergic pathophysiology in allergic fungal sinusitis. Laryngoscope 1998;108(10):1485–96.
14. Stewart AE, Hunsaker DH. Fungus-specific IgG and IgE in allergic fungal rhinosinusitis. Otolaryngol Head Neck Surg 2002;127:324–32.
15. Pant H, Kette FE, Smith WB, et al. Fungal-specific humoral response in eosinophilic mucus chronic rhinosinusitis. Laryngoscope 2005;115:601–6.
16. Luong A, Davis LS, Marple BF. Peripheral blood mononuclear cells from allergic fungal rhinosinusitis adults express a Th2 cytokine response to fungal antigens. Am J Rhinol Allergy 2009;23:281–7.
17. Collins M, Nair S, Smith W, et al. Role of local immunoglobulin E production in the pathophysiology of noninvasive fungal sinusitis. Laryngoscope 2004;114:1242–6.
18. Ahn CN, Wise SK, Lathers DM, et al. Local production of antigen-specific IgE in different anatomic subsites of allergic fungal rhinosinusitis patients. Otolaryngol Head Neck Surg 2009;141:97–103.
19. Pant H, Schembri MA, Wormald PJ, et al. IgE-mediated fungal allergy in allergic fungal sinusitis. Laryngoscope 2009;119:1046–52.
20. Pant H, Beroukas D, Kette FE, et al. Nasal polyp cell populations and fungal-specific peripheral blood lymphocyte proliferation in allergic fungal sinusitis. Am J Rhinol Allergy 2009;23:453–60.
21. Chakrabarti A, Denning DW, Ferguson BJ, et al. Fungal rhinosinusitis: a categorization and definitional schema addressing current controversies. Laryngoscope 2009;119:1809–18.
22. Ence BK, Gourley DS, Jorgensen NL, et al. Allergic fungal sinusitis. Am J Rhinol 1990;4(5):169–78.
23. Granville L, Chirala M, Cernoch P, et al. Fungal sinusitis: histologic spectrum and correlation with culture. Hum Pathol 2004;35:474–81.
24. Ferguson BJ, Barnes L, Bernstein JM, et al. Geographic variation in allergic fungal rhinosinusitis. Otolaryngol Clin North Am 2000;33(2):441–9.
25. Das A, Bal A, Chakrabarti A, et al. Spectrum of fungal rhinosinusitis; histopathologist's perspective. Histopathology 2009;54:854–9.
26. Wise SK, Ghegan MD, Gorham E, et al. Socioeconomic factors in the diagnosis of allergic fungal rhinosinusitis. Otolaryngol Head Neck Surg 2008;138:38–42.
27. Manning SC, Schaefer SD, Close LG, et al. Culture-positive allergic fungal sinusitis. Arch Otolaryngol Head Neck Surg 1991;117:174–8.
28. Gupta AK, Bansal S, Gupta A, et al. Is fungal infestation of paranasal sinuses more aggressive in pediatric population? Int J Pediatr Otorhinolaryngol 2005;70:603–8.
29. Saravanan K, Panda NK, Chakrabarti A, et al. Allergic fungal rhinosinusitis: an attempt to resolve the diagnostic dilemma. Arch Otolaryngol Head Neck Surg 2006;132:173–8.
30. Singh NN, Bhalodiya NH. Allergic fungal sinusitis-earlier diagnosis and management. J Laryngol Otol 2005;119:875–81.
31. McClay JE, Marple B, Kapadia L, et al. Clinical presentation of allergic fungal sinusitis in children. Laryngoscope 2002;112(3):565–9.
32. Manning SC, Vuitch F, Weinberg AG, et al. Allergic aspergillosis: a newly recognized form of sinusitis in the pediatric population. Laryngoscope 1989;99:681–5.

33. Meltzer EO, Hamilos DL, Hadley JA, et al. Rhinosinusitis: establishing definitions for clinical research and patient care. Otolaryngol Head Neck Surg 2004;131:S1–62.
34. Bent JP, Kuhn FA. Diagnosis of allergic fungal sinusitis. Otolaryngol Head Neck Surg 1994;111:580–8.
35. Ferguson BJ. Definitions of fungal rhinosinusitis. Otolaryngol Clin North Am 2000; 33(2):227–35.
36. Dhiwakar M, Thakar A, Bahadur S, et al. Preoperative diagnosis of allergic fungal sinusitis. Laryngoscope 2003;113:688–94.
37. Ghegan MD, Lee FS, Schlosser RJ. Incidence of skull base and orbital erosion in allergic fungal rhinosinusitis (AFRS) and non-AFRS. Otolaryngol Head Neck Surg 2006;134:592–5.
38. Wise SK, Rogers GA, Ghegan MD, et al. Radiologic staging system for allergic fungal rhinosinusitis. Otolaryngol Head Neck Surg 2009;140:735–40.
39. Campbell JM, Graham M, Gray HC, et al. Allergic fungal sinusitis in children. Ann Allergy Asthma Immunol 2006;96:286–90.
40. Reddy CE, Gupta AK, Sing P, et al. Imaging of granulomatous and chronic invasive fungal sinusitis: comparison with allergic fungal sinusitis. Otolaryngol Head Neck Surg 2010;143:294–300.
41. Aribandi M, McCoy VA, Bazan C. Imaging features of invasive and noninvasive fungal sinusitis: a review. Radiographics 2007;27:1283–96.
42. Manning SC, Merkel M, Kriesel K, et al. Computed tomography and magnetic resonance diagnosis of allergic fungal sinusitis. Laryngoscope 1997;107:170–6.
43. Zinreich SJ, Kennedy DW, Malat J, et al. Fungal sinusitis: diagnosis with CT and MR imaging. Radiology 1988;169:439–44.
44. Killingsworth SM, Wetmore SJ. Curvularia/Drechslera sinusitis. Laryngoscope 1990;100:932–7.
45. Zieske LA, Kopke RD, Hamill R. Dematiaceous fungal sinusitis. Otolaryngol Head Neck Surg 1991;105:567–77.
46. Marple BF, Mabry RL. Allergic fungal sinusitis: learning from our failures. Am J Rhinol 2000;14:223–6.
47. Hissaria P, Smith W, Wormald PJ, et al. A short course of systemic steroids in sinonasal polyposis: a double-blind, randomized, placebo controlled trial with evaluation of outcome measures. J Allergy Clin Immunol 2006;118:128–33.
48. Van Zele T, Gevaert P, Holtappels G, et al. Oral steroids and doxycycline: two different approaches to treat nasal polyps. J Allergy Clin Immunol 2010;125: 1069–76.
49. Kuhn FA, Javer AR. Allergic fungal sinusitis: a four year follow-up. Am J Rhinol 2000;14:149–56.
50. Schubert MS, Goetz DW. Evaluation and treatment of allergic fungal sinusitis. II. Treatment and follow-up. J Allergy Clin Immunol 1998;102:395–402.
51. Sohail MA, Al Khabori MJ, Hyder J, et al. Allergic fungal sinusitis: can we predict the recurrence? Otolaryngol Head Neck Surg 2004;131:704–10.
52. Joe S, Thambi R, Huang J. A systematic review of the use of intranasal steroids in the treatment of chronic rhinosinusitis. Otolaryngol Head Neck Surg 2008;139: 340–7.
53. Stjarne P, Mosges R, Jorissen M, et al. A randomized controlled trial of mometasone furoate nasal spray for the treatment of nasal polyposis. Arch Otolaryngol Head Neck Surg 2006;132:179–85.
54. Kanowitz SJ, Batra PS, Citardi MJ. Topical budesonide via mucosal atomization device in refractory postoperative chronic rhinosinusitis. Otolaryngol Head Neck Surg 2008;139:131–6.

55. Schubert MS. Antileukotriene therapy for allergic fungal sinusitis. J Allergy Clin Immunol 2001;108(3):466–70.
56. Rains BM, Mineck CW. Treatment of allergic fungal sinusitis with high dose itraconazole. Am J Rhinol 2003;17(1):1–8.
57. Weschta M, Rimek D, Formanek M, et al. Topical antifungal treatment of CRFS with nasal polyps: a randomized, double blind clinical trial. J Allergy Clin Immunol 2004;113:1122–8.
58. Calderon MA, Alves B, Jacobson M, et al. Allergen injection immunotherapy for seasonal allergic rhinitis. Cochrane Database Syst Rev 2007;1:CD001936.
59. Abramson MJ, Puy RM, Weiner JM. Allergen immunotherapy for asthma. Cochrane Database Syst Rev 2003;4:CD001186.
60. Goldstein MF, Dunksy EH, Dvorin DJ, et al. Allergic fungal sinusitis: a review with four illustrated cases. Am J Rhinol 1994;8:13–8.
61. Quinn J, Wickern G, Whisman B, et al. Immunotherapy in allergic *Bipolaris* sinusitis: a case report. J Allergy Clin Immunol 1995;95:201.
62. Mabry RL, Mabry CS. Allergic fungal sinusitis: the role of immunotherapy. Otolaryngol Clin North Am 2000;33(2):433–40.
63. Kupferberg SB, Bent JP, Kuhn FA. Prognosis for allergic fungal sinusitis. Otolaryngol Head Neck Surg 1997;117:35–41.
64. Marple B, Newcomer M, Schwade N, et al. Natural history of allergic fungal rhinosinusitis: a 4- to 10-year follow-up. Otolaryngol Head Neck Surg 2002; 127(5):361–6.

Allergy Treatment: Environmental Control Strategies

William R. Reisacher, MD

KEYWORDS

• Allergy treatment • Allergy and environment • Allergy triggers
• Allergen avoidance • Allergic asthma • Allergic rhinitis
• Inflammatory load • Dust mites • Dander

This information is designed to help physicians and allergy care providers understand:

- The role of environmental control in the treatment of allergic disease
- The concept of "the inflammatory load"
- The current studies that have been published on environmental control
- The factors that influence levels of indoor and outdoor allergens
- Different methods to decrease a patient's exposure to indoor and outdoor allergens
- The problems related to nonallergic symptom triggers
- Special considerations for school and workplace avoidance
- The role of environmental control in the prevention of allergic disease
- The various products available on the market to assist in avoidance
- How to make a plan with the patient to implement environmental control strategies.

Once the diagnosis of allergy has been made, the next step is to discuss environmental control strategies, also referred to as avoidance, with the patient. It is best to have this conversation after reviewing the results of specific allergy testing, either through skin or blood testing, but it is also reasonable to discuss these strategies based on the history alone. Most of them carry very little risk.

Nevertheless, there is often a great deal of resistance to initiating these strategies, on the part of both the physician and the patient. Discussing avoidance takes a great deal of time out of the physician's busy schedule. The physician may also not be very familiar with these strategies or has read studies that fail to demonstrate a significant benefit. Many patients are already under the erroneous impression that there is nothing that can be done for allergies, and this is compounded by the commonly

Disclosure: Phadia, Speaker's Bureau.
Department of Otorhinolaryngology, The Allergy Center, Weill Cornell Medical College, New York-Presbyterian Hospital, 1305 York Avenue, 5th Floor, New York, NY 10021, USA
E-mail address: Wir2011@med.cornell.edu

Otolaryngol Clin N Am 44 (2011) 711–725
doi:10.1016/j.otc.2011.03.019
oto.theclinics.com
0030-6665/11/$ – see front matter

Key Points: Allergy Treatment: Environmental Control

- Environmental control strategies prove a strong foundation for further allergy management
- There are many sources, besides true allergens, that may contribute to the "inflammatory load"
- Decreasing a patient's exposure to outdoor allergens is a realistic goal
- The impact of indoor allergens on the patient's symptoms should be considered, both at home and in the school or workplace
- The Focus of avoidance strategies is on "reducing" levels of allergens, rather than "eliminating" them
- Patients should be provided with a written copy of all recommendations, which should be reviewed often and kept simple.

held belief that avoidance does not work. For those patients searching for a quick and easy method to relieve their allergy symptoms, a discussion about these strategies is the last thing they want to hear.

It is universally accepted that allergen exposure is a precursor to sensitization, and there are many situations in which the benefits of environmental control are undeniable. If the allergic reaction is immediate and dramatic, the patient will intuitively link the exposure with the symptom and begin practicing environmental control strategies, such as avoiding a home where a cat is present or by staying indoors on a hot, windy day. But in other situations the reactions may be delayed, related to multiple exposures, or more difficult to recognize when symptoms are chronic.

Most of the current studies designed at quantifying the benefits of environmental control for allergic rhinitis have been low-power studies with inconsistent follow-up periods, variability in patient populations, and a lack of blinding. The 2010 review by the Cochrane Collaboration on dust mite avoidance measures concluded that they "may be of some benefit in reducing rhinitis symptoms," but the evidence was not strong.[1] In addition, most of these studies have looked at only one isolated intervention, whereas the genetic and environmental complexities of allergic rhinitis and asthma most likely require a multifaceted treatment approach.[2]

Conceptually, the management of allergies can be thought of as a pyramid with 3 levels (**Fig. 1**). The classic triad of allergy management includes environmental control,

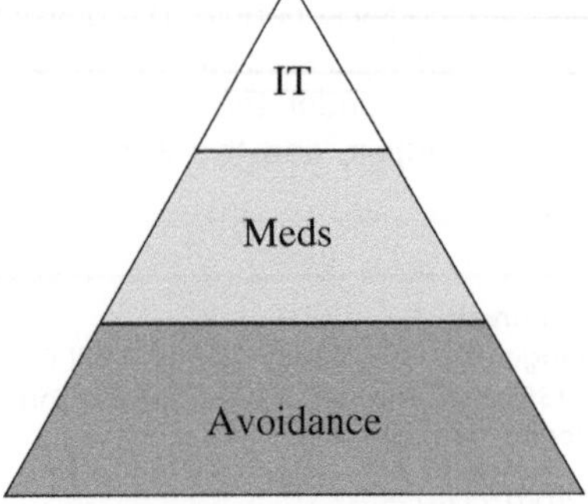

Fig. 1. The classic triad of allergy management. Environmental control strategies (Avoidance) form the foundation of this pyramid. Meds, pharmacotherapy; IT, immunotherapy.

pharmacotherapy, and immunotherapy. Environmental control forms the foundation of this pyramid, but it is actually not a treatment for allergic inflammation. Rather, it is a strategy to prevent further inflammation. Allergic symptoms may continue to gain momentum beyond the period of exposure, a phenomenon known as the "priming" effect, and for this reason avoidance alone may not seem to help at first. Every structure needs a strong foundation, but a person cannot live in the foundation alone. Environmental control sets the stage for effective treatment with pharmacotherapy and possibly immunotherapy, and for this reason, "there is no avoiding avoidance!"

CONCEPT OF THE "INFLAMMATORY LOAD"

To understand how allergen avoidance can help the allergic patient, one must first understand the concept of the "inflammatory load." The inflammatory load represents the sum of all allergens, irritants, and other immune stimulators that a patient is exposed to at any given time. When the inflammatory load is high, so are the levels of circulating allergic and inflammatory mediators. In this situation, small challenges with other stimulators may result in worsening symptoms. Direct contributors to the inflammatory load may enter the body through the respiratory tract, digestive tract, or skin. Indirect contributors to the inflammatory load include illness, stress, or problems with mucosal barriers such as high gastrointestinal permeability and IgA deficiency.

Everything that contributes to the allergic load raises the level of inflammation toward a critical threshold, much like water being added to a bucket. When the level rises above the rim, water begins to spill out and the patient becomes symptomatic. The role of avoidance is to slow down the flow of water from that source, keeping the level below the threshold. This analogy helps explain why avoiding one or two antigens can increase a patient's tolerance to other antigens that the patient is not actively avoiding. If needed, pharmacotherapy and immunotherapy may be used to increase the patient's overall threshold which, in effect, gives that patient a larger bucket.

OUTDOOR ALLERGENS

Patients are often dismayed upon learning that they are allergic to outdoor allergens because they believe that for such allergies nothing can be done. Although the outdoor environment cannot be changed, the focus for these patients is on recognizing when to enter that environment and preventing those allergens from entering the indoor environment. In order for pollen to be allergenic, it must satisfy the criteria set forth in 1931 by A.A. Thommen (**Box 1**).

Box 1
Allergenic pollen criteria

In order for pollen to produce allergic symptoms, it must:

- Come from a seed-bearing plant
- Be produced in large amounts
- Be buoyant enough to allow for airborne spread
- Be widely distributed, particularly near areas of human habitation
- Have sensitizing potential

Pollen

Pollen represents the male reproductive cells of most plants. Pollens are lightweight proteins, which may travel for many miles on the wind; they are relatively large in size, ranging from 15 to 50 μm, which does not allow them to easily penetrate the lower airway. In the Northern parts of the United States, trees pollinate from February through May, grasses pollinate from June through July, and weeds pollinate from August until the first frost of the year. Three consecutive days with temperatures above 65°F (18.5°C) allow for pollination. The pollination season is longer in warmer climates, and the phenomenon of global warming may also extend the time pollen is normally in the air.

Patients will use many names to describe their pollen allergies.

"Rose fever" is a term commonly applied to springtime allergies, but the pollen from brightly colored flowers is spread by insects and, therefore, does not enter the respiratory tract. This process is known as entemophilous spread, as opposed to airborne, or anemophilous, spread. Keep in mind that patients may still develop nasal symptoms from the odor of blooming flowers.

"Hayfever" is a term often applied to fall allergies, when hay is being harvested, but the true offender is ragweed. In the springtime, many patients notice a yellow coating of pine tree pollen on their cars and become convinced that this is what they are allergic to. This heavy pollen is actually not very allergenic because it does not remain airborne for long enough to cause symptoms. It is a clear sign, however, that pollination is actively occurring.

Patients who are allergic to pollen suffer most on hot, dry, windy days. Pollen counts tend to be highest from 5 to 10 AM. If possible, patients should shift activities, such as running or gardening, from the morning to the evening during their active season; they should limit yard work and wear a mask when working outside. Patients should also be instructed to close their windows before going to bed and open the doors and windows only for limited times during the day when necessary. Even basic air-conditioning filters are able to filter out large pollen particles, and this appliance should be used as much as possible, either on the "cool" or "vent" settings. For those patients commuting to work in the morning, they should close the car windows and use the recirculation feature of the air-ventilation system, if present.

Patients should be advised to remove their clothes and shower immediately when they return home at night, particularly after being in the park or hiking in the woods. Pollen may stick to the clothing, skin, and hair, and may be particularly problematic in patients with long hair. The clothing should be placed in a hamper or a closet that is not in the bedroom, but never placed on the bed. The bedroom needs to be the patient's "safe haven," the one place in the house where there is a low level of allergens. Washing bed sheets and pillowcases in hot water frequently during the season will help accomplish this. Outdoor pets should also be kept out of the bedroom and should be washed after spending extended time outdoors. After showering, patients should change into clothing that is not worn outdoors.

Many patients who are allergic to pollens discover that when they travel to other regions their allergies improve, and they may be tempted to relocate to that region. In the past this was one recommendation for the treatment of pollen allergies, but is generally not practical nowadays. If the patient does intend to relocate, they must be informed that the genetic ability to form allergies to pollen in the environment will surely move with them. Patients may experience relief for the first few years depending on their new environment, but this "holiday" from allergies may begin to fade as they develop new sensitivities.

Mold

Mold is a ubiquitous organism on the Earth, which is found in both the indoor and outdoor environments. Mold spores are present in the air throughout the year, unless the ground is covered by snow, and outdoor spore counts are about twice as high as indoor levels. Spores are able to survive freezing and boiling, and may range in size from 5 to 50 μm. In general, particles less than 10 μm are able to gain access to the lower airway, and this explains why mold is a potent trigger for asthma. Both the spores and the fragments of mycelia are allergenic.

Mold requires warmth, moisture, and organic debris to grow. It is attracted to damp, shady areas where decaying vegetation is present. Spore counts peak after the sun sets, and therefore cause more symptoms during the evening as opposed to the morning for pollen-allergic patients. Many patients believe that they are allergic to grass because they are symptomatic after cutting the lawn. Although the grass in the lawn is typically too short to pollinate, the clippings that stick to the blade on the underside of the lawnmower are a perfect medium for mold growth. When the lawnmower is started again, the mold particles are propelled into the air.

Although mold is a perennial allergen, there are seasonal spikes that might fool the patient and clinician into thinking that pollen is the offending allergen. In colder climates, when snow begins to thaw in the early spring, many of the mold spores that have been dormant for the entire winter suddenly become airborne. Because of the rain seen in the late spring, early summer is also a time when airborne mold spores are elevated. During the fall, the leaves decaying on the ground also serve as a perfect medium for mold growth. Mold counts are generally higher in areas near stagnant bodies of water, such as lakes or marshes.

It is not possible to eliminate mold from the outdoor environment, but performing regular surveys around the exterior home and surrounding property is a good way to recognize trouble spots. Steps should be taken to thin out dense vegetation that is close to the house or lying on the roof. Any trees and bushes that are dead or decaying near the house should be removed and leaves raked away from the foundation. Firewood should be moved away from the house. The roof must be inspected for any holes or signs of excessive wear, and any leaky gutters or improperly installed flashing repaired. Water should be diverted away from the foundation and any low-lying areas filled in. Professional masons and landscapers may be needed to get the job done properly.

INDOOR ALLERGENS

It has been estimated that a person born in the 1990s in the United States will spend more than 90% of his or her life indoors.[3] This fact is not difficult to understand when one considers all the "creature comforts" available. Between home theater, video conferencing, central air conditioning, and groceries that can be ordered over the Internet, it is surprising we leave our houses at all! Moreover, spending more time indoors provides more opportunity for exposure to multiple indoor allergens. In a cross-sectional study of representative homes in the United States, 46% had high levels of 3 or more allergens.[4]

Not only are we spending more of our time indoors, the indoor climate itself is changing. With the rising costs of energy, homes are being made more airtight and energy-efficient than ever before. Higher indoor temperature and humidity also lead to elevated levels of allergens such as dust mites and mold. For the patient this means that there is more time to become sensitized to indoor allergens as well as more time to react to their presence.

Dust

By far, dust and dust mites are the most common and important indoor allergens. In addition to dust mites, "house dust" is actually a combination of natural and synthetic fibers, organic debris, lysine sugars, pollen, mold, insect parts, food particles, and hair from pets and humans. Dust mite antigen is less allergenic than "house dust," but it is the single most representative antigen from this mixture. Dust mite is the most common allergen in children and young adults with asthma and eczema, and dust mite allergy is a predictor of asthma development. Dust mites are also a significant allergen in patients with isolated allergic rhinitis.[5]

Dust mites are microscopic members of the Arachnid family. These mites are blind and are unable to drink; they must absorb water from the air, which is why they enjoy climates that are over 50% relative humidity. Dust mites also enjoy low altitudes (lower than 3500 ft [1077 m]) and temperatures between 65° and 84°F (18.5°–29°C). Dust mites live in the same environment as humans because they feed off organic debris such as shed hair and skin cells. These mites exist in bed sheets, mattresses, pillows, carpets, furniture stuffing, stuffed animals, and real animals, to name a few. Millions of dust mites can be present in a typical mattress. The dust mite produces approximately 10 fecal balls each day containing the allergenic proteins.

The physician must be aware that informing a patient about a dust mite allergy may provoke a sensitive issue. It is important to explain to the patient that dust is not dried dirt that has been tracked into the house. Avoidance strategies for dust mites are focused primarily in the bedroom—the "safe haven" for the patient. Clutter should be reduced to provide less surface area for dust mites to adhere to. Bare floors also provide less surface area and are easier to clean. Carpets must be vacuumed twice weekly with special bags to prevent dust from escaping back into the air. Pets should be kept out of the bedroom, and certainly off the bed.

Bed sheets and pillowcases should be washed weekly in hot water. Over 130°F (54.5°C) is recommended but residential homes are limited to 120°F (49°C) to prevent scalding of children. Higher temperatures can be achieved by washing sheets and pillowcases at the Laundromat or by placing them in the sun. Stuffed animals should be put in the dryer on "High" for 15 minutes and then stored in the closet or in a cargo net. Special allergenic barriers should be purchased and placed around the pillows and mattress, underneath the regular bedding.

Animals

In the Western world, approximately 60% of households have at least one pet.[6] Among these, cat dander is an extremely important allergen and should be included in every testing battery. The majority of the allergen, Fel d 1, comes from the pelt of the animal, but is also seen in urine, sweat, and saliva. Male cats are more allergenic than females. Cat dander is very small (5 μm in diameter) and may remain airborne for long periods of time, which makes it a potential trigger for sensitized patients with asthma. The particles are very "sticky," and can accumulate in high amounts in carpeting and furniture but also on smooth floors. Because of these qualities, cat dander may be carried by humans into areas where pets are not even present or allowed. More than 90% of homes in the United States have measurable levels of cat and dog dander, whether or not a pet is present, and significant levels of dander are also found in schools, offices, public places, theaters, and airplanes.[7,8]

Dog dander is generally less allergenic than cat dander, and there is more breed to breed variability in the allergens present. Many patients who claim to be allergic to their dog may actually be allergic to other allergens that accumulate on their pelt, such as pollen, mold, dust, and even cat dander.

Bird feathers are another source of dander, and the amount of dander is related to the size of the bird. Available extracts usually consist of mixtures of chicken, duck, and goose dander. Other household sources of feathers include comforters, pillows, mattresses, and jackets. Many patients who believe that they are allergic to their pet bird may actually be reacting to the mold present at the bottom of the cage.

Without a doubt, the most effective avoidance strategy for pet allergy is to remove the pet from the home environment, but this is a very sensitive area and should be discussed very delicately with the patient. Most pets are considered a part of the family, and if the physician is insistent on breaking up this bond, the entire relationship with that patient may be damaged. Even if a pet is removed from the home, it may take several months for levels of dander to decrease to the point where the patient is no longer symptomatic.

If the animal remains in the home, it is helpful to remove carpeting and place air purifiers in the rooms the animal likes to inhabit. If possible, the pet should be restricted from going into the bedroom and particularly from sitting on the bed. After playing with the pet or sitting on furniture where the pet is present, patients should wash their hands before touching their face to prevent inoculating the dander into their eyes or nose. Washing the animal may reduce dander levels, but this has to be done every few days to be effective.

Cockroach

Cockroaches are very clever scavengers. These creatures tend to cluster around food and water sources, and populations may reach very high levels, particularly in urban settings. Cockroach sensitivity is a major risk factor for early childhood asthma and rhinitis.[5] The allergy is typically not from the living roach. After they die, their body parts become desiccated and begin to disintegrate. These shed particles are very lightweight and become airborne, where they may spread through the ventilation system of a building. For this reason many homes and buildings with significant levels of cockroach allergen have no visible evidence of infestation.

The most important strategy to prevent cockroach infestation is cleaning up food debris in the home. If roaches are seen, commercially available insecticides or boric acid powder may be used. Roach traps are minimally effective and probably not worth the money spent on them. Caulking every crack in the house might be helpful, but this is extremely difficult to achieve. If the infestation persists, the patient should not hesitate to call a professional exterminator.

Mold

Common indoor molds include *Alternaria alternata*, *Cladosporium herbarum*, *Aspergillus fumigatus*, and *Penicillium notatum*. Mold spores may enter the indoor environment through windows, doors, crawl spaces, and unsealed parts of the foundation. Cracks in the foundation may lead to excessive moisture in the basement with a characteristic odor resulting. Rooms with running water, such as the kitchen, bathrooms, and laundry room, are high-risk areas for mold growth. Other sources of mold include indoor plants, old books, furniture, and piles of newspapers. Many people come in to the office dismayed that they are allergic to their Christmas tree. This "Christmas tree syndrome" is actually caused by mold, which grows on the tree as it lies on the damp ground.

Mold may cause reactions in the body through several mechanisms. The one which is most clearly defined as "allergy" is the classic type I, IgE-mediated hypersensitivity, which is picked up on skin or via blood testing. However, skin testing often produces a delayed reaction to molds, possibly due to a type III or type IV reaction. Many people will be symptomatic because of the odor of molds or because of the direct irritation that mold spores may have on the nasal mucosa. *Stachbotrys chartarum*, a black-colored mold not particularly allergenic to humans, produces a mycotoxin when disturbed. This toxin is often released during the renovation of older structures and may produce symptoms such as congestion, rhinorrhea, and headache.

Similar to outdoor mold avoidance strategies, the quest to decrease mold in the indoor environment begins with a careful survey around the interior of the house. The patient should focus on areas of previous mold growth or water damage. Any visible evidence of mold should be cleaned with a commercially available product or a dilute solution of bleach (1 part bleach to 10 parts water). Water leaks should be fixed and a dehumidifier should be used in damp areas, such as the basement. Attics, kitchens, laundry rooms, bathrooms, and basements should always be equipped with ventilation units and exhaust fans. Indoor sources of mold, including plants, old books, magazines, and firewood should be minimized. If serious water damage is present or cracks in the foundation are discovered, a professional should evaluate the situation and recommend the proper remediation.

NONALLERGIC TRIGGERS

Airborne allergens, which are recognized by the immune system, are common sources of inflammation, but there are many other nonallergic irritants that can stimulate local inflammation without systemic effects, such as tobacco smoke. Despite public awareness of the dangers of cigarette smoking, 20.6% of adults in the United States (18 years and older) continue to smoke.[9] Exposure to maternal tobacco smoke during pregnancy and infancy is highly associated with asthma prevalence, and second-hand smoke exposure has an adjuvant effect on allergen sensitization during the first 3 years of life.[10] It is recommended that a "no-smoking" policy should be instituted in the household, and this includes the porch and garage. Clothing exposed to tobacco smoke should be put away or washed to prevent the small irritant particles (less than 1 μm) from being circulated into the air.

Chemical irritants are ubiquitous in both the outdoor and indoor living environments. Cleaning products can release high levels of alcohols, aldehydes, and benzene compounds. Likewise, products of combustion, such as carbon monoxide and nitric oxide, as well as carbon dioxide from respiration can reach toxic levels if not properly ventilated. It is important to ensure that all units in the house that use a flame, such as the furnace, stove, and fireplace, are adequately vented. Fans for fresh air ventilation should be installed, and air handlers should be adequate for the size of the house. To save money, patients may opt for a smaller unit, but this can have disastrous results. As already stated, newer homes are not as "leaky" regarding fresh air, and this may allow levels of airborne chemicals to build up very quickly.

Nonallergic stimulators to the respiratory tract may also include extremes of temperature and humidity, or rapid changes in these parameters. Patients who are sensitive to these stimuli may also react adversely to strong odors or be able to sense odors in the air that others are unable to detect. Such patients already know to stay away from the perfume counter at the department store or the scented candle store. From an evolutionary standpoint, this sensitivity probably had a selective advantage for certain humans who were able to detect dangers such as advancing storms or nearby fires.

Even the density of particles in the air can produce respiratory symptoms because of their direct irritating effect on nasal and oropharyngeal membranes. This phenomenon helps explain why patients with no detectable allergies may react on a high pollen day or when dusting the house.

SCHOOL AND WORKPLACE

Up to this point the discussion has focused on environmental control strategies at home, but this is not the only place patients inhabit. It is quite possible that some people actually spend more time in their workplace than at home. However, school and workplace avoidance poses some specific challenges. First of all, the "safe haven" is much more difficult to create, particularly if the patient is working in an open area or a cubicle setting. There may be high levels of allergens from unknown sources. Perhaps the desk is cleaned every night by a maintenance worker who is also a "cat person," or the building may have high levels of mold from a water leak or recent renovation.

Examples from the real world illustrate the point.

In one instance, several workers were becoming ill with cough and headache, particularly those who were sitting near the ventilation ducts. After an environmental engineer was called in to perform air sampling, it was determined that a maintenance worker was unknowingly storing cleaning chemicals near the air intake system of the office building.

In another instance, a child who is allergic to mold and dust was coming home every day from school with worsening respiratory symptoms and had recently to increase his asthma medication. When his mother went to speak with his teacher, she noticed that the rug on which the children gathered every day for reading time was the same one that was present when she was a student there. When the old rug was finally replaced with foam tiles, her child's asthma improved.

If a patient is suspicious that the workplace is contributing to symptoms, he or she should be asked to talk with fellow employees to see if others are having similar problems. Inquire with the management about recent problems with the building, although they may be reluctant to share this information. If the ventilation ducts have not been recently cleaned, this may be requested. Small air purifiers can be used near the patient's desk, and the desk should be kept clean and free of clutter. Have the patient inquire about moving his or her desk to another part of the office, even if the offending allergens have not yet been determined. For schools, parents should also schedule a meeting with the teachers and administrators to discuss the allergic needs of their child.

THE PREVENTION OF ALLERGIES

While environmental control strategies are designed to optimize the management of patients with allergies, do they have any role in the prevention of new sensitizations and the development of allergic disease? Studies have demonstrated an association between high allergen exposure and an increased rate of sensitization, particularly for indoor allergens.[11] Cockroaches, dust, and rat dander are early sensitizers, particularly in kids who live in the inner-city areas.[12] Data from the Childhood Asthma Management Plan demonstrated a ninefold increase in dust mite sensitization in children with asthma who lived in homes with detectable dust mite antigen, compared with those with no detectable antigen.[13] There is a strong, linear relationship between the level of sensitization and the development of asthma, allergic rhinitis, and eczema.[14]

If environmental control is used for prevention, when should it be initiated? As early as 22 weeks' gestation, fetuses of atopic mothers are capable of mounting a proliferative response to dust mite allergen, directed by maternal IgG.[15] Dust mite–specific IgE has been detected in the cord blood of fetuses whose mothers had high exposure to dust mites.[16] However, high levels of interleukin (IL)-4 and IL-5 in cord blood did not correlate with sensitization later in childhood. Serum elevation of dust mite–induced T-cell cytokines at 6 months, on the other hand, strongly correlated with sensitization by the age of 2 years.[17] This finding suggests that early childhood is a critical period for allergen sensitization.

In the Isle of Wight prevention study, 120 high-risk infants were recruited prenatally and randomized to receive either a hydrolyzed diet along with dust avoidance measures for the first year of life, or standard recommendations. The infants were monitored clinically and skin tested at ages 1, 2, 4, and 8 years. The treatment group demonstrated a significantly lower incidence of allergic rhinitis at 12 and 24 months compared with the control group, along with a reduction in positive skin-prick tests.[18] By the age of 8 years there was also a significantly lower incidence of allergic rhinitis, atopic dermatitis, and asthma in the treatment group than in the control group.[19]

The literature is controversial concerning the presence of pets in the household. It has been demonstrated in some studies that increased exposure to cat dander early in life is associated with increased sensitization, but others have failed to demonstrate this.[20,21] Two prospective studies also failed to demonstrate an association of any kind between animal exposure and the development of asthma.[20,22] It has been suggested that very high levels of cat dander may actually be protective against later allergen sensitization.[23] In houses with animals, higher levels of endotoxin, a lipopolysaccharide found in the cell wall of gram-negative bacteria, may induce a form of tolerance by producing a modified T-helper cell type 2 response, leading to IgG_4, but not IgE, antibody production. It is reasonable to recommend to expecting parents that they should not acquire new pets, but it is probably not necessary for them to eliminate their existing pets from the home.

PRODUCTS

There are a large number of products available on the market nowadays to “treat” allergies, and it is important for the physician to be knowledgable about these products. Patients will find information in catalogs and brochures, at the physician’s office, in stores, and over the Internet, but the physician must guide the patient toward the most beneficial products. For a modest-sized residence, it is not unusual to spend more than $1000 on products designed to reduce a variety of indoor allergens.[24]

Filters are used to catch allergens, and either prevent them from entering the indoor environment or remove them once they have entered. Some of the less expensive and also less efficient filters, made of such materials as fiberglass or polyester resin, are used in forced-air heating systems and as pre-filters in units containing HEPA filters. HEPA (high-efficiency particulate air) filters were originally developed by the Atomic Energy Commission to clean radioactive dust, and are able to filter 99.97% of particles larger than 0.3 μm. These filters are expensive, but will last approximately 2 to 5 years when used with a pre-filter.

The use of air purifiers increased dramatically during the 1990s. It is best for the physician not to endorse specific products or companies, but rather discuss the pros and cons of different types that are available. Air purifiers are able to decrease the airborne levels of a wide variety of allergens and irritant particles, and the patient should never be discouraged from trying one. The size of the unit purchased should depend on the size of the room in which it is being used. Of course, the patient’s “safe haven” is the best place to put this unit, but multiple units may be used

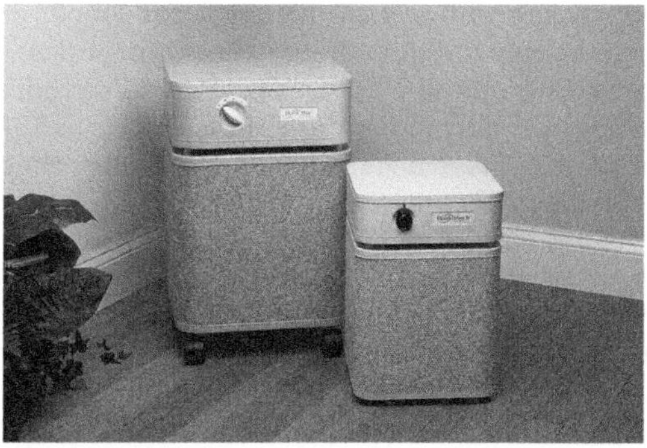

Fig. 2. Air purifiers using a high-efficiency particulate air (HEPA) filtration system. Different units are available based on the size of the room being treated. The units pictured use a 4-stage filtration process to trap allergens and absorb odors. The 360° intake system draws air in from all sides of the air purifier to trap allergens in 2 pre-filters, followed by a HEPA filter. Odors are absorbed by an activated carbon-zeolite blend. (*Courtesy of* Allergy Control Products Inc, Danbury, CT; with permission.)

throughout the home. It is best to use an air purifier in a room without carpeting. Many of the units on the market contain carbon/charcoal post-filters to remove odors, as well as ultraviolet radiation to destroy organic material without destroying the occupants or their furnishings.

The two basic types of air purifier are HEPA units and electronic precipitators. Air filters using HEPA filtration are very effective and low-maintenance units. HEPA units

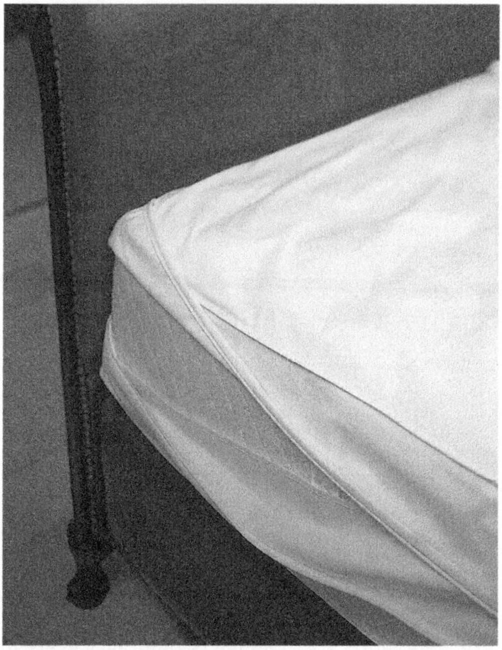

Fig. 3. Mattress encasings are made from cotton fibers that are tightly woven to a 6.8-μm pore size to protect against dust mite allergens. (*Courtesy of* Allergy Control Products Inc, Danbury, CT; with permission.)

are available as central units and in a variety of room sizes (**Fig. 2**), are used with a pre-filter, and usually come equipped with a carbon/charcoal post-filter. These purifiers do not produce any ozone. By contrast, electronic precipitators produce a small amount of ozone, as they work by charging the particles in the air and then passing them between 2 magnetic plates. These units require more maintenance because if these plates are not cleaned, their efficiency will drop dramatically. In addition, the charged particles may produce a greasy, dark residue on carpets and furniture.

Vacuum cleaners were introduced to the market in 1935. For the dust-allergic patient, it is important to vacuum carpeting twice weekly, preferably by someone else. If using a vacuum cleaner with bags, a 2- to 3-layer microfiltration bag or HEPA filtration bags should be used because dust can pass easily though the standard, single-layer bags. True HEPA vacuum cleaners are available, but less expensive and less efficient units are also sold under the names "HEPA-like" vacuum cleaners or "allergy vacuums."

Dust mite barriers, available for pillows and mattresses, are designed to entomb dust mites, essentially cutting them off from their food supply (**Fig. 3**). These barriers are made from the same tightly woven materials used to make surgical gowns and typewriter ribbons, and partial encasements for the mattress are equally as effective as total encasements. Different sizes and textures are available; it is helpful to have samples available for the patient to examine.

Acaricides may also be recommended for patients allergic to dust mites (**Fig. 4**). Tannic acid, a chemical present in tea which is also used to tan leather, denatures

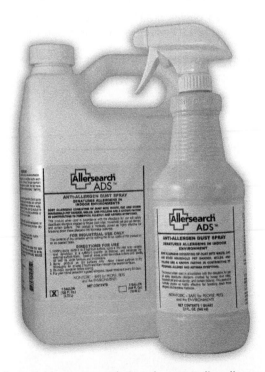

Fig. 4. Commercially available sprays are designed to neutralize allergens on contact for up to 3 months. The sprays contain tannic acid as the active ingredient, which neutralizes dust mite, pet dander, mold, and pollen allergens that can build up in carpets. (*Courtesy of* Allergy Control Products Inc, Danbury, CT; with permission.)

the dust mite antigen but does not kill dust mites. Unfortunately, this product needs frequent reapplication and may stain fabrics. Benzyl benzoate is a powder that is able to kill dust mites, but does not denature the antigen already present. The effect of this compound lasts approximately 2 to 6 months.

Table 1
Allergens and environmental control strategies

Allergens	Typical Conditions	Steps for Prevention or Post Exposure
Outdoor Allergens		
Pollen	• Hot, dry, windy days • Peak: 5–10 AM	• Close windows • Wear a mask when working outdoors • Use air conditioning • Remove exposed clothing • Shower
Mold	• Warmth + Moisture + Organic debris • Damp shady areas • Decaying leaves • Stagnant bodies of water • Peak: after sunset • Seasonal spikes: snow melt, rain	• Remove dense vegetation • Remove dead trees • Store firewood away from house • Divert water from foundation • Fill low-lying areas
Indoor Allergens		
Dust mites	• Above 50% humidity • Temperatures 65°–84°F • Low altitude (below 3500 ft) • Bed sheets, mattresses, pillows, carpets, furniture, animal fur, stuffed animals	• Bare floors less susceptible than carpet • Vacuum carpets twice weekly • Wash bed clothes over 130°F • Use allergen barriers
Animals	• Cat and dog dander • Bird feathers	• No animals in bedroom or bed • Wash hands after touching pet • Avoid down comforters, pillows, jackets
Cockroach	• Dead roach debris, not living roach	• Clean up food debris • Use insecticides or boric acid powder • Caulk house cracks • Exterminator
Mold	• Windows, doors, crawl spaces, unsealed parts of building foundation • Kitchen, bathroom, laundry, basement • Indoor plants • Old books and newspapers • Old furniture	• Clean visible evidence of mold with bleach • Fix water leaks • Use dehumidifier in damp areas • Ventilation units for attics, kitchens, laundry rooms, bathrooms, basements • Minimize indoor plants, old books, magazines, firewood
Nonallergic triggers	• Tobacco smoke • Chemical irritants • Odors	• No smoking in home • Wash clothing exposed to smoke • Fans, ventilation in home • Air purifiers

Dehumidifiers should also be considered for the dust mite–allergic or mold-allergic patient, particularly if there are rooms in the house that exceed 50% relative humidity. Relative humidity is a ratio of the absolute humidity of a space to the highest humidity level that can be achieved in that space, and may be determined with a hygrometer purchased at the local hardware or home store. The efficiency of dehumidifiers will be highest when combined with proper venting of bathroom and laundry rooms. Whole house units may be attached to a central air-conditioning system, but smaller units are also available. Humectants, containing calcium chloride to absorb moisture, can be used in small spaces such as closets.

DISCUSSING ENVIRONMENTAL CONTROL STRATEGIES

It is important to discuss avoidance strategies with the patient (**Table 1**), but the physician should not expect this to be easy and should not expect it to be over in one session. It may take several visits to finish the entire discussion, and the material needs to be repeatedly reviewed as well. Office staff and handouts may be used to help explain important points. The physician should constantly be aware of sensitive issues and avoid giving the patient a large "to do" list. A few key strategies may be chosen during each visit and prioritized for the patient. The discussion should focus on "reducing" rather than "eliminating" allergens from the environment.

The patient should receive the plan in written form and, during follow-up visits, be asked to report on progress. Rather than asking, "Have you tried the strategies we spoke about?" the physician should ask, "What have you tried since our last visit?" Environmental control is a challenging endeavor, particularly when the patient is reacting to multiple allergic and nonallergic agents. It is necessary to educate patients about their condition and encourage them every step of the way. Even if they do not see immediate results from the changes they have made, they should understand that environmental control strategies are one important component of the multimodality treatment plan for allergic disease designed to help them live a symptom-free life.

REFERENCES

1. Sheikh A, Hurwitz B, Nurmatov U, et al. House dust mite avoidance measures for perennial allergic rhinitis. Cochrane Database Syst Rev 2010;7:CD001563. Grade A.
2. Morgan WJ, Crain EF, Gruchalla RS, et al. Results of a home-based environmental intervention among urban children with asthma. N Engl J Med 2004; 351:1068–80. Grade B.
3. Tsang AM, Klepeis NE. Descriptive Statistics Tables from a Detailed Analysis of the National Human Activity Pattern Survey (NHAPS) Data, Environmental Protection Agency, Washington, DC; 1996.
4. Salo PM, Arbes SJ Jr, Crockett PW, et al. Exposure to multiple indoor allergens in US homes and relationship to asthma. J Allergy Clin Immunol 2008;121:678–84. Grade B.
5. Arshad SH. Does exposure to indoor allergens contribute to the development of asthma and allergy? Curr Allergy Asthma Rep 2010;10:49–55. Grade B.
6. Erwin EA, Wickens K, Custis NJ, et al. Cat and dust mite sensitivity and tolerance in relation to wheezing among children raised with high exposure to both allergens. J Allergy Clin Immunol 2005;115:74–9. Grade B.
7. Arbes SJ, Cohn RD, Yin M, et al. Dog allergen (Can f 1) and cat allergen (Fel d 1) in US homes: results from the National Survey of Lead and Allergens in housing. J Allergy Clin Immunol 2004;114:111–7. Grade B.

8. Abramson SL, Turner-Henson A, Anderson L, et al. Allergens in school settings: results of environmental assessments in 3 city school systems. J Sch Health 2006;76:246–9. Grade B.
9. CDC. Vital signs: current cigarette smoking among adults aged ≥18 years—United States, 2009. MMWR Morb Mortal Wkly Rep 2010;59(35):1135–40. Grade A.
10. Raherison C, Penard-Morand C, Moreau D, et al. Smoking exposure and allergic sensitization in children according to maternal allergies. Ann Allergy Asthma Immunol 2008;100:351–7. Grade B.
11. Chew GL, Perzanowski MS, Canfield SM, et al. Cockroach allergen levels and associations with cockroach-specific IgE. J Allergy Clin Immunol 2008;121: 240–5. Grade B.
12. Alp H, Yu BH, Grant EN, et al. Cockroach allergy appears early in life in inner-city children with recurring wheezing. Ann Allergy Asthma Immunol 2001;86:51–4. Grade B.
13. Huss K, Adkinson NF Jr, Eggleston PA, et al. House dust mite and cockroach exposure are strong risk factors for positive allergy skin test responses in the childhood asthma management program. J Allergy Clin Immunol 2001;107: 48–54. Grade B.
14. Arshad SH, Tariq SM, Matthews SM, et al. Sensitization to common allergens and its association with allergic disorders at age 4 years: a whole population birth cohort study. Pediatrics 2001;108:e33. Grade B.
15. Warner JA. Primary sensitization in infants. Ann Allergy Asthma Immunol 1999; 83(5):426–30. Grade B.
16. Peters JL, Suglia SF, Platts-Mills TAE, et al. Relationships among prenatal aeroallergens exposure and maternal and cord blood IgE: project ACCESS. J Allergy Clin Immunol 2009;123:1041–6. Grade B.
17. Rowe J, Kusel M, Barbara BJ, et al. Prenatal versus postnatal sensitization to environmental allergens in a high-risk birth cohort. J Allergy Clin Immunol 2007; 119:1164–73. Grade B.
18. Hide DW, Matthews S, Matthews L, et al. Effect of allergen avoidance in infancy on allergic manifestations at age two years. J Allergy Clin Immunol 1994;93: 842–6. Grade B.
19. Arshad SH, Bateman B, Sadeghnejad A, et al. Prevention of allergic disease during childhood by allergen avoidance: the Isle of Wight prevention study. J Allergy Clin Immunol 2007;119:307–13. Grade A.
20. Lau S, Illi S, Platts-Mills TAE, et al. Longitudinal study on the relationship between cat allergen and endotoxin exposure, sensitization, cat-specific IgG and development of asthma in childhood—report of the German Multicentre Allergy Study (MAS 90). Allergy 2005;60:766–73. Grade B.
21. Tariq S, Matthews S, Stevens M, et al. The prevalence of and risk factors for atopy in early childhood: a whole population birth cohort study. J Allergy Clin Immunol 1998;101:587–93. Grade B.
22. Korppi M, Hyvrinen M, Kotaniemi-Syrjnen M, et al. Early exposure and sensitization to cat and dog: different effects on asthma risk after wheezing in infancy. Pediatr Allergy Immunol 2008;19:696–701. Grade B.
23. Murray CS, Woodcock A, Custovic A. The role of indoor allergen exposure in the development of sensitization and asthma. Curr Opin Allergy Clin Immunol 2001;1: 407–12. Grade B.
24. Kattan M, Stearns SC, Crain EF, et al. Cost-effectiveness of a home-based environmental intervention for inner-city children with asthma. J Allergy Clin Immunol 2005;116(5):1058–63.

Pharmacotherapy for Allergic Rhinitis

Thuy-Anh N. Melvin, MD[a,*], Alpen A. Patel, MD[b]

KEYWORDS

• Allergic rhinitis • Allergy treatment • Allergy symptom control

Key Points: Allergic Rhinitis Pharmacotherapy

- AR can be divided into intermittent and persistent symptoms.
- Among the large array of pharmacotherapeutics available for the management of allergic rhinitis, intranasal corticosteroids and oral antihistamines are first line agents for allergic rhinitis.
- Other agents can be added in a symptom-based manner, for example, intranasal anticholinergics for rhinorrhea, intranasal decongestants for nasal obstruction, and intranasal antihistamine for pruritus.
- Anti-IgE antibody is newer class of pharmacotherapeutics that may provide better symptom control as well as downregulate IgE receptors.

Allergic rhinitis (AR) is a very common chronic respiratory disorder thought to be secondary to IgE-mediated type I hypersensitivity of the nasal mucosa to inhaled or, in some cases, to ingested allergens. It affects approximately 15% of Americans and leads to health care costs of two to five billion dollars spent per year.[1] There has been a steady rise in atopic diseases including AR.

AR has also been shown to negatively impact quality of life. Poor sleep quality is associated with AR, and daytime sleepiness can result from antihistamine medications used in the treatment of AR.[2] Decreased concentration in school children has been demonstrated,[3] and studies have shown that AR can lead to decreased productivity. AR is linked to other atopic disease states and is four to six times more likely to develop in those with asthma, which supports the link between the upper and lower airways as described by the unified airway theory.[4] AR, although frequently not life-threatening, can have significant impact on overall health status and daily life of affected individuals.

[a] Johns Hopkins Department of Otolaryngology—Head and Neck Surgery, 601 North Caroline Street, 6th Floor JHOC, Baltimore, MD 21287, USA
[b] Department of Otolaryngology, Towson Medical Center, 1447 York Road, Suite 100, Lutherville, MD 21093, USA
* Corresponding author.
E-mail address: tamelvin@gmail.com

Otolaryngol Clin N Am 44 (2011) 727–739
doi:10.1016/j.otc.2011.03.010 oto.theclinics.com

AR can be divided into seasonal (or intermittent) and perennial (or persistent). Seasonal AR is commonly known as "hay fever," although it is not caused by hay and does not present with fever. Perennial AR implicates allergen exposure on a more constant basis. AR has two phases: early-phase and late-phase inflammation. The early-phase reaction occurs usually within minutes and results in symptoms mediated by histamine. Sneezing, pruritus, nasal congestion, and rhinorrhea are some of the early-phase symptoms. Late-phase symptoms stem from eosinophils and T-cell mediated cytokines such as interleukin-4 and interleukin-5 and can present with rhinorrhea and nasal congestion.

Management of AR includes avoidance, pharmacotherapy, and immunotherapy. This article discusses the role of pharmacotherapy and reviews the wide spectrum of pharmacologic options available as well as these agents' efficacy and safety.

INTRANASAL CORTICOSTEROIDS

Topical application of corticosteroids was introduced in the early 1970s.[5] Intranasal corticosteroids are thought to work mostly locally, thereby avoiding the unwanted side effects that are associated with oral or intravenous corticosteroids such as cushingoid habitus, cataracts, osteoporosis, gastrointestinal irritation, candidiasis, and hyperglycemia, while maintaining the beneficial antiinflammatory effects that corticosteroids offer. The newer formulations of intranasal corticosteroids show even lower amounts of systemic absorption—approximately 1%. There are eight agents available currently for use in the United States (**Table 1**).

Intranasal corticosteroids are understood to be most effective against late-phase mediators in eosinophilic-dominated inflammation with some effect on the acute phase of the allergic response.[6] These agents are useful controller drugs and, therefore, should be used in a chronic manner. However, there are some data supporting its use on an as needed basis. Newer agents have been reported to have an effect as early as 24 hours after administration; however, the benefit from chronic use still seems to outweigh that of as needed use.[7]

Dexamethasone nasal drops were some of the first used topical corticosteroids. Although topically applied, they had significant adverse effects similar to those of systemic corticosteroids, partly due to its long half-life and the lack of first-pass metabolism in the liver.[5] Subsequent drugs that were first-pass metabolized included beclomethasone, which is the most extensively used in airways. Budesonide,

Table 1
Intranasal corticosteroids: generic and brand names

Generic	Brand
Beclomethasone dipropionate	Beconase Aq, Vancenase Aq
Budesonide	Rhinocort Aq
Flunisolide	Nasalide, Nasarel
Fluticasone propionate	Flonase
Mometasone furoate	Nasonex
Triamcinolone acetonide	Nasacort Aq
Newer	
Fluticasone furoate	Veramyst
Ciclesonide	Omnaris

fluticasone propionate, mometasone furoate, and triamcinolone acetonide are well studied agents that have even less bioavailability and shorter plasma half-lives than beclomethasone. The newer agents, Food and Drug Administration (FDA) approved in 2006–2007, include ciclesonide and fluticasone furoate.

Most intranasal corticosteroids are poorly lipid soluble, therefore requiring an aqueous solution used in a pump spray to suspend and deliver the drug. There appears to be a dose-dependent response to intranasal corticosteroids. Higher doses result in greater benefit. Overall, the intranasal doses tend to be smaller than those for the lung.[5]

In the treatment of seasonal AR, intranasal corticosteroids are appropriate first-line agents. Studies have demonstrated significant symptomatic relief with the use of intranasal steroids alone.[8] However, for perennial AR, management with sole intranasal corticosteroids has not proven to be as beneficial. Depending on the severity of the disease, short courses of oral corticosteroids, in addition to topical intranasal steroids, improve symptomatic relief more than intranasal steroids alone.[7]

The treatment of AR in children and in pregnant women is very similar to that of nonpregnant adults; however, because of the potential undue consequences in these two populations, practitioners may be advised to be more judicious with the administration of intranasal corticosteroids. Large pediatric studies have not shown significant adverse effects with use of intranasal corticosteroids[9] or significant systemic levels of corticosteroid absorption.[10] In pregnant women, there is always the concern for adverse effects especially to the unborn fetus, particularly cleft lip and palate development. Thus far, there have not been any reported teratogenic effects. Overall, there are not enough studies to support any definitive conclusion regarding the use of these agents in pregnancy. Therefore, careful risk-benefit analysis is recommended for mother and fetus when considering the use of intranasal corticosteroids for the treatment of AR in pregnant women. Of the intranasal corticosteroids, budesonide is the only category B drug.

Patient education regarding how to use these drugs should be highlighted. The correct method to administer a dose can vary from drug to drug and its delivery system. As mentioned previously, patients should be reminded that this medication can take some time to reach a level of maximal benefit, usually on the order of several days. After maximal benefit has been achieved, the drug can be tapered. In some cases, a 14-day course, at the onset of symptoms, is all that is needed to provide relief during an AR episode.[11]

Intranasal corticosteroids have few adverse effects. One randomized, double-blinded, controlled trial looking at pediatric subjects studied mometasone furoate and budesonide versus placebo for a short-term course of 14 days. This study showed no statistically significant difference in lower leg growth rate between groups.[9] Another study looking at intraocular pressures, conducted as a randomized, controlled, double-blinded study comparing placebo, fluticasone propionate, mometasone furoate, and beclomethasone dipropionate for 1 year, showed normal intraocular pressures across all groups.[12] However, in at least one randomized, controlled, double-blinded study, intranasal beclomethasone dipropionate was shown to have a statistically significant decrease in growth-rate for prepubertal children with perennial AR who were followed for 1 year.[13]

ANTIHISTAMINES

In the 1920s, it was discovered that histamine serves as an important mediator of pathologic allergic disease. Stemming from this basis, antihistamines were some of the first agents geared toward the treatment of atopic conditions (**Table 2**). The first

Table 2
Antihistamines: generic and brand names

Generic	Brand
First generation	
Azatadine	Optimine
Azelastine	
Brompheniramine	Dimetane
Chlorpheniramine	Chlor-Trimeton
Clemastine	Tavist
Dexchlorpheniramine	Polaramine
Hydroxyzine	Atarax
Promethazine	Phenergan
Tripelennamine	Pyribenzamine (PBZ)
Second generation	
Cetirizine	Zyrtec
Fexofenadine	Allegra
Loratadine	Claritin
Third generation	
Desloratadine	Clarinex
Levocetirizine	Xyzal

generation of antihistamines is comprised of six classes of poorly-selective histamine receptor competitive antagonists. These drugs have rapid onset and, although they are quickly efficacious, they wear off rapidly due to their short half-lives. They provide significant relief from AR symptoms such as rhinorrhea. However, this is balanced with a significant side-effect profile. The lack of selectivity for the histamine receptor results in anticholinergic effects due to unintended binding to muscarinic receptors. Consequently, adverse effects include dry mouth, blurred vision, and unwanted mucus thickening. Sedation and cognitive impairment effects stem from central histamine receptor affinity and binding. The first generation antihistamines are lipid soluble and easily cross the blood brain barrier. These medications have limited utility in light of the adverse side effects. This led to the development of second and third generation antihistamines.

Second generation antihistamines were developed in an attempt to improve selectivity and the first group of second generation antihistamines were effective at doing so; however, prolonged Q-T effects were observed in the setting of ingestion of other medications using cytochrome P450 hepatic metabolism. This adverse effect was seen in both terfenadine and astemizole, which led to their removal from the market. The next batch of second generation antihistamines did not have the hepatic side effects of the first group of second generation drugs nor the central histamine-mediated and anticholinergic side effects of first generation medications. Loratadine spearheaded this group of nonsedating H1-blockers. Although not sedating at lower doses, dose-dependent sedation has been observed.[14] Its popularity persists since it was introduced in the early 1990s. Concurrently, the development of fexofenadine followed in the footsteps of terfenadine as a nonsedating second generation antihistamine. It stands unique from loratadine due to its truly nonsedating properties even in the context of increasing dosage. Cetirizine is an active metabolite of hydroxyzine, a first generation antihistamine; therefore, it has slight blood brain barrier penetration and causes mild drowsiness. Demonstrable efficacy for AR symptoms as well as urticaria supports cetirizine as a useful drug for both respiratory and dermatologic atopic diseases. Loratadine and cetirizine are now available over-the-counter.

The third generation agents are S-isomers of the older antihistamines. Desloratadine and levocetirizine have minimal side effect profiles; however, they offer increased duration of action. Both agents have been shown to have a positive effect of nasal airflow and reduction in nasal congestion. Therefore, they may offer additional benefit to the treatment of AR[15,16] when compared with older antihistamines.

There are two topical intranasal antihistamines available in the United States: azelastine and olopatadine. Azelastine is a second generation antihistamine available for the treatment of seasonal AR. Bitter taste is the most common adverse reaction.[17] Olopatadine not only has antihistaminic properties, but it also possesses mast cell-stabilizing and antiinflammatory properties.[18] It is a new treatment approved by the FDA in 2009 for the management of AR with rapid onset and comparable efficacy to intranasal corticosteroid sprays. It is indicated for seasonal AR in patients aged 6 years or older.[19] Both agents are clinically effective on an as needed and continual basis.[20,21] In a randomized, controlled study looking at children with perennial AR, olopatadine nasal spray twice per day was significantly better than placebo.[22]

COMBINATION TOPICAL THERAPY

Studies have shown that intranasal corticosteroids when used in combination with oral antihistamines have not resulted in any further benefit for the prophylaxis of seasonal AR.[23] However, there has been new evidence that combination of topical agents, specifically topical corticosteroids and topical antihistamines, provide better symptom relief than either agent alone.[24–26] This efficacy has not been demonstrated in oral antihistamines or leukotriene antagonists when given in combination with an intranasal corticosteroid. There also may be additive benefits for treating patients with moderate-to-severe AR.[18] The safety and adverse effect profiles do not vary from that when these agents are used alone.

LEUKOTRIENE INHIBITORS

Leukotriene inhibitors target potent inflammatory mediators by competitively blocking the binding of cysteinyl leukotrienes to end-organ receptors. Montelukast is the only leukotriene inhibitor that is FDA-approved for AR, whereas zafirlukast is approved for the management of asthma. Studies have demonstrated clinical efficacy of montelukast for seasonal[27–29] and perennial[30,31] AR. Montelukast significantly reduced exhaled nitric oxide, a marker for airway inflammation, in one study comparing leukotriene inhibitors to other AR agents.[32] Montelukast works primarily through leukotriene receptors C4 and D4, which are found in the upper airways and important in the late-phase response. These agents do not primarily affect sensory nerve fibers, thus, they unlikely have a role in alleviating symptoms of itchiness and sneezing. One meta-analysis of 11 studies concluded that leukotriene receptor antagonists are modestly better than placebo, as effective as antihistamines, but less effective than nasal corticosteroids in improving symptoms and quality of life in patients with seasonal AR.[33] Because montelukast acts throughout the airway, this agent is a reasonable choice for those with concurrent asthma and AR.

Different from montelukast, zileuton acts by blocking the conversion of arachidonic acid into cysteinyl leukotrienes. Zileuton is FDA-approved for use in the treatment of asthma, and has been used in an off-label manner to treat AR and even in the treatment of nasal polyposis.

MAST CELL STABILIZERS

Cromolyn sodium is a topical over-the-counter nasal agent that works by reducing calcium influx and thereby decreasing the degranulation of histamine from mast cells. However, if the degranulation has already occurred, cromolyn sodium is theoretically not useful. Therefore, it should be used before exposure, which means it would be most useful as a preventative agent. Cromolyn has a very short half-life and therefore can require frequent dosing. The nasal spray can be used for patients aged 2 years and up, 4 to 6 times per day. Cromolyn is indicated in the management of seasonal[34] and perennial[35] AR as well as asthma.

Adverse effects are minimal due to cromolyn's poor systemic absorption. There has been reported sneezing, itching, and unpleasant taste. The safety profile is overall very good for this agent.

ANTICHOLINERGICS

Ipratropium bromide is an antimuscarinic that can be applied topically to the nasal mucosa, thereby reducing secretory output of the serous and seromucus glands. Its onset of action is relatively quick (within minutes) and, therefore, requires frequent administration throughout the day. Adverse effects include local irritation, dryness, and epistaxis. Systemic absorption is minimal; however, at high doses, systemic anticholinergic side effects can occur.[36] Ipratropium is clinically efficacious against perennial AR in both pediatric[37] and adult[38] populations. Due to the antimuscarinic properties of ipratropium, rhinorrhea is the primary symptom this drug alleviates. Therefore, its use spans all forms of rhinorrhea, including nonallergic forms. However, it has not been shown to be effective against postnasal drip.

MUCOLYTICS

Thinning out of mucus can be achieved through agents such as guaifenesin. Limited data support its efficacy, in part because clinical trials have not been performed to study its effects on the nasal airway. Lower airway studies have shown some thinning of thickened pulmonary secretions and a role in cough expectorant.[39] It is reasonable to extend these effects to the management of upper airway allergic diseases, especially given that the side effect profile is relatively good. Adverse effects include gastrointestinal upset, dry mouth, rash, and renal stones.

DECONGESTANTS

Via its effect on alpha-adrenergic receptors, decongestants can increase vasoconstriction and reduce nasal obstruction and congestion. This class of drugs is available over-the-counter in both topical (eg, oxymetazoline) and systemic (eg, phenylephrine, pseudoephedrine) forms.

Oral forms are selective for alpha-2 nasal mucosal receptors. However, they also have nonselective effects on alpha-1 and alpha-2 receptors in the central nervous, cardiovascular, and genitourologic systems. Caution should be exercised in patients with hypertension, cardiac disease, cerebrovascular disease, and urinary retention since these agents can exacerbate symptoms or trigger significant complications. Other adverse effects include insomnia, tremor, restlessness, anxiety, panic attacks, and palpitations. Due to their short half-lives, they come in time-release formulations. When metabolized, pseudoephedrine converts to methamphetamine, which has been used for recreational abuse. Therefore, access to this previously over-the-counter drug is now more controlled. In addition, this resulted in phenylephrine being used in place of pseudoephedrine in over-the-counter decongestants.

Topical decongestants offer immediate relief from nasal congestion and obstruction. For this reason, these agents can be used on an as needed basis. Adverse reactions include those listed above for systemic agents, although less common due to the relatively small systemic absorption. Prolonged use of these agents can also result in rebound rhinitis, that is, rhinitis medicamentosa. Tolerance of oxymetazoline can develop rapidly resulting in increasing doses and frequencies of application by the patient to achieve the same level of nasal symptom relief. Ultimately, this leads to increased dependence on the medication in the setting of severe nasal congestion. Patients should be advised to use this agent on a daily basis for less than 1 week straight. If rhinitis medicamentosa ultimately does develop, patients can be weaned off the topical decongestant or immediate cessation can also be advocated with the assistance of a short course of concurrent systemic and/or topical corticosteroids.

Monotherapy with decongestants is useful if the only symptom is nasal congestion. However, AR usually presents as a myriad of symptoms. In combination with antihistamines, decongestants can serve as an appropriate complement to medical management of AR. In any setting, caution must be exercised to avoid the major adverse effects of decongestants.

ANTI-IGE

One of the newer medical approaches to medical treatment of allergic disease is using humanized monoclonal anti-IgE antibodies, for example, omalizumab. This is the first of its class of drugs to be implemented for the management of atopic disease. Specifically, it is FDA-approved for the treatment of severe corticosteroid-dependent asthmatics. It binds to the Fc subunit of the IgE molecule thereby disrupting the binding of antigen to the Fab subunit of the IgE molecule. Thus, there is interference with activation of Th2-mediated cells. Although part of a novel and exciting class of drugs, omalizumab's use in the treatment of AR is currently limited by its cost—approximately $6,400 to $32,000 per year per patient. This is difficult for AR patients to afford, especially for a quality-of-life disease. Although, now that it has entered the market for the treatment of severe asthma, the estimated cost is expected to decrease with time.

Clinical studies central on the management of AR are limited for omalizumab.[40] Omalizumab has been shown to be effective for AR in both allergen challenge studies and clinical trials. Multiple randomized, double-blind, placebo-controlled studies have shown efficacy of omalizumab in seasonal[41,42] and perennial[43,44] AR. In addition, a potentially additive benefit from the use of omalizumab is the down-regulation of IgE receptors.[45]

Comparison studies between other treatment options are limited. One randomized controlled trial from Germany[46] examined safety in pediatric subjects with AR by subjecting them to immunotherapy titration phase followed by either placebo or omalizumab. Conclusions from this study supported a good safety profile for children and, although not central to their study objectives, there was data that suggested that AR symptoms were better controlled in the omalizumab arm. Another randomized, controlled study looking specifically at ragweed-sensitive AR subjects treated with either omalizumab or placebo before ragweed season showed lower nasal symptoms scores, rhinitis quality-of-life scores, and days missed from work or school in the omalizumab group. This study also showed dose-dependent reduction of serum IgE levels along with improved subjective complaints.[47] Interestingly, one randomized controlled trial looking at omalizumab versus placebo in the management of recalcitrant chronic rhinosinusitis yielded insignificant outcomes between the two groups.[48]

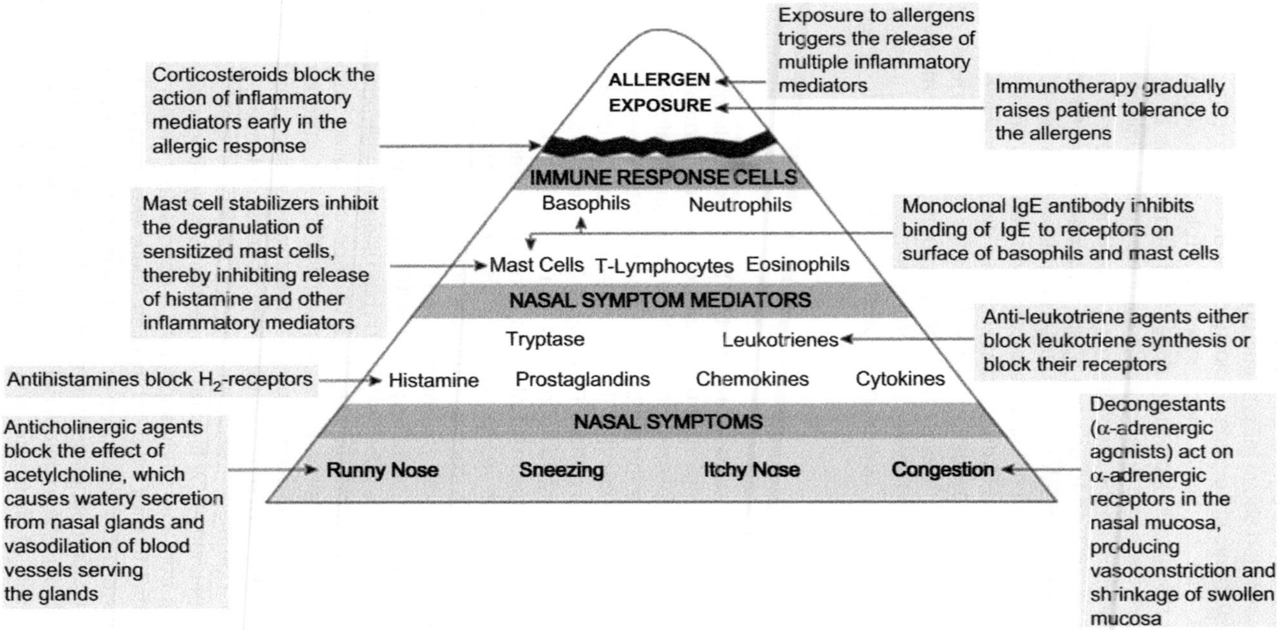

Fig. 1. Point-of-action for each drug group. (*From* Marple BF, Fornadley JA, Patel AA, et al. Keys to successful management of patients with allergic rhinitis: focus on patient confidence, compliance, and satisfaction. Otolaryngol Head Neck Surg 2007;136(Suppl 6):S107–24; with permission.)

Adverse reactions include malignancies (0.5%), life-threatening anaphylaxis in 1 to 2 of 1000 individuals, urticaria, and serum sickness.[49] Omalizumab has a short half-life, which requires passive high-dose injections every 2 to 4 weeks and therefore frequent office visits.

Research is currently being conducted on the development of active immunization against self-recognizing-IgE.[49] This could potentially reduce the side effect profile and increase the overall safety of anti-IgE therapy.

MANAGEMENT OPTIONS REVIEW

There are many options to choose from in the management of AR. They act on different points of the early and late phases of allergic reaction (**Fig. 1**). Guidelines have been established to help direct pharmacologic rationale (**Fig. 2**). For mild, intermittent AR, a single-agent of either antihistamine or leukotriene inhibitor usually offers adequate symptom relief without significant adverse reaction risk. The addition of

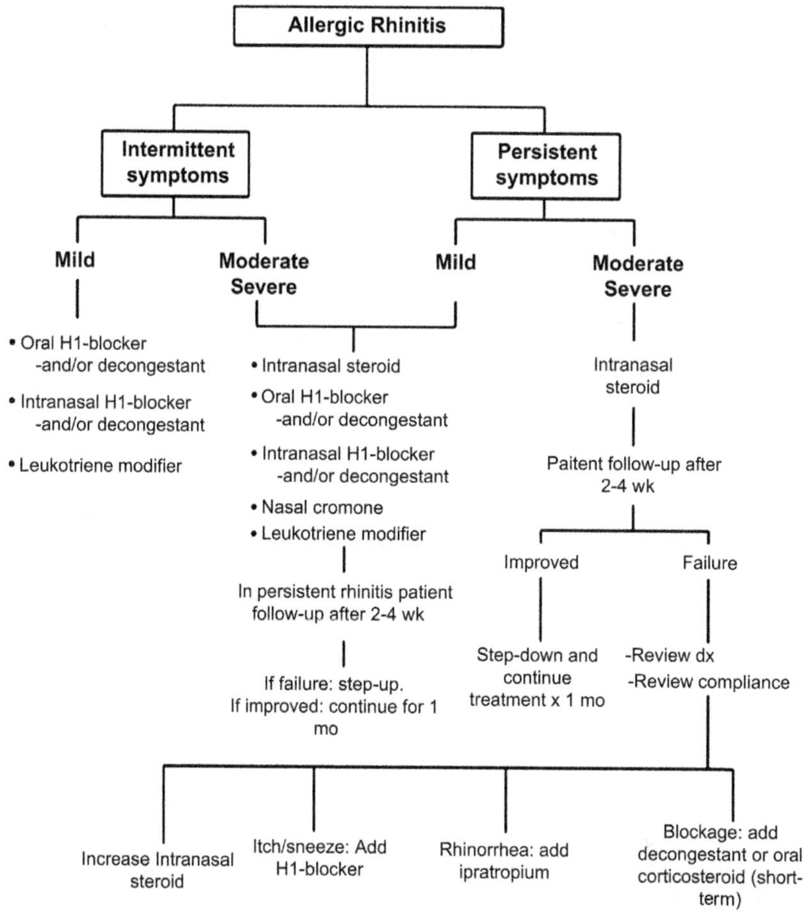

Fig. 2. Algorithm for management of AR. (*From* Greiner AN, Meltzer EO. Pharmacologic rationale for treating allergic and nonallergic rhinitis. J Allergy Clin Immunol 2006;118(5):985–96; with permission.)

a decongestant for nasal congestion or obstruction complaints can also be added to the antihistamine. For moderate-to-severe intermittent or mild persistent AR, the options are greater. Intranasal corticosteroids are the first-line of treatment; however, this regimen can be replaced by antihistamine with or without decongestant, or cromolyn alone. For moderate-severe persistent AR, intranasal corticosteroids are also the first-line treatment. Depending on the follow-up symptoms, the addition of an antihistamine for itchiness or sneezing, ipratropium for rhinorrhea, decongestant for obstruction, or increase in intranasal corticosteroid can be attempted. Some studies are now advocating the use of both topical antihistamines and intranasal corticosteroids, which can be better than each agent alone. Points to consider concerning pharmacotherapy for allergic rhinitis include (1) although avoidance is often the gold standard for management of allergic diseases, it frequently is not practical; (2) AR is a very common quality-of-life disease; (3) management starts with defining the type of allergic rhinitis, intermittent (eg, seasonal) or persistent (eg, perennial); (4) first-line therapy includes intranasal corticosteroids, which have generally shown excellent safety profile and local efficacy; (5) other agents can be used or supplement intranasal corticosteroids depending on symptomatology, such as antihistamines for itching, anticholinergics for rhinorrhea, and decongestants or systemic corticosteroids for nasal obstruction; and (6) monoclonal anti-IgE antibodies comprise a newer class of pharmacotherapeutics, although not yet FDA approved for the treatment of allergic rhinitis, may play a role in future management of AR.

SUMMARY

AR affects millions of Americans and the numbers continue to increase. Fortunately, there exists a wide array of pharmacotherapeutic options with relatively safe side effect profiles for the management of the varying subtypes of AR. Additionally, there are newer agents on the horizon for the management of AR such as anti-IgE therapy. As future, larger studies are performed, our understanding of the complicated pathophysiology of AR will continually grow and make way for improved medical management of this disease process.

REFERENCES

1. Reed SD, Lee TA, McCrory DC. The economic burden of allergic rhinitis: a critical evaluation of the literature. Pharmacoeconomics 2004;22(6):345–61.
2. Santos CB, Pratt EL, Hanks C, et al. Allergic rhinitis and its effect on sleep, fatigue, and daytime somnolence. Ann Allergy Asthma Immunol 2006;97(5):579–86.
3. Blaiss MS. Allergic rhinitis and impairment issues in school children: a consensus report. Curr Med Res Opin 2004;20(12):1937–52.
4. Krouse JH, Altman KW. Rhinogenic laryngitis, cough, and the unified airway. Otolaryngol Clin North Am 2010;43(1):111–21.
5. Mygind N, Andersson M. Topical glucocorticosteroids in rhinitis. Acta Otolaryngol 2006;126:1022–9.
6. Mygind N. Local effect of intranasal beclomethasone dipropionate aerosol in hay fever. Br Med J 1973;4:464–6.
7. Krouse JH. Allergic rhinitis—current pharmacotherapy. Otolaryngol Clin North Am 2008;41(2):347–58.
8. Siegel SC, Katz RM, Rachelefsky GS, et al. Multicentric study of beclomethasone dipropionate nasal aerosol in adults with seasonal allergic rhinitis. J Allergy Clin Immunol 1982;69:345–53.

9. Agertoft L, Pedersen S. Short-term lower leg growth rate in children with rhinitis treated with intranasal mometasone furoate and budesonide. J Allergy Clin Immunol 1999;104(5):948–52.
10. Cutler DL, Banfield C, Affrime MB, et al. Safety of mometasone furoate nasal spray in children with allergic rhinitis as young as 2 years of age: a randomized controlled trial. Pediatr Asthma Allergy Immunol 2006;19(3):146–53.
11. Rinne J, Simola M, Malmberg H, et al. Early treatment of perennial rhinitis with budesonide or cetirizine and its effect on long-term outcome. J Allergy Clin Immunol 2002;109:426–32.
12. Bross-Soriano D, Hanenberg-Milver C, Schimelmitz-Idi J, et al. Effects of three nasal topical steroids in the intraocular pressure compartment. Otolaryngol Head Neck Surg 2004;130(2):187–91.
13. Skoner DP, Rachelefsky GS, Meltzer EO, et al. Detection of growth suppression in children during treatment with intranasal beclomethasone dipropionate. Pediatrics 2000;105(2):E23.
14. Simons FE, Simons KJ. Second generation H1-receptor antagonists. Ann Allergy Asthma Immunol 1991;66:5–17.
15. Canonica GW, Tarantini F, Compalati E, et al. Efficacy of desloratadine in the treatment of allergic rhinitis: a meta-analysis of randomized, double-blind, controlled trials. Allergy 2007;62(4):359–66.
16. Bachert C, Bousquet J, Canonica GW, et al. XPERT Study Group. Levocetirizine improves quality of life and reduces costs in long-term management of persistent allergic rhinitis. J Allergy Clin Immunol 2004;114(4):838–44.
17. Shah S, Berger W, Lumry W, et al. Efficacy and safety of azelastine 0.15% nasal spray and azelastine 0.10% nasal spray in patients with seasonal allergic rhinitis. Allergy Asthma Proc 2009;30(6):628–33.
18. Kaliner MA, Oppenheimer J, Farrar JR. Comprehensive review of olopatadine: the molecule and its clinical entities. Allergy Asthma Proc 2010;31(2):112–9.
19. Roland PS, Ryan MW, Wall GM. Olopatadine nasal spray for the treatment of seasonal allergic rhinitis in patients aged 6 years and older. Expert Opin Pharmacother 2010;11(9):1559–67.
20. Roland PS, Marple BF, Wall GM. Olopatadine nasal spray for the treatment of allergic rhinitis. Expert Rev Clin Immunol 2010;6(2):197–204.
21. Kaliner MA. Azelastine and olopatadine in the treatment of allergic rhinitis. Ann Allergy Asthma Immunol 2009;103(5):373–80.
22. Okubo K, Okuda M, Magara H, et al. Olopatadine hydrochloride in children: efficacy and safety for perennial allergic rhinitis. Curr Med Res Opin 2010;26(7):1657–65.
23. Benincasa C, Lloyd RS. Evaluation of fluticasone propionate aqueous nasal spray taken alone and in combination with cetirizine in the prophylactic treatment of seasonal allergic rhinitis. Drug Invest 1994;8:225–33.
24. Hampel FC, Ratner PH, Van Bavel J, et al. Double-blind, placebo-controlled study of azelastine and fluticasone in a single nasal spray delivery device. Ann Allergy Asthma Immunol 2010;105(2):168–73.
25. LaForce CF, Carr W, Tilles SA, et al. Evaluation of olopatadine hydrochloride nasal spray, 0.6%, used in combination with an intranasal corticosteroid in seasonal allergic rhinitis. Allergy Asthma Proc 2010;31(2):132–40.
26. Bernstein JA. Azelastine hydrochloride: a review of pharmacology, pharmacokinetics, clinical efficacy and tolerability. Curr Med Res Opin 2007;23(10):2441–52.
27. Philip G, Malmstrom K, Hampel FC, et al. Montelukast for treating seasonal allergic rhinitis: a randomized, double-blind, placebo-controlled trial performed in the spring. Clin Exp Allergy 2002;32:1020–8.

28. van Adelsberg J, Philip G, Pedinoff AJ, et al. Montelukast improves symptoms of seasonal allergic rhinitis over a 4-week treatment period. Allergy 2003;58:1268–76.
29. Chervinsky P, Philip G, Malice MP, et al. Montelukast for treating fall allergic rhinitis: effect of pollen exposure in 3 studies. Ann Allergy Asthma Immunol 2004;92:367–73.
30. Chen ST, Lu KH, Sun HL, et al. Randomized placebo-controlled trial comparing montelukast and cetirizine for treating perennial allergic rhinitis in children aged 2-6 yr. Pediatr Allergy Immunol 2006;17:49–54.
31. Patel P, Philip G, Yang W, et al. Randomized, double-blind, placebo-controlled study of montelukast for treating perennial allergic rhinitis. Ann Allergy Asthma Immunol 2005;95:551–7.
32. Hung CH, Hua YM, Hsu WT, et al. Montelukast decreased exhaled nitric oxide in children with perennial allergic rhinitis. Pediatr Int 2007;49(3):322–7.
33. Wilson AM, O'Byrne PM, Parameswaran K. Leukotriene receptor antagonists for allergic rhinitis: a systematic review and meta-analysis. Am J Med 2004;116(5):338–44.
34. Meltzer EO, NasalCrom Study Group. Efficacy and patient satisfaction with cromolyn sodium nasal solution in the treatment of seasonal allergic rhinitis: a placebo-controlled study. Clin Ther 2002;24:942–52.
35. Cohan RH, Bloom FL, Rhoades RB, et al. Treatment of perennial allergic rhinitis with cromolyn sodium. Double-blind study on 34 adult patients. J Allergy Clin Immunol 1976;58:121–8.
36. Wood CC, Fireman P, Grossman J, et al. Product characteristics and pharmacokinetics of intranasal ipratropium bromide. J Allergy Clin Immunol 1995;95:1111–6.
37. Kim KT, Kerwin E, Landwehr L, et al. Use of 0.06% ipratropium bromide nasal spray in children aged 2 to 5 years with rhinorrhea due to a common cold or allergies. Ann Allergy Asthma Immunol 2005;94:73–9.
38. Kaiser HB, Findlay SR, Georgitis JW, et al. Long-term treatment of perennial allergic rhinitis with ipratropium bromide nasal spray 0.06%. J Allergy Clin Immunol 1995;95:1128–32.
39. Smith SM, Schroeder K, Fahey T. Over-the-counter medications for acute cough in children and adults in ambulatory settings. Cochrane Database Syst Rev 2008;1:CD001831.
40. Morjaria JB, Polosa R. Off-label use of omalizumab in non-asthma conditions: new opportunities. Expert Rev Respir Med 2009;3(3):299–308.
41. Casale TB. Anti-IgE (Omalizumab) therapy in seasonal allergic rhinitis. Am J Respir Crit Care Med 2001;164(Suppl):S18–21.
42. Adelroth E, Rak S, Huahtela T, et al. Recombinant humanized mAb-E25, an anti IgE mAb, in birch pollen-induced seasonal allergic rhinitis. J Allergy Clin Immunol 2000;106:253–9.
43. Chervinsky P, Casale T, Townley R, et al. Omalizumab, an anti-IgE antibody, in the treatment of adults and adolescents with perennial allergic rhinitis. Ann Allergy Asthma Immunol 2003;91:160–7.
44. Vignola AM, Humbert M, Bousquet J, et al. Efficacy and tolerability of anti-immunoglobulin E therapy with omalizumab in patients with concomitant allergic asthma and persistent allergic rhinitis: SOLAR. Allergy 2004;59:709–17.
45. Storms W. Allergens in the pathogenesis of asthma: potential role of anti-immunoglobulin E therapy. Am J Respir Med 2002;1(5):361–8.
46. Kamin W, Kopp MV, Erdnuess F, et al. Safety of anti-IgE treatment with omalizumab in children with seasonal allergic rhinitis undergoing specific immunotherapy simultaneously. Pediatr Allergy Immunol 2010;21(1 Pt 2):e160–5.

47. Stokes J, Casale T. Anti-IgE therapy. In: Atkinson NF, Bochner BS, Busse WW, et al, editors. Middleton's allergy: principles and practice. 7th edition. St Louis (MO): Mosby; 2008. p. 1679–89.
48. Pinto JM, Mehta N, DiTineo M, et al. A randomized, double-blind, placebo-controlled trial of anti-IgE for chronic rhinosinusitis. Rhinology 2010;48(3):318–24.
49. Peng Z. Vaccines targeting IgE in the treatment of asthma and allergy. Hum Vaccin 2009;5(5):302–9.

Immunotherapy – Traditional

Yekaterina A. Koshkareva, MD, John H. Krouse, MD, PhD*

KEYWORDS

• Allergy • Allergens • Immunotherapy • Inhalant • Treatment

Key Points: Immunotherapy for Allergy

- Allergy immunotherapy involves the sequential administration of antigen to patients with symptomatic, atopic conditions to induce tolerance to the offending antigens.
- Numerous well-controlled studies have documented the efficacy of immunotherapy in the treatment of both allergic rhinitis and asthma.
- Although subcutaneous immunotherapy can be rarely associated with serious adverse systemic reactions, it is generally safe and well tolerated.
- Immunotherapy is associated with decreased health care costs.

Between 30 and 60 million Americans are diagnosed with allergic rhinitis (AR) annually. AR affects between 10% and 30% of adults, and as many as 40% children. The current management options include environmental control; pharmacologic therapy including oral and intranasal antihistamines, steroids, and decongestants, and antileukotriene receptor antagonists and mast cell stabilizers; and allergen immunotherapy. Immunotherapy is a fascinating area of research and an attractive choice of therapy because it is the only option with the potential to change the natural course of allergy.[1]

The first documented description of clinical application of allergy immunotherapy dates back to the early 20th century. In 1911, Noon and Freeman[2] reported the successful treatment of patients with hay fever using pollen injections. Since then, protocols and techniques have evolved, although core concepts have remained the same. Specific immunotherapy (SIT) involves a series of controlled exposures to escalating doses of allergen, which alter immune system pathways and downregulate the allergic response, thereby decreasing the allergic symptoms associated with exposure to environmental allergens.

Temple University School of Medicine, Department of Otolaryngology-Head and Neck Surgery, 3440 North Broad Street, Kresge West # 300, Philadelphia, PA 19140, USA
* Corresponding author.
E-mail address: jkrouse@temple.edu

Otolaryngol Clin N Am 44 (2011) 741–752
doi:10.1016/j.otc.2011.03.011
oto.theclinics.com

MECHANISM

Despite intense research in the areas of immunology and allergy, a precise and detailed mechanism of immunotherapy remains to be elucidated. It is known, however, that immunotherapy induces several in vitro changes at molecular and cellular levels. The first immunologic difference can be detected as early as 7 days after initiation of immunotherapy, as manifested by a rise in cytokine interleukin (IL)-10.[3] IL-10 has been shown to play a central role in tolerance induction and immunologic change with immunotherapy (**Fig. 1**).

Shortly after beginning SIT, a slight increase in IgE is noted. Levels of IgE subsequently decrease, and a rise in IgG and IgA levels occurs, particularly IgG4 and IgA2.[4] The rise in IgG can be seen at as early as 5 weeks, and is predictive of response to immunotherapy at 1 year.[5] The simultaneous decline in IgE levels and increase in IgG levels have been described as a "scissors effect" and have led to development and popularization of a blocking antibody concept. IgG antibodies were once believed to prevent binding of allergen to mast cell and basophil-bound IgE, thereby blocking degranulation of these modulators of allergic response.[6] Recent evidence, however,

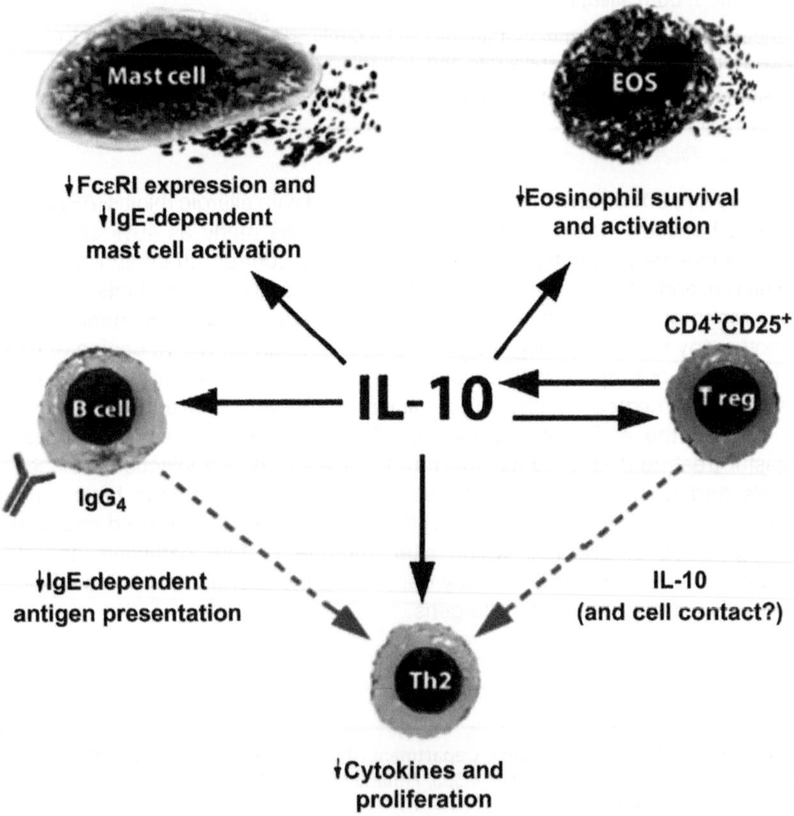

Fig. 1. The antiallergenic properties of IL-10 on different limbs of the allergic immune response. T-reg, T-regulatory cell; EOS, eosinophil. (*Reproduced from* Till SJ, Francis JN, Nouri-Aria K, et al. Mechanisms of immunotherapy. J Allergy Clin Immunol 2004;113:1029; with permission.)

suggests that the shift in antibody levels is a mere effect of immunotherapy, not the driving mechanism.[7]

In the early 1980s thymus-derived effector and helper lymphocytes were identified as the key components of hypersensitivity. T-helper 1 (Th1) cells are primarily involved in Gell and Coombs type 4 delayed reactions, and T-helper 2 (Th2) cells are predominant in Gell and Coombs type 1 immediate hypersensitivity reactions. Th2 cells produce IL-4, IL-5, and IL-13, which direct B lymphocytes to switch to IgE production. IL-5 also promotes eosinophil activity in the peripheral tissues. Th1 cytokines, such as interferon gamma, transforming growth factor β, and IL-10, inhibit IgE production and are involved in Th2 regulation.[8,9] In atopic conditions, such as allergic rhinoconjunctivitis and asthma, the T-cell balance is shifted toward proallergic Th2, with subsequent increase in proinflammatory agents.[10] Early observations of decreased expression of the Th2 cytokines IL-4 and IL-5 and increased levels of the Th1 cytokines IL-2 and IL-12 led to the belief that immunotherapy works through restoring the normal Th1/Th2 balance (**Fig. 2**).[7]

How this balance is restored remains unclear; although it is probably an end result of a complex interaction of different modulators at both cellular and molecular levels. Currently, thymic lymphocytes known as T-regulatory cells (T-reg) are known to play a key role (**Fig. 3**). T-reg cells constitute 10% of circulating lymphocytes and have been shown to regulate tolerance to both self (internal) and non-self (external) antigens.[10] The increase in T-reg cell levels can be detected as early as 6 hours after administration of SIT and is directly correlated with the Th2 to Th1 shift.[11]

On repetitive presentation with an allergen, T-reg cells are able to differentiate into T-reg 1 subtype, capable of producing IL-10 or transforming growth factor β. Both are known to modulate T-cell activity, favoring Th1 proliferation. B-cell phenotype is also affected as isotype switching toward IgG4 and IgA is promoted, resulting in suppression of IgE. Finally, activation and migration of eosinophils and mast cells to target tissues are diminished.[11–13]

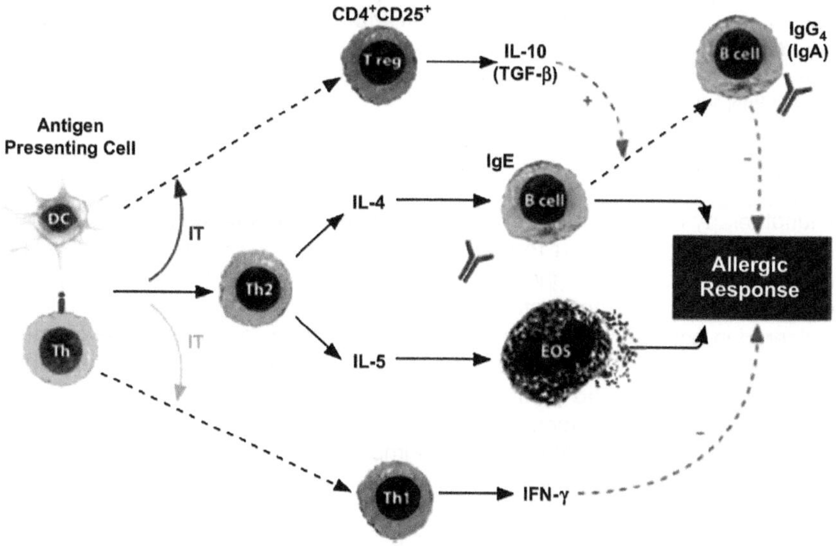

Fig. 2. Immunotherapy readdressed the balance between Th1/Th2 responses. An increase in IL-10 producing T cells and regulatory T cells is also seen. T-reg, T-regulatory cell; DC, dendritic cell; EOS, eosinophil. (*Reproduced from* Till SJ, Francis JN, Nouri-Aria K, et al. Mechanisms of immunotherapy. J Allergy Clin Immunol 2004;113:1028; with permission.)

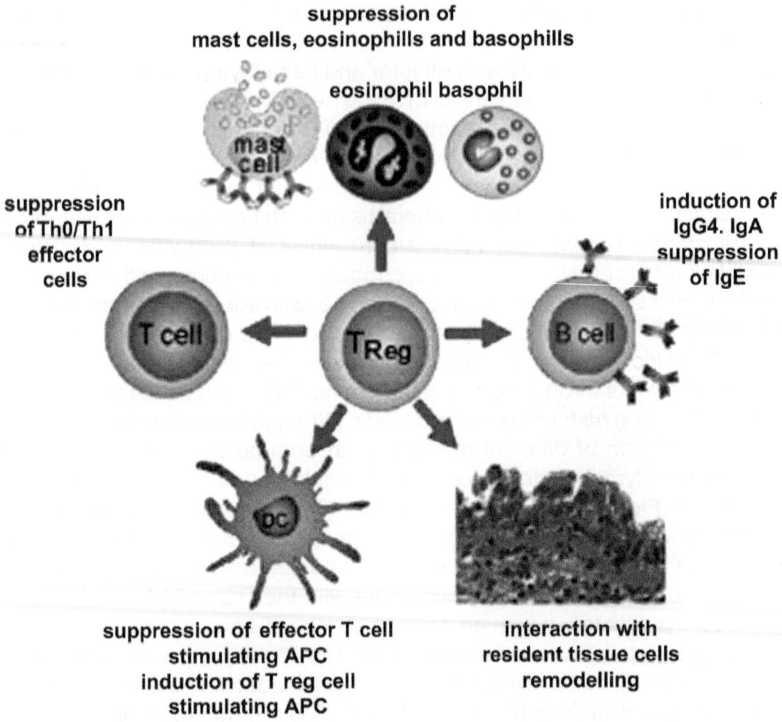

Fig. 3. T-reg cells contribute to the control of allergen-specific immunotherapy in five major ways: (1) suppression of antigen-presenting cells *(APC)* that support the generation of effector Th2 and Th1 cells; (2) suppression of Th2 and Th1 cells; (3) suppression of allergen-specific IgE and induction of IgG4, IgA, or both; (4) suppression of mast cells, basophils, and eosinophils; and (5) interaction with resident tissue cells and remodeling. (*Reproduced from* Akdis M, Blaser K, Akdis CA. T regulatory cells in allergy: novel concepts in the pathogenesis, prevention, and treatment of allergic diseases. J Allergy Clin Immunol 2005;116:966; with permission.)

PATIENT SELECTION

Immunotherapy targets a particular patient population, in whom symptoms of allergy are induced through exposure to identifiable allergens. The degree of response to prior environmental modulation and maximal pharmacologic treatment, duration and severity of symptoms, and patient compliance must be reviewed. SIT should be considered in patients who do not experience response to or are unable to tolerate the side effects of conventional therapy. Alternatively, allergic immunotherapy should be offered to patients who wish to avoid long-term dependence on pharmacologic agents or are seeking a potential cure for their disease.[1]

According to the Allergic Rhinitis and its Impact on Asthma (ARIA) guidelines, indications for immunotherapy in adults and children older than 5 years of age include[14]:

1. Patients with symptoms induced predominantly by allergen exposure.
2. Patients with a prolonged season or with symptoms induced by succeeding pollen season.
3. Patients with rhinitis and symptoms from the lower airways during peak allergen exposure.

4. Patients in whom antihistamines and moderate-dose topical glucocorticoids insufficiently control symptoms.
5. Patients who do not want to be on constant or long-term pharmacotherapy.
6. Patients in whom pharmacotherapy induces undesirable side effects.

In addition to clinical symptoms, objective evidence of the presence of IgE antibodies specific to those allergens must be identified and documented in the form of either in vitro testing, such as radioallergosorbent test (RAST) or enzyme-linked immunosorbent assay (ELISA), or in vivo testing, such as intradermal, prick, or combined skin testing. Alternatively, the testing can be classified as qualitative and quantitative. The goal of qualitative testing is to identify the offending allergen. Quantitative testing attempts to detect both presence and degree of sensitivity. Intradermal skin end point titration (SET) and modified quantitative testing (MQT) are considered the standard quantitative methods. SET involves intradermal injections of serial fivefold dilutions of antigen into the skin, until the end point, or the extent of sensitivity, is determined. MQT is a more efficient form of intradermal testing. It uses percutaneous technique at the initial stage to estimate the level of sensitivity, followed by selected intradermal tests to assess a more precise level of response. Because of this blended method, MQT results in shorter testing time with less expense.[7]

To maximize patient safety, immunotherapy based on qualitative testing must be initiated at very dilute concentrations, because the degree of sensitivity is not determined, and significant adverse events can occur with treatment. Immunotherapy based on quantitative methods, however, has an excellent index of safety.[15] Experts have also suggested that patients managed with SIT based on quantitative testing experience clinical improvement sooner. The hypothesis behind this observation is that higher concentrations of allergen can be delivered at the initial stages of immunotherapy.[7]

As stated by Haydon and Gordon,[16] "the only absolute contraindication to immunotherapy is failure to prove that a relevant allergy exists." However, immunotherapy is strongly discouraged in patients whose medical status would preclude them from surviving a systemic adverse reaction or its treatment .[17] Several relative contraindications also exist, the most serious being poorly controlled asthma, because the risk of anaphylaxis is greater in patients with reduced pulmonary function. Patients on β-blocker drugs are considered high risk because the systemic reaction may be more severe and more resistant to management with adrenergic agents, such as epinephrine.

Pregnant patients also deserve special consideration. Although initiating or escalating the schedule in a pregnant patient is not recommended, continuing the maintenance dosing is considered safe. Other patients who requiring careful management are those with established autoimmune abnormalities, because development of autoimmune disease has been reported in patients being treated with SIT.[16]

ALLERGEN SELECTION

The most commonly used allergen extracts are derived from dust mites, cat and dog dander, cockroach, molds, and pollens of trees, grasses, and weeds. Extracts are prepared in aqueous, alum-precipitated, or lyophilized solutions. Standardized extracts are supplied in concentrations expressed in allergen units (AU) or bioequivalent allergy units (BAU). In the process of standardization, the biologic activity of the allergen is calibrated to the concentration units through the use of intradermal skin testing in selected reference populations.[9] The U.S. Food and Drug Administration currently endorses 19 standardized allergen preparations.[18]

One challenging decision for clinicians is how many allergens to treat. Proponents of the blocking antibody theory argue for using all offending allergens, so that a specific antibody is formed for each one of them. However, the effectiveness of immunotherapy can be compromised through the use of too many antigens, because each individual component can become too dilute to exert effect. Furthermore, in accordance with the currently accepted theory that immunotherapy normalizes immune system mechanisms, treating for the few prominent offenders should be sufficient to induce overall immune tolerance. Treatment patterns therefore vary among allergists practicing in the United States, and between domestic and international allergists.

A literature review by Nelson[19] concluded that concurrent delivery of multiple properly identified antigen extracts in adequate quantities is clinically effective. In the author's opinion, several prominent allergens should be selected for treatment based on the patient's past medical history with respect to exposure to the suspected allergens, results of allergy testing, and patterns of allergens' seasonal and geographic distribution.

TIMING OF ADMINISTRATION

Haydon[16] describes the technical aspects of conventional immunotherapy administration. In general, immunotherapy involves biphasic subcutaneous injections of offending allergen extracts over several years.

During the incremental phase, also known as *build-up* or *induction*, escalating doses of an allergen are administrated until the maintenance dose is reached. The conventional build-up phase involves weekly injections and commonly takes between 10 and 13 weeks.[8] The 1-week interval is based on historic experience, as recalled by Freeman[20]: "Inoculations were given weekly merely because our out-patients at St Mary's Hospital were in the habit of coming every week."

Accelerated build-up schedules have been developed to save time and allow patients to experience the benefits of immunotherapy more rapidly, in hopes of improving compliance. Patient inconvenience was shown to be the most common reason for discontinuing immunotherapy, with the greatest inconvenience occurring during the incremental phase because of the frequency of visits.[21] In a cluster immunotherapy model, two to three injections are administered per day, on nonconsecutive days, which shortens the time frame for reaching the maintenance dose to 4 to 8 weeks. In a rush schedule, the escalating allergen doses are administered at intervals between 15 and 60 minutes over several days. Safety is a concern with accelerated escalation, with evidence showing that the risk of systemic reactions is higher with rush and cluster models. In a recent study by Pfaar and colleagues,[22] none of the adverse events encountered in their treatment of 157 adult patients was life-threatening nor resulted in alteration of the titration schedule. In addition, a literature review by Cox[23] concluded that premedication with antihistamines lowers this risk to the levels encountered with conventionally scheduled immunotherapy.

The frequency of injections is reduced from weekly to once or twice monthly during the maintenance phase. The maintenance dose tends to be between 5 and 20 μg of the allergen per injection, which translates to a number between 1000 and 2000 BAUs. In patients who are unable to tolerate the projected maintenance dose because of local or systemic side effects, the highest tolerated concentration is used as the maintenance dose. It no clinical benefits are observed after 1 year of treatment, immunotherapy should be discontinued. However, no firm guidelines exist on the duration of SIT if improvement is obvious. Most authorities recommend a 3- to 5-year treatment duration.[9] The literature review by Cox and Cohn[24] concluded that because no reliable tests are available to predict which patients will remain in remission after discontinuing SIT, the plan to terminate the treatment should individualized, based on patient's severity of symptoms, degree of improvement as a result of SIT, and the convenience of immunotherapy to the patient.

EFFICACY OF IMMUNOTHERAPY IN ADULTS

Immunotherapy has been shown to be an effective treatment option in adults with inhalant allergies caused by pollen, animals, and dust mites.[1] The 2007 Cochrane meta-analysis that reviewed 51 trials comprising 2871 patients with seasonal AR addressed the allergens ragweed, mixed grass, timothy, parietana, birch, orchard, cedar, Bermuda, juniperus ashei, and cocos. Among the studies, 15 showed clinical benefits of immunotherapy in patients with seasonal AR, using reduced symptom scores as the primary outcome measure. Furthermore, 13 studies reported reduced medication use scores in patients undergoing immunotherapy.[25] Passalacqua and Durham[26] reviewed recent studies (2000–2006) involving patients with AR treated with immunotherapy. The reduced need for medication and diminished clinical symptoms were confirmed in the patient group receiving immunotherapy.

In addition to reducing symptom and medication use scores, immunotherapy has been shown to improve quality of life in patients with AR. Frew and colleagues,[27] for example, followed up 410 patients with grass pollen–induced seasonal rhinitis. In their study, patients treated with immunotherapy had a marked improvement in quality of life compared with a well-matched control group. This finding parallels earlier literature outcomes.[28]

Immunotherapy has been shown to be effective in patients with allergic rhinoconjunctivitis caused by cat allergy. Marked reduction in symptoms on cat exposure, and in skin sensitivity to cat hair and dander extract, were shown in patients treated with immunotherapy.[5,29] In addition, Varney and colleagues[29] reported diminished skin sensitivity to house dust mite in patients treated with immunotherapy for cat allergy, further supporting the idea that immunotherapy induced overall immune tolerance.

In the early 1980s, Bousquet and colleagues[30,31] reported on the efficacy of immunotherapy in patients with asthma caused by house dust mite allergy. More recently, Varney and colleagues[32] were able to show a decline in symptom diary card scores, reduced use of rescue medication, and diminished skin prick sensitivity to *Dermatophagoides pteronyssinus* extract in patients with AR.

In summary, immunotherapy benefits have been thoroughly investigated and confirmed in adult patients with seasonal AR. Data on perennial allergic rhinitis exist in the form of multiple truncated reports. A protocol for systematic review of injection immunotherapy in perennial AR was submitted to the Cochrane Library in 2008 and is currently under review.[33]

The data on the efficacy of SIT in children with inhalant allergy remain conflicting. According to van Wijk,[34] "neither the efficacy not the ineffectiveness of subcutaneous immunotherapy in children has been proven." Based on the recent systematic review by Roder and colleagues,[35] the last placebo-controlled trial of immunotherapy in a pediatric population was in 1986. Of the six studies of SIT reviewed, five were of low quality and only two showed efficacy. The historic and evidence-based efficacy of SIT in adults has led to immunotherapy use in the pediatric population, with extrapolation from the adult data and without extensive investigation. Well-designed, powerful studies are needed to show the effects of immunotherapy in children.

LONG-TERM OUTCOMES

Eng and colleagues[36,37] presented the longest controlled follow-up studies of grass pollen sensitivity in children treated with immunotherapy. They were able to show that the clinical symptom score and use of medication remained low 6 and 12 years after a 3-year course of specific immunotherapy. In addition, the rates of new sensitization to unrelated antigens remained lower in children treated with immunotherapy compared with controls. This finding suggests that immunotherapy can modulate the natural course of allergy.

Durham and colleagues[38] showed long-term efficacy of immunotherapy in grass pollen–allergic adults 3 years after discontinuation of treatment. After a 3- to 4-year immunotherapy course, half of the participants continued with conventional immunotherapy, whereas the other half received placebo injections for another 3 years. Allergy symptom and medication use scores, and late skin responses, remained low in both patients who continued immunotherapy and those who stopped. Similarly, Tella and colleagues[39] found improvement in clinical scores in adults with AR and asthma treated with 3 to 5 years of immunotherapy. However, no significant difference in development of new sensitivities was identified. According to Ebner and colleagues,[40] about a third of patients experienced symptomatic relapse after a successful course of immunotherapy within the first 3 years of discontinuation. The risk of relapse after 3 years seems to be small.

In addition to improvement of clinical condition and possible prevention of onset of new sensitivities, immunotherapy seems to reduce the risk of development of asthma in patients with AR. Approximately one-third of individuals with AR develop asthma within 10 years.[6] Jacobsen and colleagues[41] followed up a group of adult patients with tree pollen allergy for 6 years after a 3-year immunotherapy treatment period. They found that 86% of the patients with AR and 68% with asthma maintained clinical benefit over the 6-year follow-up. In addition, none of the patients with AR developed asthma within that period.

RISKS

Similar to any therapeutic management option, immunotherapy is not without side effects, both local and systemic. Early side effects manifest within 20 to 30 minutes of injection, and late side effects after 30 minutes, most commonly after 6 to 24 hours. Local reactions present as edema, erythema, tenderness, and pruritis at the site of injection. Systemic side effects include rhinitis, dyspnea, fever, fatigue, angioedema, urticaria, and anaphylactic shock.[42]

In general, the reported incidences for local side effects range from 1% to 40% of injections.[42,43] Rogala and colleagues[42] found that patients with both chronic rhinitis and bronchial asthma are at risk of experiencing more-severe local reactions. The frequency and severity of local reactions tend to decrease with the duration of treatment.

The incidence of serious systemic reactions with conventional subcutaneous immunotherapy is considerably less, with most studies reporting it among fewer than 2% of injections.[15,42,44] According to Toubi and colleagues,[45] more than two-thirds of systemic reactions are encountered during the escalation phase of treatment. Major systemic side effects, such as wheezing, chest tightness, angioedema, and urticaria, tend to occur within 20 minutes of injection. The most commonly reported risk factors for major reactions include escalation phase of immunotherapy, active asthma, and first injection from a newly prepared vial.[8,15,44] Other cited factors for anaphylaxis include β-blockers, a high degree of skin test reactivity, and injections given during times of symptom exacerbations.[46] Less-serious systemic reactions, such as rhinorrhea, fever, and fatigue, tend to occur later. **Box 1**[42] illustrates factors commonly associated with adverse reactions to SIT. Overall, 24 cases of fatal anaphylactic shock caused by immunotherapy were reported in the United States between 1945 and 1985, and 26 were reported in the United Kingdom between 1957 and 1986.[47,48]

COST

The economic advantages of allergen immunotherapy over conventional pharmacologic treatment of allergy have been reported by many groups in both American and European health care systems. This finding applies to both adult and pediatric populations affected by AR.[49–52] The cost-effectiveness of immunotherapy was shown in multiple areas of health care economics. Particularly, Hankin and colleagues[51] reported that children receiving immunotherapy had lower medical per-patient total health care costs ($3247 vs $4872), outpatient costs not related to immunotherapy ($1107 vs $2626), and pharmacy costs ($1108 vs $1316).

FUTURE DIRECTIONS

Areas for future development and novel discoveries in the field of immunotherapy are nicely summarized by Passalacqua and colleagues[53] in their recent report. New indications for immunotherapy are being investigated, including food allergy, atopic dermatitis, and latex allergy. New routes of administration are also being studied. Liposomes are being tested as the vehicles for allergen administration. A new needle-free method of nanoparticle administration is being applied to immunotherapy. Finally, intralymphatic administration of allergen extracts is being tested with the hope of improving the efficacy of immunotherapy at lower doses.

Immunotherapy injections themselves are also being improved. Recombinant forms have been developed for many antigenic proteins. This approach provides the theoretical possibility of improving the effectiveness of immunotherapy through injecting relevant molecules only. Additionally, adjuvant nonantigenic elements are being

Box 1
Factors associated with adverse reactions to SIT

- Early months of treatment (induction course)
- Dosage errors
- Intravenous injection of dose (inadvertent)
- History of previous systemic reaction
- Extreme sensitivity to allergen
- Vigorous exercise before injection
- Change of vial
- Febrile illness
- Uncontrolled asthma
- Environmental exposure to allergen (eg, during the pollen season)
- Administration of β-blocker drugs

Data from Frew AJ, Norman PS, Golden DB, et al. Immunotherapy. In: Holgate ST, Church MK, Lichtenstein LM, editors. Allergy. 2nd edition. London: Mosby; 2001. p. 175–88.

investigated as potential augmentation of the immunologic effects of allergen injections. Monophosphoryl-lipid A (a mixture of bacterial cell wall phospholipids capable of inducing a Th1 response) has been shown to produce significant improvement in patients with grass pollen allergy. Finally, the area of genic immunotherapy is focusing on administering genes encoding for allergens via DNA vehicles, such as plasmids.

SUMMARY

Specific immunotherapy has been a safe and effective treatment option for a carefully selected population of patients with inhalant allergies for many decades. Despite the great advances in understanding of how immunotherapy exerts its effects, the detailed mechanism remains to be elucidated. Because of the lack of uniform guidelines for allergen selection and administration, each patient must be approached as a unique case, and collaboration between physician and patient is crucial for treatment success.

SUMMARY POINTS

- Immunotherapy has been shown to be a safe and efficacious treatment of atopic airway diseases such as AR and asthma.
- Successful immunotherapy involves induction of tolerance through immunologic change coordinated by T-regulatory lymphocytes and IL-10.
- Treatment with immunotherapy will evolve as new methods and mechanisms for inducing immunogenicity are developed and implemented.

REFERENCES

1. Wallace DV, Dykewicz MS, Bernstein DI, et al. The diagnosis and management of rhinitis: an updated practice parameter. J Allergy Clin Immunol 2008;122:S1–84.
2. Noon L, Cantab BC. Prophylactic inoculation against hay fever. Lancet 1911;10: 1572–3.
3. James LK, Durham SR. Update on mechanisms of allergen injection immunotherapy. Clin Exp Allergy 2008;38(7):1074–88.
4. Peng ZK, Naclerio RM, Norman PS, et al. Qualitative IgE and IgG subclass responses during and after long-term ragweed immunotherapy. J Allergy Clin Immunol 1992;89(2):519–29.
5. Nanda A, O'Connor M, Anand M, et al. Dose dependence and time course of the immunologic response to administration of standardized cat allergen extract. J Allergy Clin Immunol 2004;114(6):1339–44.
6. Yang X. Does allergen immunotherapy alter the natural course of allergic disorders? Drugs 2001;61(3):365–74.
7. Krouse JH, Krouse HJ. Modulation of immune mediators with MQT-based immunotherapy. Otolaryngol Head Neck Surg 2006;134:746–50.
8. Frew AJ, Norman PS, Golden DB, et al. Immunotherapy. In: Holgate ST, Church MK, Lichtenstein LM, editors. Allergy. 2nd edition. London: Mosby; 2001. p. 175–88.
9. Portnoy JM. Immunotherapy for inhalant allergies. Postgrad Med 2001;109(5):89–106.
10. Osguthorpe JD. Immunotherapy. Curr Opin Otolaryngol Head Neck Surg 2010; 18:206–12.
11. Pipet A, Botturi K, Pinot D, et al. Allergen-specific immunotherapy in allergic rhinitis and asthma. Mechanisms and proof of efficacy. Respir Med 2009;103:800–12.
12. Schmidt-Weber CB, Blaser K. Immunological mechanisms in specific immunotherapy. Springer Semin Immunopathol 2004;25:377–90.

13. Till SJ, Francis JN, Nouri-Aria K, et al. Mechanisms of immunotherapy. J Allergy Clin Immunol 2004;113(6):1025–34 [quiz: 1035].
14. Bousquet J, Khaltaev N, Cruz AA, et al. Allergic Rhinitis and its Impact on Asthma (ARIA) 2008 update (in collaboration with the World Health Organization, GA(2) LEN and AllerGen). Allergy 2008;63(Suppl 86):8–160.
15. Hurst DS, Gordon BR, Fornadley JA, et al. Safety of home-based and office allergy immunotherapy: a multicenter prospective study. Otolaryngol Head Neck Surg 1999;121:553–61.
16. Haydon RC, Gordon BR. Aeroallergen immunotherapy. In: Krouse JH, Chadwick SJ, Gordon BR, et al, editors. Allergy and immunology: an otolaryngic approach. Philadelphia: Lippincott Williams and Wilkins; 2002. p. 151–84.
17. Cox L, Li J, Nelson HS, et al. Allergen immunotherapy: a practice parameter second update. J Allergy Clin Immunol 2007;120:S25–85.
18. Slater JE. Standardized allergen vaccines in the United States. J Clin Allergy Immunol 2008;21:273–82.
19. Nelson HS. Multiallergen immunotherapy for allergic rhinitis and asthma. J Allergy Clin Immunol 2009;123:763–9.
20. Freeman J. "Rush inoculation," with special reference for hay fever treatment. Lancet 1930;215:744–7.
21. Cohn JR, Pizzi A. Determinants of patient compliance with allergen immunotherapy. J Allergy Clin Immunol 1993;91(3):734–7.
22. Pfaar O, Klimek L, Fischer I, et al. Safety of two cluster schedules for subcutaneous immunotherapy in allergic rhinitis or asthma patients sensitized to inhalant allergens. Int Arch Allergy Immunol 2009;150:102–8.
23. Cox L. Accelerated immunotherapy schedules: review of efficacy and safety. Ann Allergy Asthma Immunol 2006;97:126–38.
24. Cox L, Cohn JR. Duration of allergen immunotherapy in respiratory allergy: when is enough, enough? Ann Allergy Asthma Immunol 2007;98:416–26.
25. Calderon MA, Alves B, Jacobson M, et al. Allergen injection immunotherapy for seasonal allergic rhinitis. Cochrane Database Syst Rev 2007;1:CD001936.
26. Passalacqua G, Durham SR. Allergic rhinitis and its impact on asthma update: allergen immunotherapy. J Allergy Clin Immunol 2007;119(4):881–91.
27. Frew AJ, Powell RJ, Corrigan CJ, et al. Efficacy and safety of specific immunotherapy with SQ allergen extract in treatment-resistant seasonal allergic rhinoconjunctivitis. J Allergy Clin Immunol 2006;117(2):319–25.
28. Walker SM, Pajno GB, Lima MT, et al. Grass pollen immunotherapy for seasonal rhinitis and asthma: a randomized controlled trial. J Allergy Clin Immunol 2001; 107(1):87–93.
29. Varney VA, Edwards J, Tabbah K, et al. Clinical efficacy of specific immunotherapy to cat dander: a double-blind placebo-controlled trial. Clin Exp Allergy 1997;27(8):860–7.
30. Bousquet J, Calvayrac P, Guerin B, et al. Immunotherapy with a standardized Dermatophagoides pteronyssinus extract. I. In vivo and in vitro parameters after a short course of treatment. J Allergy Clin Immunol 1985;76(5):734–44.
31. Bousquet J, Hejjaoui A, Clauzel AM, et al. Specific immunotherapy with a standardized Dermatophagoides pteronyssinus extract. II. Prediction of efficacy of immunotherapy. J Allergy Clin Immunol 1988;82(6):971–7.
32. Varney VA, Tabbah K, Mavroleon G, et al. Usefulness of specific immunotherapy in patients with severe perennial allergic rhinitis induced by house dust mite: a double-blind, randomized, placebo-controlled trial. Clin Exp Allergy 2003; 33(8):1076–82.

33. Calderon MA, Carr VA, Jacobson M, et al. Allergen injection immunotherapy for perennial allergic rhinitis. Cochrane Database Syst Rev 2008;2:CD007163.
34. Van Wijk RG. When to initiate immunotherapy in children with allergic disease? Lessons from the paediatric studies. Curr Opin Allergy Clin Immunol 2008;8: 565–70.
35. Roder E, Berger MY, De Groot H, et al. Immunotherapy in children and adolescents with allergic rhinoconjuntivitis: a systematic review. Pediatr Allergy Immunol 2008;19:197–207.
36. Eng PA, Reinhold M, Gnehm HP. Long-term efficacy of preseasonal grass pollen immunotherapy in children. Allergy 2002;57:306–12.
37. Eng PA, Borer-Reinhold M, Heijnen IA, et al. Twelve-year follow-up after discontinuation of preseasonal grass pollen immunotherapy in childhood. Allergy 2006;61:198–201.
38. Durham SR, Walker SM, Varga EM, et al. Long-term clinical efficacy of grass-pollen immunotherapy. N Engl J Med 1999;341(7):468–75.
39. Tella R, Bartra J, San Miguel M, et al. Effects of specific immunotherapy on the development of new sensitizations in monosensitized patients. Allergol Immunopathol 2003;31(4):221–5.
40. Ebner C, Kraft D, Ebner H. Booster immunotherapy (BIT). Allergy 1994;49(1): 38–42.
41. Jacobsen L, Nuchel Petersen B, Wihl JA, et al. Immunotherapy with partially purified and standardized tree pollen extracts: IV. Results from long-term (6-year) follow-up. Allergy 1997;52(9):914–20.
42. Rogala B, Markiewics-Bendkowska IB, Brzoza Z, et al. Side-effects of injective allergen immunotherapy administered to intermittent or persistent allergic rhinitis patients. Rhinology 2007;45:134–9.
43. Tamir R, Levy I, Duer S, et al. Immediate adverse reactions to immunotherapy in allergy. Allergy 1992;47(3):260–3.
44. Nettis E, Giordano D, Pannofino A, et al. Safety of inhalant allergen immunotherapy with mass units-standardized extracts. Clin Exp Allergy 2002;32:1745–9.
45. Toubi E, Kessel A, Blant A, et al. Follow-up after systemic adverse reactions of immunotherapy. Allergy 1999;54(6):617–20.
46. Bousquet J, Lockey R, Malling HJ. Allergen immunotherapy: therapeutic vaccines for allergic diseases. A WHO position paper. J Allergy Clin Immunol 1998;102(4 Pt1):558–62.
47. Lockey RF, Benedict LM, Turkeltaub PC, et al. Fatalities from immunotherapy (IT) and skin testing (ST). J Allergy Clin Immunol 1987;79(4):660–77.
48. Committee on Safety in Medicine. Desensitizing vaccines. Br Med J 1986;293:948.
49. Berto P, Frati F, Incorvaia C. Economic studies of immunotherapy: a review. Curr Opin Allergy Clin Immunol 2008;8(6):585–9.
50. Omnes LF, Bousquet J, Scheinmann P, et al. Pharmacoeconomic assessment of specific immunotherapy versus current symptomatic treatment for allergic rhinitis and asthma in France. Eur Ann Allergy Clin Immunol 2007;39(5):148–56.
51. Hankin CS, Cox L, Lang D, et al. Allergen immunotherapy and health care cost benefits for children with allergic rhinitis: a large-scale, retrospective, matched cohort study. Ann Allergy Asthma Immunol 2010;104(1):79–85.
52. Schadlich PK, Brecht JG. Economic evaluation of specific immunotherapy versus symptomatic treatment of allergic rhinitis in Germany. Pharmacoeconomics 2000; 17(1):37–52.
53. Passalacqua G, Compalati E, Canonica GW. Advances in allergen-specific immunotherapy. Curr Drug Targets 2009;10:1255–62.

Sublingual Immunotherapy

Sandra Y. Lin, MD[a,*], Bryan Leatherman, MD[b]

KEYWORDS

- Sublingual immunotherapy • Allergen-specific immunotherapy
- Allergic rhinitis • Subcutaneous immunotherapy • Asthma

Key Points: Sublingual Immunotherapy for Allergy

- SLIT has been show in multiple studies to be efficacious in allergic rhinitis for adults and children.
- SLIT has also been shown to be helpful in asthma and in preventing the development of new sensitivities to allergens.
- Studies have shown immunologic changes in SLIT that are similar to SCIT, suggesting a similar mechanism of action.
- SLIT enjoys a good safety profile, allowing for the convenience of dosing in the home and in individuals unable to tolerate injections, such a young children, although a few cases of anaphylaxis have been reported.
- The majority of literature has been published in Europe, with multiple factors making the translation of dosing to the United States difficult. Future studies will help continue to clarify optimal dosing and schedule in the United States.

The incidence of allergic disease has increased significantly over the past 40 years.[1] Allergic rhinitis is a very common health problem associated with considerable decreases in quality of life, and affects 5% to 22% of Americans.[2] Although it is typically not a life-threatening disease, medical management costs are substantial. More than $1 billion are spent on management of allergic rhinitis every year in the United States.[3] If the apparent trend of increasing atopy continues, a growing number of patients will be affected by the decreased quality of life associated with allergic rhinitis, and the increasing societal economic burdens associated with treatment of the disease and losses in worker productivity.

The mainstays of treatment for allergic rhinitis include avoidance of allergen, pharmacotherapy, and immunotherapy. Immunotherapy involves administering increasing

[a] Department of Otolaryngology-Head & Neck Surgery, Johns Hopkins School of Medicine, 601 North Caroline Street, #6254, Baltimore, MD 21287, USA
[b] Coastal Ear, Nose and Throat Associates, Coastal Sinus and Allergy Center, 1213 Broad Avenue, Suite 4, Gulfport, MS 39501, USA
* Corresponding author.
E-mail address: Slin30@jhmi.edu

Otolaryngol Clin N Am 44 (2011) 753–764
doi:10.1016/j.otc.2011.03.012 oto.theclinics.com
0030-6665/11/$ – see front matter

concentrations of allergen to sensitized individuals to reduce allergic symptoms caused by natural exposures to these allergens. When immunotherapy is administered over an adequate duration, the body gradually adapts the immune response to the sensitized allergen and allows for increased tolerance.

Immunotherapy is an alternative for individuals who are refractory to avoidance of allergens or medical therapy. Unlike pharmacotherapy or avoidance, allergen-specific immunotherapy has the advantage of providing potential continued symptom suppression after discontinuation of therapy, preventing or halting progression of asthma, and preventing the development of new allergies.[4–6] Currently, the most common form of allergen-specific injection immunotherapy in the United States is subcutaneous injection immunotherapy (SCIT), which not only has been proven to be efficacious in reducing symptoms but also effects measurable immunologic changes in individuals who have undergone this treatment.[7]

Allergen-specific injection immunotherapy was introduced approximately 100 years ago, and currently 7 to 10 million allergy immunotherapy injections are administered annually in the United States.[8] However, injection immunotherapy is associated with rare but real risks of anaphylaxis and death. Injection immunotherapy must be administered in an appropriately supervised physician's office on a repeated basis, from once a week to once a month over several years. For many young children, needle-phobic patients, and areas with limited access to specialists, injection immunotherapy is not a realistic treatment option.

Over the years, different routes of allergen-specific immunotherapy administration have been investigated as alternatives to injection immunotherapy.[9] Previous studies of oral immunotherapy found that this route was not efficacious, and the same is true of bronchial immunotherapy, which also confers a high risk of bronchospasm. Local nasal immunotherapy has been shown to significantly improve allergy symptoms and decrease the need for allergy medications. However, local nasal immunotherapy must be carefully administered to prevent bronchospasm, and it frequently provokes rhinitis on administration. None of these alternative dosing routes has gained popularity in the clinical arena. Sublingual immunotherapy (SLIT), in which the allergen is held under the tongue for an interval and then either swallowed or spit out, was first introduced in the United States in the 1940s, but it did not gain widespread acceptance at that time.

Concerns over safety, patient convenience, and patient tolerability of injection allergen immunotherapy led to renewed interest in alternative forms of immunotherapy. In 1986, the British Committee for the Safety of Medicine questioned the risk–benefit ratio of SCIT after several deaths occurred.[10] Although subsequent investigation found the deaths to be from avoidable human error, this report greatly increased interest in developing alternative routes of immunotherapy. Interest in SLIT steadily increased after sublingual administration of dust mite allergen was reported in 1986.[11] Since the early reports more than 2 decades ago, investigators have published increasing data on the safety and efficacy of SLIT, primarily in Europe. Data supporting the clinical use of SLIT began to increase, and in 1998 the World Health Organization (WHO) concluded that SLIT was an acceptable means of immunotherapy.[12] Further publications by the European Academy of Allergy and Immunology and the Allergic Rhinitis and Its Impact on Asthma (ARIA) treatment guideline support the use of SLIT in allergen desensitization in children and adults.[7,13]

The use of SLIT in clinical practice has increased in Europe over the past 2 decades. The European clinical experience includes SLIT in the form of oral aqueous and tablet formulations. Its excellent safety profile has allowed it to be administered in the convenience of the home, and the lack of needles makes it an attractive option in the pediatric population. Interest in SLIT has also been increasing in the United States, with some clinicians offering this treatment modality to patients. However, because no sublingual allergens are currently approved by the U.S. Food and Drug Administration (FDA), these practitioners are using allergens approved for injection immunotherapy in an off-label route of administration.

IMMUNOLOGIC RESPONSE

Several articles have addressed the immunologic effects of SLIT, both local and systemic. Experts believe the interaction of the allergen in the sublingual mucosa may be important in the mechanism of action. A study involving radiolabeled SLIT found evidence of radioactivity in the oral cavity for 2 to 20 hours after initial administration of SLIT; this is thought to possibly be caused by the local uptake of antigen by dendritic cells.[14] Other studies have focused on potential local immune changes in the oral submucosa. A study comparing sublingual mucosal biopsies of subjects receiving SLIT with those of controls found no difference in CD3+, CD1a+, or CD68+ cell counts.[15] However, another study found that sublingual salivary eosinophil cationic protein was significantly reduced after 7 months of SLIT.[16]

A larger number of studies have focused on the systemic immunologic responses induced by SLIT, particularly examining changes in serum inflammatory mediators. Several studies have shown that one of the most consistent changes in inflammatory mediators is the reduction of serum eosinophil cationic protein (ECP). This decrease has been seen in both children and adults after 6 to 24 months of treatment with SLIT.[17–20] The decrease in ECP was found to correspond with a decrease in serum eosinophil counts.[21] The most widely studied antibody responses to SLIT include changes in IgE and IgG4. Studies show decreases in antigen-specific IgE after treatment with SLIT; antigen-specific serum IgG4 has shown a dose–response increase to SLIT after the first year of use, and then a plateau in levels.[22–24] SLIT has also been shown to suppress skin prick test after treatment,[23,25,26] although this seems to be affected by duration of treatment, with suppression in skin responses seen after 18 to 24 months of use.

The immunologic changes seen after SLIT administration are similar to those seen after administration of SCIT. Both induce changes in skin testing, increases in allergen-specific IgG4, and decreases in antigen-specific IgE. These findings suggest a similar mechanism underlies both routes of immunotherapy. SCIT induces changes in regulatory T cells that lead to increased tolerance of antigen, and SLIT probably acts in a similar manner.[27]

EFFICACY

Several recent large reviews and meta-analyses discuss the efficacy of SLIT. In 2005, Wilson and colleagues[28] published the first large-scale meta-analysis entitled "Sublingual Immunotherapy for Allergic Rhinitis," which examined 979 pediatric and adult subjects pooled from 22 randomized, double-blind, placebo-controlled studies of SLIT. This meta-analysis found significant reductions in symptom and medication scores with SLIT, and concluded that it was effective in treating allergic rhinitis. The authors acknowledged, however, the large heterogeneity in dosages and treatment schedules among the studies.

In 2006, the American Academy of Allergy, Asthma and Immunology (AAAAI) and the American College of Allergy, Asthma, and Immunology (ACAAI) formed a task force that was charged with providing a comprehensive, updated report on SLIT for the North American Allergy community.[29] The ACAAI/AAAAI task force reviewed

104 articles addressing SLIT dosing, efficacy, immunologic response, and safety. The doses used in the studies varied by 30,000-fold, with frequency ranging from daily to weekly; few comparative studies were found regarding optimal dosing and schedules. Of the 47 studies that met criteria for clinical efficacy, most showed some evidence of this. Studies suggested a dose–response effect, but a consistent relationship among treatment dose, duration, and efficacy was not found. Although the task force found evidence for the efficacy of SLIT in treating allergic rhinitis, many questions remain regarding SLIT, including was is the effective dose and schedule.

Other SLIT studies have examined efficacy in specific subpopulations, such as asthmatics. In 2006, Calamita and colleagues[30] performed a systematic review of the efficacy of SLIT in asthma. This review included randomized controlled clinical trials involving adult and pediatric patients and conducted from 1974 to 2005; 1706 patients from 25 studies met study inclusion criteria. The authors found that SLIT was beneficial for asthma treatment in terms of symptoms, medication use, lung function, and bronchial provocation. However, the authors concluded that the effects, although statistically significant, were small in scale.

The pediatric population is another subgroup in which the efficacy of SLIT is studied frequently. In 2006, Penangos and colleagues[31] published a meta-analysis focusing on the use of SLIT in patients aged 3 to 18 years. Ten studies met selection criteria, and 484 patients from these studies were evaluated. The authors found a significant reduction in symptoms and medication use after SLIT. Subset analysis showed a greater improvement related to seasonal allergens as opposed to perennial, and for patients receiving therapy for greater than 18 months. The authors concluded that SLIT was an effective form of therapy for allergic rhinitisin the pediatric population. An updated review in 2008 found evidence of efficacy with SLIT for grass allergies in children, but the evidence of efficacy in dust mite allergy was inconsistent.[32]

Other pediatric studies have examined the potential protective effects of SLIT on the pediatric population. For example, Novembre and colleagues[33] studied whether short-term coseasonal SLIT for grass allergen would benefit children compared with a control group taking standard allergy and asthma medications. The SLIT group underwent 3 years of therapy. At the conclusion of the study, the control group was found to be 3.8 times more likely to have developed asthma than the SLIT-treated group. The authors concluded that SLIT not only improved seasonal allergic rhinitis symptoms but also reduced the development of seasonal asthma in children with grass pollen allergy.

Another study by Marogna and colleagues[34] in 2008 also focused on the preventative effects of SLIT in children. In this study, 216 children were randomized to receive either medications alone or SLIT plus medications for 3 years. New sensitizations to allergens were found in 34.8% of controls compared with 3.1% receiving SLIT. Mild persistent asthma also occurred less frequently in the SLIT group. The number of children with positive methacholine challenge tests decreased significantly after 3 years in the SLIT group only, suggesting that SLIT reduces both new sensitizations and bronchial hyperreactivity. Di Rienzo and colleagues[35] also evaluated the duration of these positive SLIT effects in children The children in this study received either 4 to 5 years of SLIT (n = 35) or allergy medications (n = 25). The patients were evaluated at baseline, end of SLIT, and 4 to 5 years after SLIT discontinuation. The SLIT group was found either to be less likely to have asthma or to have improved asthma. The positive clinical effects were maintained for 4 to 5 years after discontinuation of SLIT.

Several recent publications have focused on the efficacy of a specific form of SLIT, the grass tablet.[36,37] The sublingual grass antigen tablet is currently available in Europe, and efforts seem to be underway to bring it to the United States. These multicenter, double-blind, and placebo-controlled studies have shown a significant reduction in allergy symptoms in grass-sensitized patients. The grass tablet has also decreased the need for medication, improved asthma, and improved disease-specific quality of life. Efficacy seems to be greater if the grass tablet is given preseason. Administration of the grass tablet has also led to corresponding immunologic changes seen with allergen-specific immunotherapy, such as an increase in antigen-specific IgG.

Similar to the grass tablet studies, most SLIT studies have been single allergen studies; however, most allergic patients in the United States are polysensitized. In the United States, most practitioners use multiantigen treatment when using allergy-specific immunotherapy to treat polysensitized patients. Of the few studies performed on the use of SLIT in polysensitized patients, one published in the United States in 2009 evaluated the quality of life using multiantigen SLIT.[38] Patients undergoing multiantigen SLIT were found to have statistical improvement in 12 of 14 domains of the Mini Rhinoconjunctivitis Quality of Life Questionnaire. This study, although small, offered encouraging pilot results of multiantigen SLIT. A subsequent larger European study of SLIT in polysensitized subjects found similar gains in disease-specific quality of life.[39]

The literature has attempted to answer the important question of how SLIT compares with SCIT in terms of efficacy. Although studies have found both modalities to be efficacious,[40–43] no agreement has been reached on which treatment is more effective. In a double-blind, placebo-controlled study performed in 2004[43] comparing SLIT and SCIT in birch pollen–sensitive subjects, both therapies decreased symptoms and medication scores compared with placebo. Although SLIT had a higher safety profile, a nonsignificant greater improvement occurred in the SCIT group. Among the varied findings in multiple studies, no clear cut answer seems to exist regarding the efficacy of SLIT versus SCIT; this is an area that would benefit from future, large-scale, randomized, placebo-controlled studies.

SAFETY

The safety profile of SLIT compared with traditional SCIT is one of the reasons for increased interest in the sublingual dosing route. In Europe, SLIT has been dosed at the patient's home rather than the physician's office because of its perceived improved safety profile. However, there have been reported side effects and adverse reactions to SLIT. SLIT studies have typically broken down the adverse events into local and systemic reactions. Local reactions include oral irritation and itching, with an estimated prevalence of 0.68 per 1000 doses.[29] Reported systemic reactions to SLIT include asthma, urticaria, gastrointestinal symptoms, and other systemic reactions that have been severe enough to require hospitalization, according to a recent large review.[29] This review of SLIT also examined safety of SLIT comparison with SCIT; in 1,019,826 SLIT doses, 14 serious adverse events were reported. The rate of systemic reactions was 0.6% for SCIT versus 0.056% SLIT, and the prevalence of death was 1 per 2.5 million for SCIT versus no reported deaths for SLIT. These findings indicate an improved safety profile of SLIT over SCIT.

However, as the use of SLIT has increased in Europe over the past 20 years, severe systemic and anaphylactic reactions have been reported in clinical use. The first report of anaphylaxis in Europe was in an asthmatic child undergoing SLIT with a dust mite and pollen mix at maintenance dosing.[44] This reaction occurred during peak spring pollen season. Other reports of anaphylaxis in the Netherlands involved the use of the sublingual grass tablet; two individuals who had previous reactions to SCIT experienced severe systemic reactions to their first dose of grass tablet.[45] The authors suggested that the first dose of grass tablet be given to patients in a supervised setting in a physician's office. Finally, a report of SLIT anaphylaxis in the United States[46] occurred in a patient with asthma who was being treated with multiantigen therapy while in the escalation phase. Large-scale reviews of SLIT have been unable to find consistent relationships between adverse events and dose, or whether these occur in escalation versus maintenance therapy.[29] However, a recent clinical study did not find skin test sensitivity, asthma, gender, or age to be risk factors predictive of adverse events.[47]

Although SLIT has a good safety profile that appears to be better than SCIT, and has been dosed in Europe in the home for 20 years, serious reactions have been reported, suggesting that clinicians offering SLIT should perform some common sense safety precautions. For example, patient vials should be labeled with more than one patient identifier to avoid distribution to the wrong patient. Mixing should be performed in a quiet environment where no outside distractions can lead to errors in mixing. Patients must be thoroughly educated on how to perform proper dosing at home, and consideration given to administering the first dose in the office. Patients receiving allergen-specific immunotherapy should be instructed on the signs and symptoms of anaphylaxis. Patients should be trained on how to use an epinephrine auto injection device and should be given a prescription for the device. These steps and precautions may provide increased safety for patients receiving SLIT.

DOSING

Although different dosing techniques are available for SCIT, fairly standard techniques for escalation and maintenance doses have been adopted and taught by the major allergy associations in the United States. The optimal dosage, timing of administration, and optimal length of treatment with SLIT are not as clearly defined. One of the earliest references to SLIT dosing in the otolaryngology literature is found in a training manual written by French Hansel and Jack Anderson in the late 1950s.[48] Most modern dosing information available in the literature comes from European studies using antigens that are not available in the United States. Multiple factors make it difficult to compare the effective doses used in these published studies. A direct correlation has been difficult to establish between the antigen content of sublingual preparations used in most published European studies and the antigen content of products available in the United States. These factors have made the effective dose of SLIT using the liquid-based antigen preparations available in the United States more difficult to establish. Fortunately, more information is becoming available, and some general insight can be obtained from the large number of sublingual studies available in the literature, providing some basis for determining an effective dose. One fairly consistent finding from previous studies is that higher doses of antigen are necessary for SLIT than for SCIT. It is also clear that a level of safety has been shown over wide variations in dosing amounts for SLIT. Furthermore, several larger studies conducted in North America within the past few years give some measure of what is an effective dose.

Correlations should be attempted between the antigen units reported in studies conducted outside the United States and those currently available in the United States to establish a comparable dosing strategy. Larenas-Linnemann and Cox[49] published their efforts to determine the antigen content in the SLIT products used in many of the European sublingual studies and available on the European pharmaceutical market. Determining the true antigen content is often challenging, and they concluded that they were unable to accurately determine the microgram allergen contents sufficiently to correlate with allergen products available in the United States. This conclusion has some limitations, however. The major allergen content of many of the sublingual products from European antigen suppliers is identified in the study. The study mentions that these should not be compared directly with micrograms of antigen available in United States because of differences in the technique used to determine major allergen content. This same limitation would therefore also need to be applied to SCIT. Recommendations have been made on target microgram doses for SCIT based on studies using antigens from one allergen manufacturer.[50] Given the cost limitations in replicating large dose–response studies to include multiple allergen extract providers, it is reasonable to make some correlations with an established effective microgram dose and apply that microgram dose for treatment using extract from a separate manufacturer, both for SCIT and SLIT. However, more dose–response studies are needed for both SLIT and SCIT to evaluate what dose of antigen produces good results without producing excessive risk.

Most algorithms use daily dosing. Variation exists in the duration of dosage escalation, but the overall trend is toward very short periods of escalation or no escalation at all.[51] Sambugaro and colleagues[52] published an induction phase comparison in 2003. The randomized open study included three different induction schedules (8-, 15-, and 20-day inductions, respectively) and a control group. All three groups had a once-daily maintenance phase for a total treatment duration of 2 years. The authors found no significant difference in the rate of adverse events with the three different induction groups. Reviews of substantial numbers of clinical trials have not shown a correlation between adverse events and different durations of escalation.[29,53] The tablet-based SLIT products available in Europe do not use dose escalation, but rather start at the maintenance dose with the first dose. Once the maintenance dose is achieved, it is continued daily in most clinical trials. The target sublingual maintenance dose has not been established for any commercially available allergen product in the United States, but recent data allow some generalizations to be made.

Although no dosing schedule can be found on the product labels for antigens available in the United States, several practical observations can be made. The maintenance dose used in clinical trials has ranged from 3 to 500 times the typical SCIT injection dose for the given study center.[53] Most of the European antigen manufacturers' recommendations for monthly maintenance SLIT dose are between 5 and 45 times the dose they recommend for SCIT maintenance treatment with their products.[49] Several recent North American–based SLIT studies can provide some insight into potential effective dose ranges. Greer Laboratories conducted a study evaluating the efficacy of SLIT for short ragweed using their liquid short ragweed antigen product currently labeled for SCIT use.[54] The study showed a reduction in rhinoconjunctivitis symptoms and antiallergy medication use scores for both the 4.8 and 48 Amb a 1 unit doses versus placebo. The reduction only reached statistical significance for the higher dose. Compared with other recent studies, the Greer study included a relatively low number of participants. Nonetheless, the study did not produce as vigorous improvements as desired, and did not allow for inclusion of SLIT dosing on the short ragweed product label. The study does at least provide a target dosing range within which improvements were observed.

The results of two large North American studies using tablet-based timothy grass SLIT were recently reported. The first study was conducted in the pediatric population[55] and showed a significant reduction in total combined symptom and medication scores (26% reduction) and individual daily symptom (25% reduction) and medication use scores (66% reduction). This study replicated the previous findings with the product in similar studies conducted at European centers. The maintenance dose used in this study was approximately 15 μg of Phl p 5 timothy antigen. A study in the adult population[56] using the same timothy grass tablet resulted in a significant reduction in total combined symptom and medication scores, individual daily symptom scores, and daily medication use scores (20%, 18%, and 26% reductions, respectively). However, approximately 85% of the patients in both of these studies were multisensitized to other nongrass antigens but were treated only for timothy grass. Although these studies show significant efficacy for a tablet-based SLIT product that is not currently available commercially in the United States, they provide a reasonable maintenance microgram target dose for timothy grass SLIT that can be prepared with currently available liquid antigen products, with reasonable expectations of safety and efficacy. More large studies are underway at European centers evaluating the efficacy of tablet-based SLIT for house dust mite and birch antigens. These studies will provide more insight into approximate microgram dosing ranges necessary for efficacy for other antigens.

The timing of SLIT has also been a topic of discussion and study. In different clinical trials, the antigen has been delivered perennially, preseasonal, and coseasonal, and coseasonal alone. Perennial administration of SCIT for 3 to 5 years is generally preferable for long-term maintenance of the improvement after immunotherapy completion. A recent study[57] evaluated the use of a five grass sublingual mixture delivered coseasonally only for three consecutive grass pollen seasons. The study showed a significant reduction in combined symptom and medication scores, and individual daily symptom scores. The reduction seen in daily medication scores did not reach significance. These patients were also followed up for 3 years after completion of the active treatment. A continued reduction in all three parameters was seen, but only daily symptom scores maintained statistically significant reductions. This study shows that SLIT given only during the season at least may generate improvements, which may improve the willingness of some patients to use the treatment. Another study evaluated the efficacy of dust mite SLIT given intermittently versus continually over a year.[58] One group was given SLIT treatment daily for a year, and a second group alternated between 2 months of active treatment and 2 months off treatment. Both treatment groups showed a significant reduction in allergy symptoms and overall quality of life measures. This study was only preliminary, but at least showed that improvement could be achieved with intermittent dosing schedules. The long-term effect is unknown with this type of dosing schedule. Another publication investigated the efficacy of coseasonal and perennial SLIT.[59] The authors performed an independent patient data meta-analysis of three open, prospective, observational studies of SLIT using standardized allergen extracts in patients with allergic rhinoconjunctivitis with and without asthma to compare the effectiveness of perennial and coseasonal treatments, and ultra-rush and standard titrations. A total of 1052 patients were assessed, and symptom improvement was seen in all treatment groups, with no significant difference between perennial, coseasonal, ultra-rush, and standard titration protocols. This study is obviously limited by a lack of controls, but does show that multiple options may be available for sublingual dosing that can be tailored to the needs of individual patients.

Durham and colleagues[60] recently published a report analyzing the sustained effect of 3 years of active SLIT with timothy grass tablets in 257 subjects who had previously shown significant improvement in daily symptom and medication scores during a 3-year trial of sublingual timothy grass tablets. One year after completing active SLIT treatment, these subjects were reevaluated during grass season and were found to maintain a significant reduction in allergy symptoms (26% reduction) and medication use (29% reduction) scores compared with the placebo group. The study is important because it involves a large number of patients in a well-designed and controlled study who showed significant sustained improvement in both symptom and medication use scores at least 1 year posttreatment after the active SLIT treatment was given perennially for 3 years.

A large collection of world literature now supports the efficacy and safety of SLIT, and this treatment modality has been advocated as effective by the WHO,[12] the World Allergy Association,[61] the European Academy of Allergy and Clinical Immunology,[62] and the ARIA study.[7] Although an FDA-approved SLIT allergen extract product is not currently available in the United States, this does not indicate that SLIT cannot be effective in the United States, especially after it has shown efficacy in multiple other countries. Although the optimal dose of SLIT prepared with liquid-based antigen extract products available in the United States needs to be clarified, the amount of information available allows physicians to make reasonable estimations of possible effective doses for appropriate patients. The great safety profile shown with SLIT allows a cushion of safety while the most effective sublingual dose is determined for different antigens. It is certainly reasonable for physicians to extrapolate the existing data to offer SLIT to patients. Numerous physicians are offering SLIT to their patients across the United States, with anecdotal good success in improving allergic disease. Many medications are commonly used in an FDA off-label manner when a physician determines this to be appropriate for an individual patient. In fairness, much of the SCIT doses in use are extrapolated from limited amounts of dose–response data for a limited number of antigens. All of the antigen extracts available in the United States have FDA labeling for single-antigen use, but allergists more commonly deliver these antigens in multiallergen vials. The use of multiallergen SCIT is an off-label use of an FDA-approved product. In addition, no data support that the same amount of antigen is required to produce symptom improvement with SCIT when given in combination with other antigens versus giving the antigen by itself; therefore, either greater or lesser amounts may be required for each individual antigen when delivering multiantigen immunotherapy. Experts have generally assumed and placed into practice that the same amount of antigen should be delivered whether single or multiantigen immunotherapy is used. To exclude SLIT as a reasonable treatment option because of the lack of an FDA-approved dose would be selectively applying the standard to SLIT, while not requiring it for SCIT. All of these limitations should be discussed with patients undergoing immunotherapy. The hope is that more information will become available about the optimal dose of antigen for SLIT for different antigen preparations available in the United States, or that an FDA-approved product will become commercially available. In the meantime, individual physicians must evaluate the appropriateness of SLIT for individual patients in their practice, and use the best information currently available to determine what dose of antigen to deliver.

REFERENCES

1. Howarth PH. Is allergy increasing?—early life influences. Clin Exp Allergy 1998; 28(Suppl 6):2–7.
2. Bellanti JA, Wallerstedt DB. Allergic rhinitis update: epidemiology and natural history. Allergy Asthma Proc 2000;21(6):367–70.
3. Nathan RA. The burden of allergic rhinitis. Allergy Asthma Proc 2007;28(1):3–9.
4. Durham SR, Walker SM, Varga EM, et al. Long-term clinical efficacy of grass-pollen immunotherapy. N Engl J Med 1999;341:468–75.
5. Purello-D'ambrosio F, Gangemi S, Merendino RA, et al. Prevention of new sensitizations in monosensitized subjects submitted to specific immunotherapy or not. A retrospective study. Clin Exp Allergy 2001;31:1295–302.
6. Polosa R, Al-Delaimy WK, Russo C, et al. Greater risk of incident asthma cases in adults with allergic rhinitis and effect of allergen immunotherapy: a retrospective cohort study. Respir Res 2005;6:153.

7. Bousquet J, Van Cauwenberge P, Khaltaev N. Allergic rhinitis and its impact on asthma. J Allergy Clin Immunol 2001;108:S147–334.
8. Lockey R. Adverse skin reactions associated with skin testing and immunotherapy. Allergy Proc 1995;16(6):292–6.
9. Canonica GW, Passalcqua AG. Noninjection routes for immunotherapy. J Allergy Clin Immunol 2003;111:437–48.
10. Medicines CotSo. CMS update: desensitizing vaccines. Br Med J 1986;292:984.
11. Scadding GK, Brostoff J. Low dose sublingual therapy in patients with allergic rhinitis due to house dust mite. Clin Allergy 1986;16:483–91.
12. Bousquet J, Lockey R, Maling H. World Health Organization Position paper: allergen immunotherapy: therapeutic vaccines for allergic diseases. Allergy 1998;53:1–14.
13. Malling H, Abreu-Noguera J, Alvarez-Cuesta E, et al. EAACI/EXPACI position paper on local immunotherapy. Allergy 1998;53:933–44.
14. Bagnosco M, Mariani G, Passalacqu G, et al. Absorption and distribution kinetics of the major Parietaria judaica allergen (Par j 1) administered by noninjectable routes in healthy human beings. J Allergy Clin Immunol 1997;100:122–9.
15. Lima M, Wilson D, Pitkin L, et al. Grass pollen sublingual immunotherapy for seasonal rhinoconjunctivitis: a randomized controlled trial. Clin Exp Allergy 2002;32:507–14.
16. Marcucci F, Sensi L, Frate F, et al. Sublingual tryptase and ECP in children treated with grass pollen sublingual immunotherapy (SLIT): safety and immunologic implications. Allergy 2001;56:1091–5.
17. Passalacqua G, Albano M, Fregonese L, et al. Randomized controlled trial of local allergoid immunotherapy on allergic inflammation in mite induced rhinoconjunctivitis. Lancet 1998;351:629–32.
18. Ippoliti F, De Santis W, Volterrani A, et al. Immunomodulation during sublingual therapy in allergic children. Pediatr Allergy Immunol 2003;14:216–21.
19. Sanchez Palacios A, Shcamann F, Garcia JA. Sublingual immunotherapy with cat epithelial extract. Personal experience. Allergol Immunopathol (Madr) 2001;29:60–5.
20. Durham SR, Yang WH, Pedersen MR, et al. Sublingual immunotherapy with once-daily grass allergen tablets: a randomized controlled trial in seasonal allergic rhinoconjunctivitis. J Allergy Clin Immunol 2006;117:802–9.
21. Bahceciler NN, Arikan C, Taylor A, et al. Impact of sublingual immunotherapy on specific antibody levels in asthmatic children allergic to house dust mites. Int Arch Allergy Immunol 2005;136:287–94.
22. Bufe A, Aiegler-Kirbach E, Stoeckmann E, et al. Efficacy of sublingual swallow immunotherapy in children with severe grass pollen allergic symptoms: a double-blind placebo-controlled study. Allergy 2004;59:498–504.
23. La Rosa M, Ranno C, Andre C, et al. Double blind placebo-controlled evaluation of sublingual-swallow immunotherapy with standardized Parietaria judaica extract in children with allergic rhinoconjunctivitis. J Allergy Clin Immunol 1999;104:425–32.
24. Smith H, White P, Annila I, et al. Randomized controlled trial of high-dose sublingual immunotherapy to treat seasonal allergic rhinitis. J Allergy Clin Immunol 2004;114(4):831–7.
25. Tonnel AB, Sherperrl A, Douay B, et al. Allergic rhinitis due to house dust mites: evaluation of the efficacy of specific sublingual immunotherapy. Allergy 2004;59:491–7.
26. Tari MG, Mancino M, Monti G. Efficacy of sublingual immunotherapy in patients with rhinitis and asthma due to house dust mite. A double blind study. Allergol Immunopathol (Madr) 1990;18:277–84.

27. Tari MG, Mancino M, Madonna F, et al. Immunologic evaluation of 24 month course of sublingual immunotherapy. Allergol Immunopathol (Madr) 1994;22(5):209–16.
28. Wilson DR, Torres LI, Durham SR. Sublingual immunotherapy for allergic rhinitis. Cochrane Database Syst Rev 2003;2:CD002893.
29. Cox LS, Linnemann DL, Nolte H, et al. Sublingual immunotherapy: a comprehensive review. J Allergy Clin Immunol 2006;117:1021–35.
30. Calamita Z, Saconato H, Pela AG, et al. Efficacy of sublingual immunotherapy in asthma: systematic review of randomized-clinical trials using the Cochrane Collaboration method. Allergy 2006;62(10):1162–72.
31. Penangos M, Compalati E, Tarantini F, et al. Efficacy of sublingual immunotherapy in the treatment of allergic rhinitis in pediatric patients 3 to 18 years of age: a meta-analysis of randomized, placebo-controlled, double-blind trials. Ann Allergy Asthma Immunol 2006;97(2):141–8.
32. Larenas-Linnemann D. Subcutaneous and sublingual immunotherapy in children: complete update on controversies, dosing, and efficacy. Curr Allergy Asthma Rep 2008;8(6):465–74.
33. Novembre E, Galli E, Landi F, et al. Coseasonal sublingual immunotherapy reduces the development of asthma in children with allergic rhinoconjuntivitis. J Allergy Clin Immunol 2004;114(4):851–7.
34. Marogna M, Tomassetti D, Bernasconi A, et al. Preventive effects of sublingual immunotherapy in childhood: an open randomized controlled study. Ann Allergy Asthma Immunol 2008;101(2):206–11.
35. Di Rienzo V, Marcucci F, Puccinelli P, et al. Long-lasting effect of sublingual immunotherapy in children with asthma due to house dust mite: a 10 year prospective study. Clin Exp Allergy 2003;33(2):206–10.
36. Wahn U, Tabar A, Kuna P, et al. Efficacy and safety of 5-grass-pollen sublingual immunotherapy tablets in pediatric allergic rhinoconjunctivitis. J Allergy Clin Immunol 2009;123(1):160–6.
37. Bufe A, Eberle P, Franke-Beckmann E, et al. Safety and efficacy in children of an SQ-standardized grass allergen tablet for sublingual immunotherapy. J Allergy Clin Immunol 2009;123(1):167–73.
38. Wise SK, Woody J, Koepp S, et al. Quality of life outcomes with sublingual immunotherapy. Am J Otolaryngol 2009;30(5):305–11.
39. Ciprandi G, Cadario G, Valle C, et al. Sublingual immunotherapy in polysensitized patients: effect on quality of life. J Investig Allergol Clin Immunol 2010;20(4):274–9.
40. Quirino T, Iemoli E, Seciliana E, et al. Sublingual versus injective immunotherapy in grass pollen allergic patients: a double blind (double dummy) study. Clin Exp Allergy 1996;26:1253–61.
41. Mungan D, Misirligil Z, Gurbuz L. Comparison of the efficacy of subcutaneous and sublingual immunotherapy in mite-sensitive patients with rhinitis and asthma—a placebo controlled study. Ann Allergy Asthma Immunol 1999;82:485–90.
42. Bernadis P, Agnoletto M, Puccinelli P, et al. Injective versus sublingual immunotherapy in Alternaria tenuis allergic patients. J Investig Allergol Clin Immuno 2000;10:142–8.
43. Kinchi MS, Poulsen LK, Carat F, et al. Clinical efficacy of sublingual and subcutaneous birch pollen allergen-specific immunotherapy: a randomized placebo-controlled, double blind, double dummy study. Allergy 2004;59:45–53.
44. Eifan AO, Keles S, Bahceciler NN, et al. Anaphylaxis to multiple pollen allergen sublingual immunotherapy. Allergy 2007;62:567–8.
45. de Groot H, Bijl A. Anaphylactic reaction after the first dose of sublingual immunotherapy with grass pollen tablet. Allergy 2009;64(6):963–4.

46. Dunsky EH, Goldstein MF, Dvorin DJ, et al. Anaphylaxis to sublingual immunotherapy. Allergy 2006;61:1235.
47. Esch RE, Bush RK, Peden D, et al. Sublingual-oral administration of standardized allergenic extracts: phase I safety and dosing results. Ann Allergy Asthma Immunol 2008;100:475–81.
48. Hansel FK, Anderson JR. Allergy in otolaryngology. Am Acad Ophthalmol Otolaryngol 1959;186 (American Academy of Ophthalmology and Otolaryngology Home Study Courses, Section on Instruction).
49. Larenas-Linnemann D, Cox LS; Immunotherapy and Allergy Diagnostics Committee of the American Academy of Allergy, Asthma and Immunology. European allergen extract units and potency: review of available information. Ann Allergy Asthma Immunol 2008;100(2):137–45.
50. Cox L, Li JT, Nelson H, et al. Allergen immunotherapy: a practice parameter second update. J Allergy Clin Immunol 2007;120:S25–85.
51. Frati F, La Grutta S, Bernardini R, et al. Sublingual immunotherapy: administration, dosages, use. Int J Immunopathol Pharmacol 2009;22(Suppl 4):13–6.
52. Sambugaro R, Puccinelli P, Burastero SE, et al. The efficacy of sublingual immunotherapy for respiratory allergy is not affected by different dosage regimens in the induction phase. Allergol Immunopathol (Madr) 2003;31:329–37.
53. Leatherman BD, Owen S, Parker M, et al. Sublingual immunotherapy: past, present, paradigm for the future? a review of the literature. Otolaryngol Head Neck Surg 2007;136:S1–20.
54. Skoner D, Gentile D, Bush R, et al. Sublingual immunotherapy in patients with allergic rhinoconjunctivitis caused by ragweed pollen. J Allergy Clin Immunol 2010;125(3):660–6.
55. Blaiss M, Maloney J, Nolte H, et al. Efficacy and safety of timothy grass allergy immunotherapy tablets in North American children and adolescents. J Allergy Clin Immunol 2011;127(1):64–71, e1–4.
56. Nelson HS, Nolte H, Creticos P, et al. Efficacy and Safety of Timothy Grass Allergy Immunotherapy Tablet (AIT) in North American Adults. J Allergy Clin Immunol 2011;127(1):72–80, e1, e2.
57. Ott H, Sieber J, Brehler R, et al. Efficacy of grass pollen sublingual immunotherapy for three consecutive seasons and after cessation of treatment: the ECRIT study. Allergy 2009;64(1):179–86.
58. Cadario G, Ciprandi G, Larosa M, et al. Comparison between continuous or intermittent schedules of sublingual immunotherapy for house dust mites: effects on compliance, patient satisfaction, quality of life and safety. Int J Immunopathol Pharmacol 2008;21(2):471–3.
59. Sieber J, Koberlein J, Mosges R. Sublingual immunotherapy in daily medical practice: effectiveness of different treatment schedules—IPD meta-analysis. Curr Med Res Opin 2010;26(4):925–32.
60. Durham SR, Emminger W, Kapp A, et al. Long-term clinical efficacy in grass pollen-induced rhinoconjunctivitis after treatment with SQ-standardized grass allergy immunotherapy tablet. J Allergy Clin Immunol 2010;125(1):131–8.
61. Canonica GW, Bousquet J, Casale T, et al. Sub-lingual immunotherapy world allergy organization position paper 2009. Allergy 2009;64(Suppl 91):1–59.
62. Alvarez-Cuesta E, Bousquet J, Canonica GW, et al. Standards for practical allergen-specific immunotherapy. Allergy 2006;61(Suppl 82):1–20.

The Allergic March: Can We Prevent Allergies and Asthma?

Bruce R. Gordon, MA, MD[a,b,c,*]

KEYWORDS

- Allergic march • Atopic march • Hygiene hypothesis
- Eczema • Asthma • Probiotics • Chemical pollution
- Inhalant allergen immunotherapy

A common question, often asked by both parents and by physicians, is: will this child develop asthma? The follow-up question is: if asthma is likely, how can it be prevented? Until very recently, it was impossible to give a precise answer to either query, but increasing knowledge of the allergic (or atopic) march has now made it possible to give partial answers to both. The goals of this article are to explain the allergic march concept, review the available evidence, describe attempts to prevent the march, and, finally, outline possible intervention options for allergists and parents.

The allergic march is a postulated progression of atopic disease in infants with eczema to subsequently develop asthma, and then allergic rhinoconjunctivitis. The march was identified by many clinical observations during the 20th century, yet the first meta-analysis of this subject was prepared just 11 years ago.[1] In this article, Catani summarized the available information on age of onset for allergic diseases. Eczema begins in the first year of life in 80% of children, with specific food allergies detected: cow's milk allergy in 73%, egg allergy in 71%, and fish allergy in 51%. Asthma has a later onset, with only 42% evident in the first year, and 49% in the second year, but 92% develop symptoms before age 8. Rhinoconjunctivitis occurs even later, with 35% in year 1, and only 59% by age 5. The march can be visualized graphically (**Fig. 1**).[2] Evidence for developing food allergies generally occurs synchronously with signs and symptoms of eczema, and, in most allergic children, both precede respiratory symptoms.

No funding support.
The author has no conflicts to disclose.

[a] Department of Surgery, Cape Cod Hospital, 27 Park Street, Hyannis, MA 02601, USA
[b] Department of Otolaryngology, Massachusetts Eye and Ear Infirmary, 243 Charles Street, Boston, MA 02114, USA
[c] Department of Laryngology and Otology, Harvard Medical School, 25 Shattuck Street, Boston, MA 02115, USA
* Cape Cod ENT, 65 Cedar Street, Hyannis, MA 02601.
E-mail address: docbruce@comcast.net

Otolaryngol Clin N Am 44 (2011) 765–777
doi:10.1016/j.otc.2011.03.006 **oto.theclinics.com**
0030-6665/11/$ – see front matter

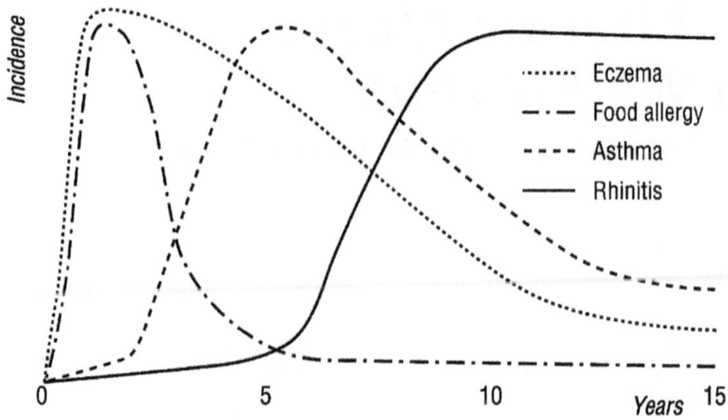

Fig. 1. Allergic march: progression with age from eczema to asthma to rhinoconjunctivitis. (*Adapted from* Barnetson RS, Rogers M. Childhood atopic eczema. BMJ 2002;324:1376; with permission.)

EVIDENCE FOR THE ALLERGIC MARCH

Clinical observations of the eczema-to-asthma-to-rhinitis progression were originally from cross-sectional studies that are subject to recall bias. Birth cohort studies have recently been done, and generally confirm the march concept. But, the initial idea of a uniform progression, in all patients, from eczema to asthma, has not been confirmed.[3] At least 3 clinical variants occur: (1) a normal allergic march from eczema to asthma to rhinitis,[4] (2) a reverse allergic march from asthma to eczema,[5] (3) and a purely respiratory allergic march of rhinitis to asthma, without any eczema. The allergic march also is not restricted to children, but can occur at any age. The relative risks for eczema progressing to asthma and rhinoconjunctivitis have been calculated for 250 infant eczema patients, followed for as long as 22 years.[6] Incidences of both asthma and rhinoconjunctivitis rise steadily with age, and by age 18, 34% develop asthma, and 66% rhinoconjunctivitis, while eczema declines to 42%. The severity of eczema is proportional to the risk of developing asthma, with the most severe eczema cases having 4.8 times the risk of mild cases ($P = .001$). The risk of developing rhinoconjunctivitis is similarly increased 3.2 times by prior development of asthma in these children.

RISK FACTORS FOR DEVELOPING ASTHMA

In a systematic review of 26 eczema follow-up studies from 1950 to 2006, about 30% of all eczema patients develop asthma by age 6,[7] and those eczema patients who are atopic are much more likely to develop asthma. For example, children with eczema and early wheezing but no atopy (defined by no positive allergy tests) have a lower risk of later asthma (odds ratio [OR] 2.84), compared with similar patients who are allergen sensitized (OR 6.68).[8] Infant wheezing is also a risk for adult asthma. Fifty-nine patients who wheezed before age 2 were re-evaluated at age 26 to 29, and 41% had asthma versus 10% of controls (OR 13.3).[9] Family history is significant, since the presence of sibling asthma increases asthma risk (OR 5.68).[9] In addition to the effects of atopic status and family history, in children of all ages, food allergy is an independent risk for asthma. Severe or multiple food allergies further increase the risk.[10]

ALLERGIC MARCH VARIATIONS

A reverse allergic march has been reported by Canonica and Passalacqua's group, in a study of 692 child asthmatics without either food allergy or eczema.[5] During the 9-year follow-up, 20% developed eczema. Mite monosensitization was more common in those who developed eczema.

Settipane made the first clinical observations of a purely respiratory allergic march in a 23-year follow-up of 738 atopics who had no eczema and were allergy tested as college students. The incidence of both allergic rhinitis and asthma continued to increase with age in these patients. Similar to eczema patients, positive allergy tests were a risk factor for asthma development ($P = .001$), but in addition, so was the presence of allergic rhinitis ($P = .002$).[11] Two other long-term studies, a 20-year follow-up of 252 infant eczema patients,[6] and a 40-year follow-up of 2100 adult rhinitis patients,[12] have confirmed that allergic rhinitis is an independent risk factor for developing asthma (independent of eczema). A recent 467-member birth cohort study has also confirmed, using Allergic Rhinitis and its Impact on Asthma (ARIA) criteria,[13] that at least to age 13, the prevalence of allergic rhinitis continues to increase, and there is a clear genetic risk component. In this cohort, symptomatic allergic rhinitis occurs in 44% of patients with at least 1 allergic parent versus 24% with no parental allergy.[14]

The last variation of the allergic march is possible sex specificity. A surprising finding of a large birth cohort study[3] of children with an atopic family history, studied from birth to age 7, was that eczema in the first 2 years predicts asthma in boys (OR 2.45), but not girls (OR 0.88). There were no changes in the conclusions if the data were adjusted for early allergy sensitization or wheezing, and these results remain unexplained.

ROLE OF FOOD ALLERGENS IN TRIGGERING THE ALLERGIC MARCH

The average age of sensitization to various allergens varies substantially, and this has a bearing both on which allergens are more likely to trigger the allergic march, and where preventative measures should be focused. Egg and milk food allergies are among the very first allergies to appear, often before 12 months,[14] while sensitivity to other staple foods usually begins in the second year, and does not reach the same prevalence level until around age 5.[15] Sensitivity to indoor inhaled allergens (mites and animals) also is rare before age 2, and increases thereafter similarly to staple foods. Sensitivity to outdoor pollen allergens also is rare before age 2, and increases markedly only after age 3. As a result of these data, both egg and milk allergy have been scrutinized closely for possible roles as allergic march and asthma triggers. A subgroup of allergic rhinitis patients has been found to have food allergy-mediated rhinitis.[16] In one study, open oral food challenge positive, cow's milk allergic infants, who had only rhinitis and no positive inhalant tests, were followed from age 1 to 5 years. During this time, milk allergy decreased from 100% to 14%, while asthma increased from 0% to 72%, identifying another large asthma risk factor.[17] Ricci and colleagues[6] similarly identified a very strong risk for later asthma and allergic rhinitis associated with early sensitization to eggs.

Independent risk factors for developing asthma are therefore: early eczema, eczema severity, atopy (allergic sensitization), early persisting wheezing, allergic rhinitis, male sex, and food allergy, especially allergy to cow's milk and chicken's egg.

RELATIONSHIP OF ENVIRONMENTAL AND GENETIC FACTORS TO ECZEMA PREVALENCE

National eczema prevalences range from 0.3% to 20.5%, are highest in Scandinavia, Canada, Australia, Chile, and the United States, and lowest in the tropics and Russia.[4]

Eczema is increasing in 70% of nations, where the prevalence correlates directly with national per capita income. The very rapid rate of change in eczema prevalence strongly suggests environmental, rather than purely genetic, factors are involved. There is also good evidence for genetic influence, since atopic children are much more likely to develop eczema than nonatopics. This genetic influence is seen most strongly in affluent nations, where many eczema cases are positively correlated to atopy (OR 2.69). However, only in 15% of poor nations is correlation with atopy found, which supports the existence of environmental influences on eczema, influences that vary with economic status.[4] One possible explanation for the difference in eczema cases seen in different nations can be inferred from longitudinal studies in locales that are undergoing urbanization, such as in Africa. There, atopy is increasing everywhere with national income level. In South African cities, the rise in atopy correlates both with assuming an urban, Western diet, and with less exposure to infections.[18] Several environmental factors have now been postulated to be affecting eczema and the allergic march, including the hygiene hypothesis, vitamin D levels, maternal nutrition, infant feeding practices, chemical pollution, and antibiotic and anti-inflammatory drugs.

HYGIENE HYPOTHESIS

This is the most frequently considered hypothesis to explain historic increases in atopic diseases during 20th century, including the allergic march.[19] Newborns have a predominately Th2, allergic immune response, and acquire Th1 responses by infection exposures. Environmental changes have been dramatic in the 20th century: small families, cleaner, almost entirely indoor living, processed and sanitized foods with chemical additives, infection prevention and antibiotic treatments, and world-wide pollution. These changes either directly reduce exposure to pathogens, or can alter immune functioning, so the hygiene hypothesis posited that these environmental influences caused a shift in the balance between Th1- and Th2-mediated immunity to favor a continued allergic, Th2 state, rather than the development of a normal balance between Th1 and Th2 responses.

This simple paradigm is not entirely correct, because

- Th2 responses to parasitic infestations protect from allergies
- Th1 autoimmune diseases are increasing at the same time allergies are
- Both Th1 and Th2 diseases may occur in the same patients
- High-dose exposures to allergens that generate a Th2 response can cause tolerance, rather than sensitization.[19]

Furthermore, at the time the hygiene hypothesis was first proposed, the full extent of the T-cell network was not known, including the existence of Th17, a third class of CD4+ helper T-lymphocytes, and Treg, a class of regulatory T- lymphocytes.[20] In light of these points, a modified hygiene hypothesis has been proposed: that the modern increase in allergic diseases is due to an imbalanced, misregulated, or inappropriate T-cell response, which leads to excessive immune stimulation from Th1, Th2, and/or Th17 classes of T helper cells.

EVIDENCE FOR THE HYGIENE HYPOTHESIS

One of the observations providing strong support for the hygiene hypothesis is that farm life protects from atopy, allergic rhinitis, and asthma, either when infants or their pregnant mothers are exposed to farm living. When farm children are compared with carefully matched controls, early exposure (under 1 year) or prolonged exposure (until age 5) is strongly protective. Key antiallergy factors are exposure to stables and drinking unpasteurized milk.[21] Mothers living on a farm have significantly higher levels of the cytokines transforming growth factor beta (TGF-β) and interleukin (IL)-10 (P = .05 for both) in their colostrum and mature milk, compared with control nonfarm rural mothers. TGF-β helps establish innate immunity, and IL-10 has broad antiallergic activity, which may influence the infant's immune balance away from allergy.[22]

A second area of support for the hygiene hypothesis comes from the effects of early life infections. Attending group daycare or having many older siblings reduces the risk of developing atopy or asthma, presumably because of increased infections.[19] The role of specific viruses is not as clear, since, in some reports, certain viruses protect, but human rhinoviruses and respiratory syncytial virus normally initiate or aggravate asthma.[23,24] In a birth cohort study, infections (colds, diarrhea with fever, or any fever) in the first 3 months of life increased wheezing risk by age 2 years.[25]

Intestinal flora and infections have also been studied. Early oro–fecal exposure, as measured by exposure to hepatitis A, toxoplasmosis, or parasite infestations, protects from asthma, as does administration of many types of probiotic bacteria. Reducing gut levels of lactobacilli and bifidobacteria (eg, by antibiotic use) increases the risk, as does abnormal intestinal microbial balance, for example, when pathogenic bacteria like *Clostridium difficile* predominate.[19] Neonatal antibiotic use is statistically correlated with later asthma, and there is a dose effect, with more courses of antibiotics increasing asthma risk, but the overall increase in risk, in 1 study, is only about 15%.[26]

A final group of supportive studies involves birth-related infections. Elective cesarian section decreases asthma risk (OR 0.34), and a lengthy time of ruptured membranes (>3 hours) before delivery increases asthma risk (OR 6.7). These reports are believed to be due to varying degrees of infant exposure to vaginal flora, including *Ureaplasma* and staphylococci, which are known to be associated with subsequent asthma development.[27]

A meta-analysis of 46 papers reporting the effects of early life exposures on the risk of triggering the allergic march has been done. Exposure to pets (n = 27) slightly reduces risk, dog exposure being better than cat (OR 0.84, confidence interval [CI]: 0.73–0.96). Exposure to endotoxin (n = 13) slightly reduces risk, (OR 0.90 CI: 0.78–1.0). Drinking unpasteurized milk (n = 7) reduces risk (OR 0.68 CI: 0.61–0.76). Finally, livestock exposure (n = 8) produces a sizable risk reduction, (OR 0.58 CI: 0.39–0.87).[28] Tse and Horner believe, based on their studies, that normal levels of respiratory exposure to a variety of allergens found in house dusts are naturally tolerogenic. But, intermittent high exposures can break through this normal tolerance, to cause symptomatic allergic disease.[28]

EFFECTS OF VITAMIN D ON THE ALLERGIC MARCH

Vitamin D has broad immune effects, since vitamin D receptors are present in the nucleus of B- and T-lymphocytes, monocytes, macrophages, and dendritic cells, where vitamin D modulates cytokine levels, including thymic stromal lymphopoetin (TSLP), IL-2, 4, 5, and 13, interferon gamma (IFN-γ), and many others.[29] Vitamin D deficiency increases infections, all allergic diseases, and autoimmunity risk. The effects on allergy depend on both vitamin D dose and patient age. Vitamin D supplements may have a steroid-sparing effect in asthma, and high levels are associated with better lung function. High maternal vitamin D is associated with less wheezing in those mother's children, but, there is evidence that the dose–response curve may be U-shaped, so that both low and very high vitamin D levels may increase allergy risk.

Vitamin D should benefit eczema because of its known biologic effects of increasing keratinocyte proliferation, promotion of wound healing, stimulation of skin antimicrobial canthelicidins, and suppression of skin inflammation. In a small study, vitamin D supplements improved winter eczema.[29]

EFFECTS OF MATERNAL NUTRITION ON THE ALLERGIC MARCH

Three recent reports agree that insufficient maternal nutrition during pregnancy increases the risk for children to develop allergies, eczema, and asthma. The studies focused on different aspects of nutrition, but found that increased maternal zinc and antioxidant intake are protective, and that vitamin E, citrus fruits, and green and yellow vegetables are possibly protective.[30]

EFFECTS OF CHEMICAL POLLUTION ON THE ALLERGIC MARCH

Chemical pollutants are associated with increased risk of both atopy and asthma. Respiratory exposure to natural gas cooking fumes and tobacco smoking both increase only asthma,[31,32] while traffic exhaust increases eczema, asthma, and rhinitis.[33] In a prenatal birth cohort study, the active fractions in traffic pollution were identified as polyaromatic cyclic hydrocarbons (PAH) and ultrafine particulates, and both maternal prenatal and infant postnatal exposure were found to be important. Traffic exhaust may injure the lung surface barrier, increasing pulmonary sensitization.[34]

EFFECTS OF ANTI-INFLAMMATORY DRUGS ON THE ALLERGIC MARCH

Anti-inflammatory drugs have long been suspected of increasing atopic diseases, but evidence from human observational studies has been conflicting. Recently, a mouse model system found that aspirin drives Th17 T-cell responses to Th2, and increases eosinophilic lung injury, which gives a plausible mechanism by which these drugs could influence the allergic march.[35] The most recent birth cohort study, 7 years in duration, and very carefully controlled, shows no other factors except acetaminophen exposure can account for the observed asthma risk increase.[36] Finally, a very large multi-center study in Spain showed that the proallergic effects of acetaminophen in children are additive to, and independent of, the effects of antibiotic use.[37]

ORIGIN OF THE ALLERGIC MARCH: MOLECULAR BIOLOGY OF ECZEMA

Understanding of eczema has changed dramatically with the discovery of the role of filaggrin, the filament-aggregating protein in the epidermis. Filaggrin is a late-acting epidermal differentiation protein that is essential to form a functional, waterproof, infection-resistant epidermal barrier, by aggregating and cross-linking keratin.[38] Light microscopy with antifilaggrin antibody staining demonstrates that eczema patients show extensive physical barrier disruption.[39] Loss-of-function filaggrin mutants are common, occurring in about 10% of people in most ethnic groups. In a cohort of infants with identified filaggrin mutations, who were followed until school age, the loss-of-function mutants increased eczema by age 1 (P = .0003), asthma attacks by age 1 (P = .01), allergic sensitization by age 4 (P = .00007), and persistent asthma by age 5 (P = .03).[40] Allergic rhinitis is also significantly increased.[4] The reason filaggrin mutants increase allergies is because the poor keratin cross-linking causes epithelial barrier dysfunction with water loss, increased allergen and irritant absorption, and decreased infection resistance. The barrier dysfunction leads to local epidermal Th2 inflammation, and then to systemic inflammation, with involvement of cytokines, eosinophils, TSLP, and Th17 activation.[4] This eosinophilic inflamation has now been detected in pediatric bronchial lavage specimens from 2 to 5 years before the recognized onset of asthma symptoms.[41]

ECZEMA: EVIDENCE FOR SYSTEMIC INFLAMMATORY EFFECTS

These human observations have been expanded in a mouse model of repeated skin exposure to *Aspergillus fumigatus*. Mold exposure induces a Th2 response with local eczema, followed by rhinitis and bronchial hyper-reactivity. Elevated *Aspergillus*-specific immunoglobulin (Ig)E, IgG1, and increased IL-4, but not IFN-γ, hallmarks of Th2 allergy, are all present.[42] Other mouse models show both normal allergic march progression from eczema to asthma and also respiratory allergic march progression from rhinitis to asthma. In both variants, T-cell dependent systemic sensitization with requirements for TSLP, vitamin D, and IL-17 (required for bronchial hyper-reactivity) was found.[4] Human clinical studies and mouse models also show that atopy may be maternally inherited from prenatal epigenetic changes, especially DNA methylation, similar to the known effects of prenatal tobacco smoke exposure.[43]

ATTEMPTS TO INTERVENE IN THE ALLERGIC MARCH

There have been numerous attempts to prevent or stop the allergic march, including trials of drugs, dietary microbial supplements, infant feeding strategies, and immunotherapy.

Medications

Pharmacologic prevention initially appeared to be helpful. Eczema patients, 1 to 2 years old, were treated with cetirizine for 18 months, and observed for another18 months. The onset of asthma symptoms was delayed in pollen-sensitive (P = .002) and mite-sensitive (P = .005) children, and benefits persisted for 3 years in some.[44] Unfortunately, attempted replication of this study was not significant for the primary endpoint of asthma prevention. Several subsequent attempts to use inhaled steroids to prevent asthma were also unsuccessful, as was a trial of pimecrolimus cream to prevent eczema from progressing to asthma.[4]

Probiotics

On the other hand, many studies now show prenatal prebiotics or probiotics are effective for eczema prevention, although fewer studies show benefits with established allergic disease.[45] In 1 study, mothers were probiotic treated daily for the final month of pregnancy, and infants were treated for 6 months. At 2 years, eczema (OR 0.41) and all allergies (OR 0.38) were reduced by treatment. Infant cytokine profiles showed low-grade inflammation, with elevated IgE, IgA, and IL-1 similar to levels seen in helminth infestation.[46] A second study evaluated *Lactobacillis* F19 supplements during weaning, and reduced eczema to half the control incidence (P = .05).[47] In a third study, probiotic treatment of mothers during pregnancy and lactation decreased child eczema at age 2 years by two-thirds (OR 0.32, P = .0098).[48] Probiotics can also have very prolonged beneficial effects, with treatment at birth decreasing allergies up to 20 years later.[49] Probiotics are also effective for preventing eczema in cesarian section babies (OR 0.47, P = .035, at age 5 years).[50]

A few studies have shown that certain probiotics or use schedules are not effective or are possibly harmful. For example, when newborns were treated daily for 6 months with *Lactobacillus acidophilus* (LAVRI-A1), at 6 months there was no difference in eczema, but the experimental group had an increased number of positive allergy tests compared with controls.[51] And, when mothers were treated for the final 4 to 6 weeks of pregnancy and the next 6 months with *Lactobacillus* GG (ATC 53,103), at 18 months there was no difference in eczema, but the treated mother's children had 2.85 times more infant wheezing and bronchitis.[52]

There have been several recent reviews of dietary probiotics, including a structured review of the effects of probiotics for eczema prevention or treatment.[53] Of the double-blinded, placebo-controlled studies that were robust enough to include, 6 of 9 showed significant eczema reduction, and 1 showed a favorable trend. According to Tang, Lahtinen, and Boyle: "Probiotic bacteria represent the most promising intervention for primary allergy prevention that has been studied to date...."[45] Other reviews indicate that probiotics are effective for normalizing intestinal barrier function and reducing production of allergic inflammatory cytokines, and therefore, probiotics are potentially useful, and may be effective for treatment or prevention of food allergy, eczema, and allergic rhinitis.[54,55] In summary, current evidence supports consideration of using probiotics before giving birth in several situations:

Allergic mothers, especially with personal history of eczema, asthma, or severe persistent allergic rhinitis
Mothers who have prior children with food allergy, eczema, or asthma
Allergic mothers with a scheduled cesarian section, or history of early rupture of membranes, or history of recent intestinal bacterial infection.

Infant Feeding

Breast feeding has been studied as a possible means of interrupting the allergic march, and it has been found that breast milk contains immune components that may be allergy-protective. A systematic review of TGF-β levels in breast milk found that both TGF-β1 and TGF-β 2 are present, and two-thirds of studies show high levels of TGF-β protect from development of allergies.[56] A recent report found that TSLP is also present in colostrum and early milk, where it may influence gastrointestinal sensitization.[57] Finally, breast milk contains protective bifidobacter probiotic bacteria, but allergic mothers have low counts, and transfer fewer beneficial bacteria to their infants than do normal mothers.[58] Formula feeding also influences the allergic march. For example, cesarian section children are more likely to become cow's milk allergic because of the greater frequency of formula feeding in these infants (OR 10.9). Risk for cow's milk allergy is also increased by using formula supplements while breast feeding (OR 2.86), and also, surprisingly, by extending the period of exclusive breast feeding (delayed weaning) beyond 2 months (OR 4.14).[59] If cesarian section babies are exclusively breast fed, then they are less likely to develop cow's milk allergy (OR 0.42). Cow's milk allergy can also be prevented by exclusively feeding an extensively hydrolyzed casein formula (eg, Nutramigen or Pregestamil) (OR 0.44). Sánchez-Valverde and colleagues[59] comment that: "Feeding [only] one or two bottles of cow's milk in the first few days of life is related to the development of IgE-mediated cow's milk allergy. (Unless exclusively breast-feeding), a diet of an extensively hydrolyzed, high grade formula appears to be the best choice to avoid the antigenic stimulus (and the subsequent Allergic March)."

The American Academy of Pediatrics has published evidence-based recommendations for infant feeding.[60] Found to be not useful are maternal diet restrictions during pregnancy or lactation, and delaying the introduction of solid foods beyond 4 to 6 months of age. Useful practices are:

Breast feeding for at least 4 months (prevents or delays the occurrence of cow's milk allergy, eczema, and wheezing)

Use of hydrolyzed formulas, in not exclusively breast fed infants, for 4 to 6 months (may delay or prevent onset of atopic disease)

Extensively hydrolyzed formulas (have better protective benefits than less hydrolyzed or unhydrolyzed formulas).

Immunotherapy

Inhalant allergen immunotherapy has also been found to interrupt the allergic march. In a large 3-year, parallel group subcutaneous immunotherapy (SCIT) study of mildly asthmatic adults with or without allergic rhinitis, SCIT decreased asthma progression risk, while pharmacotherapy alone did not.[61] In a second 3-year SCIT treatment study of children with allergic rhinitis but no asthma, SCIT decreased asthma progression risk for at least 10 years (OR 0.4 at 3 years, OR 0.3 at 5 years, OR 0.4 at 10 years).[62] Sublingual immunotherapy (SLIT) is also effective. In a 3-year, parallel group study of mono grass-allergic children with allergic rhinitis and not more than mild intermittent asthma, the SLIT-treated children had fewer symptoms and less medication use in the second and third years, and had 3.8 times less persistent asthma at the conclusion of the study.[63] A second pediatric SLIT parallel group study showed that 4 to 5 years after completing a 4 to 5-year SLIT treatment course, there was persisting suppression of asthma in the treated group, compared with the control group ($P = .001$). Peak expiratory flows and medication use were also were statistically better in the SLIT group.[64]

THE ALLERGIC MARCH: CONCLUSIONS

The allergic march is a progression of atopic disease from eczema to asthma, and then to allergic rhinoconjunctivitis. This can occur at any age, and does not always follow the classic sequence of illnesses. Based on both human clinical data and mouse models, the march appears to be caused by a regional allergic response that then initiates systemic allergic inflammation. There are many known predisposing environmental factors to developing the allergic march, including the effects of infectious agents (hygiene hypothesis), vitamin D levels, maternal nutrition, chemical pollution exposures, antibiotic and anti-inflammatory drug exposures, and infant feeding practices. When eczema is the initial allergic illness, the currently understood pathway to developing systemic inflammation is initiated by epithelial barrier dysfunction resulting from filaggrin loss-of-function mutations. The breached permeability barrier increases skin exposure to irritants, pollutants, contact allergens, and microbes, and, combined with food allergy in susceptible atopics, initiates local Th2 inflammation, which progresses to systemic inflammation, and then to rhinitis and/or asthma.

Knowing this, is enough known to interrupt the march to prevent allergy, and especially, to prevent asthma? There are limited, but very promising data to support 4 different possible interventions: (1) supplements of dietary probiotics, (2) exclusive breast feeding during the first few months of life, or, alternatively, (3) use of extensively hydrolyzed infant formulas, and finally, (4) treatment with inhalant allergen immunotherapy by either SCIT or SLIT methods. From current data, if these strategies were widely employed, there would probably be a substantial reduction in future asthma cases.

ACKNOWLEDGMENTS

For expert research assistance, the author thanks the staff from Frazier-Grant Medical Library, Cape Cod Hospital: Jeanie Vander Pyl, MLIS, director, June Bianchi, library assistant, and Judy Donn, MLS, library assistant.

REFERENCES

1. Cantani A. The growing genetic links and the early onset of atopic diseases in children stress the unique role of the atopic march: a meta-analysis. J Investig Allergol Clin Immunol 1999;9(5):314–20.
2. Barnetson RS, Rogers M. Childhood atopic eczema. BMJ 2002;324:1376–9.
3. Lowe AJ, Carlin JB, Bennett CM, et al. Do boys do the atopic march while girls dawdle? J Allergy Clin Immunol 2008;121(5):1190–5.
4. Spergel M. Epidemiology of atopic dermatitis and atopic march in children. Immunol Allergy Clin North Am 2010;30:269–80.
5. Barberio G, Pajno GB, Vita D, et al. Does a reverse atopic march exist? Allergy 2008;63(12):1630–2.
6. Ricci G, Patrizi A, Baldi E, et al. Long-term follow-up of atopic dermatitis: retrospective analysis of related risk factors and association with concomitant allergic diseases. J Am Acad Dermatol 2006;55(5):765–71.
7. van der Hulst AE, Klip H, Brand PL. Risk of developing asthma in young children with atopic eczema: a systematic review. J Allergy Clin Immunol 2007;120(3):565–9.
8. Ker J, Hartert TV. The atopic march: what's the evidence? Ann Allergy Asthma Immunol 2009;103(4):282–9.
9. Ruotsalainen M, Piippo-Savolainen E, Hyvarinen MK, et al. Adult asthma after wheezing in infancy. Allergy 2010;65:503–9.
10. Schroeder A, Kumar R, Pongracic JA, et al. Food allergy is associated with an increased risk of asthma. Clin Exp Allergy 2009;39:261–70.
11. Settipane RJ, Hagy GW, Settipane GA. Long-term risk factors for developing asthma and allergic rhinitis: a 23-year follow-up study of college students. Allergy Proc 1994;15(1):21–5.
12. van den Nieuwenhof L, Schermer T, Bosch Y, et al. Is physician-diagnosed allergic rhinitis a risk factor for the development of asthma? Allergy 2010;65(8):1049–55.
13. Cruz AA, Popov T, Pawankar R, et al. Common characteristics of upper and lower airways in rhinitis and asthma: ARIA update, in collaboration with GA(2)LEN. Allergy 2007;62(Suppl 84):1–41.
14. Keil T, Bockelbrink A, Reich A, et al. The natural history of allergic rhinitis in childhood. Pediatr Allergy Immunol 2010;21(6):962–9.
15. Kulig M, Bergmann R, Klettke U, et al. Natural course of sensitization to food and inhalant allergens during the first 6 years of life. J Allergy Clin Immunol 1999; 103(6):1173–9.
16. Wang DY, Gordon BR, Chan YH, et al. Potential non-IgE mediated food allergies: comparison of open challenge and DBPCFC. Otolaryngol Head Neck Surg 2007; 137(5):803–9.
17. Huang SW. Follow-up of children with rhinitis and cough associated with milk allergy. Pediatr Allergy Immunol 2007;18(1):81–5.
18. Obeng BB, Hartgers F, Boakye D, et al. Out of Africa: what can be learned from the studies of allergic disorders in Africa and Africans? Curr Opin Allergy Clin Immunol 2008;8(5):391–7.
19. Gore C, Custovic A. Protective parasites and medicinal microbes? The case for the hygiene hypothesis. Prim Care Respir J 2004;13(2):68–75.
20. Chaplin DD. Overview of the immune response. J Allergy Clin Immunol 2010;125: S3–23.
21. Riedler J, Braun-Fahrländer C, Eder W, et al. Exposure to farming in early life and development of asthma and allergy: a cross-sectional survey. Lancet 2001; 358(9288):1129–33.

22. Peroni DG, Pescollderungg L, Piacentini GL, et al. Immune regulatory cytokines in the milk of lactating women from farming and urban environments. Pediatr Allergy Immunol 2010;21(6):977–80.
23. Chi B, Dickensheets HL, Spann KM, et al. Alpha and lambda interferon together mediate suppression of CD4 T cells induced by respiratory syncytial virus. J Virol 2006;80(10):5032–40.
24. Wong T, Hellermann G, Mohapatra S. The infectious march: the complex interaction between microbes and the immune system in asthma. Immunol Allergy Clin North Am 2010;30:453–80.
25. Mommers M, Thijs C, Stelma F, et al. Timing of infection and development of wheeze, eczema, and atopic sensitization during the first 2 yr of life: the KOALA Birth Cohort Study. Pediatr Allergy Immunol 2010;21(6):983–9.
26. Korppi M. Bacterial infections and pediatric asthma. Immunol Allergy Clin North Am 2010;30:565–74.
27. Keski-Nisula L, Karvonen A, Pfefferle PI, et al. Birth-related factors and doctor-diagnosed wheezing and allergic sensitization in early childhood. Allergy 2010; 65(9):1116–25.
28. Tse K, Horner AA. Allergen tolerance versus the allergic march: the hygiene hypothesis revisited. Curr Allergy Asthma Rep 2008;8(6):475–83.
29. Searing DA, Leung DYM. Vitamin D in atopic dermatitis, asthma, and allergic diseases. Immunol Allergy Clin North Am 2010;30:269–80.
30. Miyake Y, Sasaki S, Tanaka K, et al. Consumption of vegetables, fruit, and antioxidants during pregnancy and wheeze and eczema in infants. Allergy 2010;65(6): 758–65.
31. Wang HY, Pizzichini MMM, Becker AB, et al. Disparate geographic prevalences of asthma, allergic rhinoconjunctivitis and atopic eczema among adolescents in five Canadian cities. Pediatr Allergy Immunol 2010;21:867–77.
32. Wong GW, Ko FW, Hui DS, et al. Factors associated with difference in prevalence of asthma in children from three cities in China: multicentre epidemiological survey. BMJ 2004;329:486–90.
33. Jedrychowski WA, Perera FP, Maugeri U, et al. Intrauterine exposure to polycyclic aromatic hydrocarbons, fine particulate matter and early wheeze. Prospective birth cohort study in 4-year olds. Pediatr Allergy Immunol 2010;21:e723–32.
34. Gehring U, Wijga AH, Brauer M, et al. Traffic-related air pollutionand the development of asthma and allergies during the first 8 years oflife. Am J Respir Crit Care Med 2010;181:596–603.
35. Moon HG, Tae YM, Kim YS, et al. Conversion of Th17-type into Th2-type inflammation by acetyl salicylic acid via the adenosine and uric acid pathway in the lung. Allergy 2010;65(9):1093–103.
36. Shaheen SO, Newson RB, Smith GD, et al. Prenatal paracetamol exposure and asthma: further evidence against confounding. Int J Epidemiol 2010;39(3):790–4.
37. Garcia-Marcos L, Gonzalez-Diaz C, Garvajal-Urueña I, et al. Early exosure to paracetamol or to antibiotics and eczema at school age: modification by asthma and rhinoconjunctivitis. Pediatr Allergy Immunol 2010;21(7):1036–42.
38. Sandilands A, Sutherland C, Irvine AD, et al. Filaggrin in the front line: role in skin barrier function and disease. J Cell Sci 2009;122:1285–94.
39. Nemoto-Hasebe I, Akiyama M, Nomura T, et al. Clinical severity correlates with impaired barrier in filaggrin-related eczema. J Invest Dermatol 2009;129:682–9.
40. Bønnelykke K, Pipper CB, Tavendale R, et al. Filaggrin gene variants and atopic diseases in early childhood assessed longitudinally from birth. Pediatr Allergy Immunol 2010;21(6):954–61.

41. Thavagnanam S, Williamson G, Ennis M, et al. Does airway allergic inflammation pre-exist before late onset wheeze in children? Pediatr Allergy Immunol 2010; 21(7):1002–7.
42. Akei HS, Brandt EB, Mishra A, et al. Epicutaneous aeroallergen exposure induces systemicTH2 immunity that predisposes to allergic nasal responses. J Allergy Clin Immunol 2006;118(1):62–9.
43. Shaheen SO, Adcock IM. The developmental origins of asthma: does epigenetics hold the key? Am J Respir Crit Care Med 2009;180(8):690–1.
44. Warner JO, Etac Study Group. Early Treatment of the Atopic Child. A double-blinded, randomized, placebo controlled trial of cetirizine in preventing the onset of asthma in children with atopic dermatitis. J Allergy Clin Immunol 2001;108(6): 929–37.
45. Tang ML, Lahtinen SJ, Boyle RJ. Probiotics and prebiotics: clinical effects in allergic disease. Curr Opin Pediatr 2010;22(5):626–34.
46. Marschan E, Kuitunen M, Kukkonen K, et al. Probiotics in infancy induce protective immune profiles that are characteristic for chronic low-grade inflammation. Clin Exp Allergy 2008;38(4):611–8.
47. West CE, Hammarström ML, Hernell O. Probiotics during weaning reduce the incidence of eczema. Pediatr Allergy Immunol 2009;20(5):430–7.
48. Rautava S, Kalliomäki M, Isolauri E. Probiotics during pregnancy and breast-feeding might confer immunomodulatory protection against atopic disease in the infant. J Allergy Clin Immunol 2002;109(1):119–21.
49. Lodinová-Zádníková R, Cukrowska B, Tlaskalova-Hogenova H. Oral administration of probiotic Escherichia coli after birth reduces frequency of allergies and repeated infections later in life. Int Arch Allergy Immunol 2003;131(3):209–11.
50. Kuitunen M, Kukkonen K, Juntunen-Backman K, et al. Probiotics prevent IgE-associated allergy until age 5 years in cesarean-delivered children but not in the total cohort. J Allergy Clin Immunol 2009;123(2):335–41.
51. Taylor AL, Dunstan JA, Prescott SL. Probiotic supplementation for the first 6 months of life fails to reduce the risk of atopic dermatitis and increases the risk of allergen sensitization in high-risk children: a randomized controlled trial. J Allergy Clin Immunol 2007;119(1):184–91.
52. Kopp MV, Hennemuth I, Heinzmann A, et al. Randomized, DBPC trial of probiotics for primary prevention: no clinical effects of Lactobacillus GG supplementation. Pediatrics 2008;121(4):e850–6.
53. Betsi GI, Papadavid E, Falagas ME. Probiotics for the treatment or prevention of atopic dermatitis: a review of the evidence from randomized controlled trials. Am J Clin Dermatol 2008;9(2):93–103.
54. del Giudice MM, Rocco A, Capristo C. Probiotics in the atopic march: highlights and new insights. Dig Liver Dis 2006;38(Suppl 2):S288–90.
55. Singh M, Ranjan DR. Probiotics for allergic respiratory diseases–putting it into perspective. Pediatr Allergy Immunol 2010;21:e368–76.
56. Oddy WH, Rosales F. A systematic review of the importance of milk TGF-beta on immunological outcomes in the infant and young child. Pediatr Allergy Immunol 2010;21:47–59.
57. Macfarlane TV, Seager AL, Moller M, et al. Thymic stromal lymphopoietin is present in human breast milk. Pediatr Allergy Immunol 2010;21:e454–6.
58. Grönlund MM, Gueimonde M, Laitinen K, et al. Maternal breast milk and intestinal bifidobacteria guide the compositional development of the *Bifidobacterium* microbiota in infants at risk of allergic disease. Clin Exp Allergy 2007;37(12): 1764–72.

59. Sánchez-Valverde F, Gil F, Martinez D, et al. The impact of caesarean delivery and type of feeding on cow's milk allergy in infants and subsequent development of allergic march in childhood. Allergy 2009;64(6):884–9.
60. Greer FR, Sicherer SH, Burks AW. Effects of early nutritional interventions on the development of atopic disease in infants and children: the role of maternal dietary restriction, breastfeeding, timing of introduction of complementary foods, and hydrolyzed formulas. Pediatrics 2008;121(1):183–91.
61. Marogna M, Spadolini I, Massolo A. Rhinitis and asthma comorbidity in respiratory allergy due to house dust mite: results of an observational open controlled parallel group study in real-life setting. Eur Ann Allergy Clin Immunol 2005; 37(4):135–42.
62. Jacobsen L, Niggemann B, Dreborg S, et al. Specific immunotherapy has long-term preventive effect of seasonal and perennial asthma: 10-year follow-up on the PAT study. Allergy 2007;62(8):943–8.
63. Novembre E, Galli E, Landi F, et al. Coseasonal sublingual immunotherapy reduces the development of asthma in children with allergic rhinoconjunctivitis. J Allergy Clin Immunol 2004;114(4):851–7.
64. Di Rienzo V, Marcucci F, Puccinelli P, et al. Long-lasting effect of sublingual immunotherapy in children with asthma due to house dust mite: a 10-year prospective study. Clin Exp Allergy 2003;33(2):206–10.

The Surgical Management of Allergic Rhinitis

Nipun Chhabra, MD[a], Steven M. Houser, MD[b,*]

KEYWORDS

- Allergic rhinitis • Nasal obstruction • Submucous resection
- Septoplasty • Inferior turbinate hypertrophy

Key Points: Allergic Rhinitis: Surgical Management

- Allergic rhinitis is a widespread condition, and nasal obstruction is a defining and bothersome symptom.
- Allergic rhinitis that is refractory to medical therapy may necessitate surgical intervention.
- Reduction of the inferior turbinate is the primary means of augmenting the nasal airway in allergic rhinitis patients.
- A variety of procedures exist for the surgical reduction of inferior turbinate tissue, including outfracture, submucous resection, laser vaporization, radiofrequency ablation, and coblation.
- Septoplasty alone has little role in the treatment of nasal obstruction for allergic rhinitis.
- Endoscopic sinus surgery is an important treatment method for allergic rhinitis when it contributes to chronic sinusitis, nasal polyposis, or allergic fungal disease.
- No single operation has evolved as the gold standard for treatment of nasal obstruction in allergic rhinitis; instead the surgeon should be familiar and facile with several approaches.

Allergic rhinitis (AR) is a widespread condition that affects millions of patients yearly, and the hallmark complaint of nasal obstruction accounts for one of the most common reasons for outpatient otolaryngologic visits. Comorbid conditions often seen with AR include asthma, otitis media, atopic disease, and various forms of rhinosinusitis. The

Disclosure(s): The authors have no funding, financial relationships, or conflicts of interest to disclose.

[a] Department of Otolaryngology, Head and Neck Surgery, Case Western Reserve University & University Hospitals Case Medical Center, 11100 Euclid Avenue, LKS 5045, Room 4535, Cleveland, OH 44106, USA
[b] Department of Otolaryngology, Head and Neck Surgery, MetroHealth Medical Center, Case Western Reserve University, 2500 MetroHealth Drive, Cleveland, OH 44109, USA
* Corresponding author.
E-mail address: shouser@metrohealth.org

Otolaryngol Clin N Am 44 (2011) 779–795
doi:10.1016/j.otc.2011.03.007 oto.theclinics.com

differentiation between rhinosinusitis and AR is often based on clinical history, associated perennial symptoms, nasal cytology, and response to different medical or surgical therapies.[1] Many interventions exist for the treatment of AR, but the most common surgical interventions are aimed at reducing nasal obstruction to better augment the nasal airway.

BACKGROUND

Allergic rhinitis has been described as the "total rhinologic disease," and requires comprehensive otolaryngologic care.[1,2] Treatment of patients with AR can be challenging, and has the goal of reducing perennial symptoms while improving quality of life. The disease process can contribute to chronic rhinosinusitis, nasal polyposis, and chronic rhinitis, and therefore AR may be difficult to differentiate from these associated conditions. Patients with chronic AR may also present with fungal disease of the paranasal sinuses or persistent acute sinus exacerbations, often caused by secondary ostial obstruction from edematous sinonasal mucosa (**Fig. 1**). These coexisting conditions may further complicate patient care.

The incidence of AR is steadily increasing, with up to 24% of the general population having this condition, including approximately 30% of the adult population and 40% of children.[3,4] More than 600 million patients worldwide are afflicted, making AR the most prevalent atopic disorder.[5] The total direct and indirect cost associated with AR treatment exceeds $5 billion annually.[6] The hallmark symptoms include nasal obstruction, sneezing, seromucosal rhinorrhea, and nasal pruritus.[7] Symptoms may show seasonal or perennial variations, and medical therapy is generally implemented early in the disease process. Systemic symptoms or conditions may also be present with AR, including asthma, bronchitis, pneumonia, and atopic dermatitis. Clinical history is of central diagnostic value, and helps to delineate etiologic factors. Additional allergen testing or serum diagnostics are often used in the workup of patients and to confirm and help direct therapy.

The origin of AR has many contributing factors. The mucosa of the nose and paranasal sinuses is continuous with the lower airway, with only microscopic changes on different levels.[1] Based on this membrane continuum, the association among asthma, certain pulmonary conditions, and AR can be understood. Seasonal variations are often attributed to external factors, such as trees, grass, weeds, and molds. Skin prick, nasal allergen provocation or challenge, intradermal, or in vitro serum–specific testing can delineate allergens and narrow therapeutic regimens. Occupational

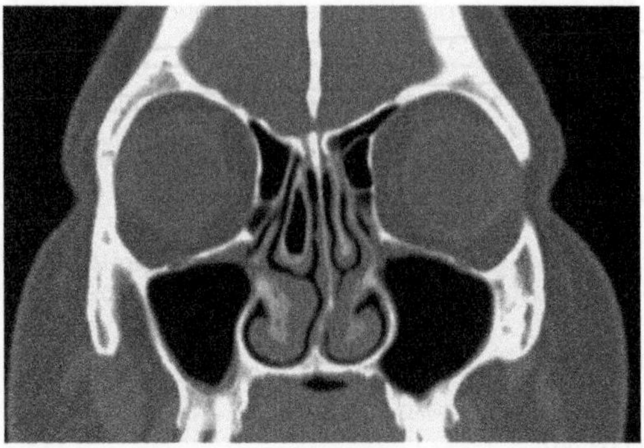

Fig. 1. A coronal CT scan showing bilateral maxillary ostial edema and closure from AR.

exposures often contribute to episodic AR, and common triggers include wood dust, latex, spores, or certain chemical irritants. Perennial disease is often caused by indoor allergens, but certain outdoor allergens that are present year-round can also be contributing factors.[8] House dust mites, specifically *Dermatophagoides farinae* and *Dermatophagoides pteronyssinus*, pets, and cockroaches are common culprits of perennial AR.[9]

Allergen responses in the nasal mucosa are mediated by a variety of complex interactions among inflammatory markers. IgE is the main mediator of the allergen-allergic response and the resulting sequelae. Mast cells are present in ample quantities in the nasal mucosa, and IgE-mediated binding of allergens initiates a cascade of inflammatory mediator release, both immediate and delayed. Histamine, tryptase, kinins, leukotrienes, and prostaglandins are included in the array of mediators and lead to rhinorrhea.[10] The effects include mucous gland stimulation and increased vascular permeability, resulting in increased secretions, edema, and exudate. Vasodilation leads to engorgement of nasal mucosa and structures, especially the inferior turbinates, thereby causing nasal obstruction, congestion, and discomfort. Inflammation of neuroepithelium and sensory nerve endings cause nasal pruritus and bothersome sneezing. The effects continue in a delayed fashion, causing recruitment and migration of inflammatory cells, including macrophages, neutrophils, and eosinophils. This late phase may persist for hours or days.

The sequence of events initiated by the allergen also causes secondary sinus ostia closure, which results in negative pressure within the sinus cavities and sets the stage for bacterial invasion.[11] Further reduction in ciliary function leads to accumulation of secretions, bacterial stasis, or biofilm formation. A cycle of sinusitis may ensue and quality of life can be significantly impaired (**Fig. 2**). First-line treatment includes aggressive nasal hygiene, parenteral therapy, and topical nasal corticosteroids. More complex or persistent disease may benefit from immunotherapeutic desensitization or surgical intervention. Additionally, certain patients are refractory to even long-term medical management, and repeated physician visits for immunotherapy may not be feasible.

The literature agrees that nasal obstruction is the symptom in AR that is most refractory to medical management. It is also perhaps the most important symptom in

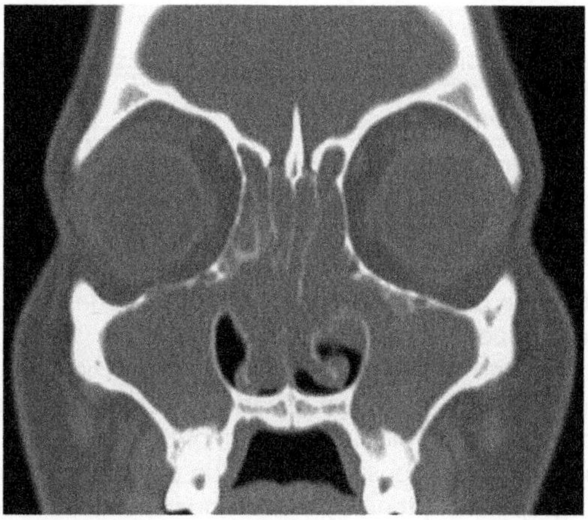

Fig. 2. Pansinusitis in a patient with AR.

improving quality of life for these patients. Surgical intervention may be necessary to address this issue, and also to reduce fixed obstruction and aid in dynamic compliance of the nasal airway. Although surgery will not eliminate the inflammation central to AR, additional patency of the nasal fossa reduces the effects of edematous mucosa and may alleviate symptoms. Before the era of endoscopic sinus techniques, septoplasty and inferior turbinate reduction were the classic surgical interventions for the treatment of AR. Neurectomy and selective nasal tissue reduction have been used, though limited data is available to support their routine use. Endoscopic sinus surgery has gained increasing popularity in the past decade and has proven useful, especially when AR contributes to chronic sinusitis, fungal disease, or polyposis. Still, inferior turbinate reduction is perhaps the most common and widely used procedure for treating nasal obstruction in AR that is refractory to medical therapy.

The Role of the Inferior Turbinate in AR

Hypertrophy of the inferior turbinates has long been established as the central cause of symptomatic nasal obstruction in AR. Allergic inflammation causes vasoreactive engorgement of turbinate tissue and associated inflammation of the mucosal lining. The mucosal epithelium of the inferior turbinates has been regarded as the central site for IgE-mediated reactions and nasal eosinophilia.[12] Topical intranasal corticosteroid therapy targets the inferior turbinate epithelium to help attenuate the allergic inflammatory response. In certain refractory cases or in chronic rhinosinusitis, surgical reduction/removal of turbinate tissue may help alleviate symptoms.

The effect of reducing allergic symptoms using surgical reduction of turbinate tissue can best be understood through histologic and anatomic considerations of the inferior turbinate. The lower turbinates have a very important role in nasal physiology and airway compliance. They are bony structures lined with mucosa consisting of ciliated pseudostratified columnar epithelium.[13] The submucosal lamina propria supports this superficial epithelial layer and contains key histologic elements, including parasympathetic nerve fibers, mucous glands, Goblet cells, and abundant vasculature.[13,14] Hyperplasia of glandular elements within the submucosal layer of the turbinate may worsen nasal obstruction and rhinorrhea in AR.[13] The inferior turbinates modulate inhaled air temperature and nasal resistance, while sharing important mucociliary functions with surrounding nasal tissue. The first points of contact for allergens are the lower turbinates, and deposition in these areas results in localized inflammation stemming from submucosal structures. The goal of surgery of the inferior turbinate is to minimize allergen effects through reducing bulky inflammatory tissue or inducing scar formation, while enhancing patency of the nasal fossa.

Inferior Turbinate Reduction in AR

Over the years, total turbinectomy has become significantly less common and essentially obsolete, partly because of fear of complications such as atrophic rhinitis or empty nose syndrome (ENS).[15] Radical turbinectomy also compromises ciliary function and reduces nasal resistance and humidification. Additionally, technological advances have led to the development of a broader and less-traumatic armamentarium of surgical techniques for turbinoplasty.

Mechanisms accounting for symptomatic improvement in patients with AR after turbinate surgery are likely a combination of various factors. The net mucosal surface may be slightly decreased after volume reduction of the turbinates, thereby reducing available contact points for allergens.[16] Scar tissue develops within the submucosal layer after surgical manipulation, thereby destroying vasculature and glandular structures while impeding regrowth through fibrosis. The reduced volume of the inferior turbinate results in increased nasal patency, allowing the nasal fossa to accommodate swelling of the turbinate from AR. The net effect is improved quality of life through decreased nasal obstruction.

Many techniques are available for turbinate reduction, including classic lateral outfracture techniques, submucosal resection, radiofrequency ablation, coblation, and laser reduction.

Lateralization Outfracture of the Inferior Turbinate

Lateral outfracture of the inferior turbinates has a longstanding history in the otolaryngologic treatment of nasal obstruction. The anterior and inferior portions of the lower turbinate are the main determinants of nasal resistance, and hence are the target of outfracture. Poiseuille's law states that the laminar flow rate of air along a pipe is proportional to the fourth power of the pipe's radius.[17,18] Therefore, small changes in the inferior turbinate will dramatically affect nasal airflow, which is the physiologic basis on which reduction of lower turbinate tissue rests.

Of all the turbinate reduction techniques, outfracture lateralization is the most surgically conservative and considered the least traumatic to mucosa and surrounding nasal structures. The outfracture procedure was first described by Killian in 1904 as an alternative and replacement to the more historic radical turbinectomy.[17] The risk of nasal adhesions is negligible and there is a minimal chance of developing atrophic rhinitis. Historically, outfracture techniques were thought to produce only short-lasting benefits with a modest increase in nasal patency that is not predictable, especially because the turbinate may medialize over time and symptoms may recur.[19,20] The classic method is displacement of the inferior turbinate in a lateral, then superior, and then inferior fashion until a crunching sound is heard (**Fig. 3**). Minor variations exist; some authors prefer to first displace the turbinate in an inferomedial direction, whereas others will add chiseling to the lateral wall attachment to facilitate anterior lateralization.

Aksoy and colleagues[17] evaluated the effectiveness of bilateral turbinate outfracture in 40 patients as a function of the angles and distances between the inferior turbinate and lateral nasal sidewall on paranasal coronal CT scans. They found statistically significant reductions in the angle and distance between the inferior turbinate bone and lateral nasal wall and the area lateral to the inferior turbinate. This reduction was sustained at 6 months postoperatively, leading the authors to conclude that medialization does not occur in at least the first 6 months after outfracture. In general, lateralization outfracture of the inferior turbinate is a safe and simple method of enhancing nasal patency and can be accomplished with routine instrumentation. Additionally, there is virtually no disruption of mucosa and sensory afferents or risk of damage to surrounding structures, including the nasolacrimal system. Further studies with large patient populations are needed to evaluate the long-term efficacy of lateralization outfracture.

Laser Vaporization of the Inferior Turbinate

Six basic laser systems are available for the treatment of hypertrophic inferior turbinates: carbon dioxide (CO_2), diode, neodymium-yttrium aluminum garnet (Nd:YAG), potassium-titanyl phosphate (KTP), argonion, and holmium-yttrium aluminum garnet (Ho:YAG) lasers.[21] Each laser differs slightly in depth of penetration and the optimum chromophore. Cited benefits of laser therapy include enhanced hemostasis, reduced postoperative pain, and improved healing.

The concept of laser therapy is to prevent excessive mucosal damage or bony exposure while inducing fibrosis and reducing turbinate bulk and surface area.

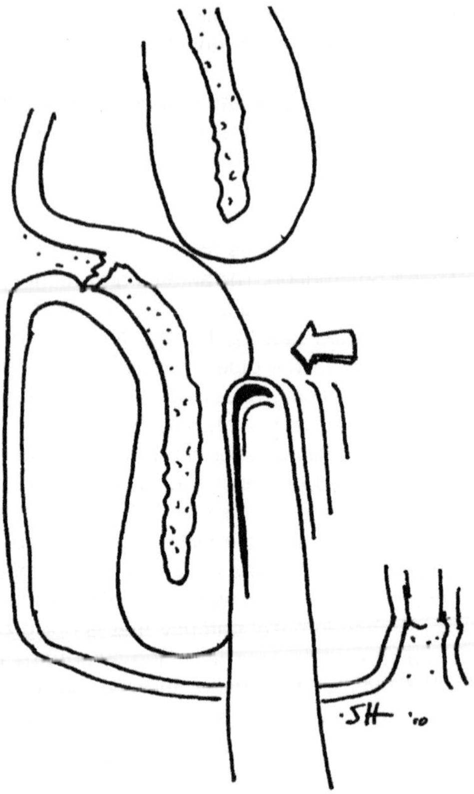

Fig. 3. Schematic representation of outfracture lateralization of the right inferior turbinate.

Vaporization of the entire turbinate has been reported but is not widespread.[22] The laser may be applied in a linear fashion, anterior-to-posterior stripes, cross-hatching across the entire mucosal surface, or along only the anterior or inferior aspect of the turbinate.[23] Spot treatment based on obvious areas of edema or inflammation or any combination of these techniques may also be used for increased efficacy.

The effect of laser therapy on allergen-mediated responses of the inferior turbinates has been studied in histochemical models. Elwany and Abel Salaam[24] reported on 15 patients undergoing CO_2 laser ablation turbinoplasty. Biopsy specimens taken 1 month after laser treatment showed many disorganized seromucinous acini in a background of dense fibrous stoma. Electron microscopy showed an overall reduction in the number of active nasal glands, likely accounting for the postoperative reduction in nasal rhinorrhea. Although this study included specimens only up to 1 month postoperatively, other authors have verified the long-term histologic changes induced by the laser.[25]

Caffier and colleagues[26] recently reported on the effects of diode laser turbinoplasty on 40 subjects, both seasonal and perennial sufferers. Some patients had concomitant septal or middle turbinate pathology that was also addressed, but overall, 95% of patients had diode laser inferior turbinoplasty. The investigators noted statistically significant improvements in both objective rhinomanometry and subjective scores for nasal obstruction, rhinorrhea, sneezing, and nasal pruritus. The improvement was greatest in symptomatic nasal obstruction and was initially higher in perennial patients, but was more sustained in the seasonal rhinitis population. No significant group differences were seen in symptoms of rhinorrhea, sneezing, or itching. Overall, 80% and 65% of patients experienced a stable, nonmedicated course at 1 and 2 years, respectively.[26] In some cases, bony exposure of septal crests or spurs occurred, but no significant long- or short-term adverse outcomes were seen.

Takeno and colleagues[27] prospectively compared CO_2 laser partial turbinectomy in perennial and seasonal patients, and noted initially less-pronounced improvement in sneezing and rhinorrhea in the seasonal group and greater cross-sectional enlargement of nasal cavity volume in the perennial group. These findings led the authors to conclude that laser therapy may be beneficial for acute seasonal exacerbations, but the effects may not be maximally therapeutic until later in the allergy season. Supiyaphun and colleagues[28] found no statistically significant differences in total airway resistance assessed by rhinomanometry after KTP turbinoplasty, although improvements in total inspired nasal airflow were noted.

Overall, symptomatic improvement from laser turbinoplasty and turbinectomy is varied in the literature, from 50% to 100% effectiveness. Proponents advocate less postoperative pain, better hemostasis, and more precise delivery of focused energy to achieve results. Additionally, the use of in-office lasers obviates the need for general anesthesia. Although lasers have a very low side-effect profile, the equipment can be expensive, bulky, and unavailable in many medical centers. Complications include crusting, synechiae formation, and bony exposure of nasal structures.

The Role of Submucosal Resection

The classic procedure of submucous resection involved an incision and the raising of a mucosal flap on the medial/septal side of the lower turbinate, followed by resection of bone with forceps (**Fig. 4**). The mucosa overlying the inferior meatus on the lateral aspect of the inferior turbinate was often also removed, and the medially conserved mucosa was then redraped over the resection site. Over time, the term *submucous resection* has become somewhat unclear and is now used throughout the literature in reference to a variety of techniques, including thermal ablation of cavernous submucosal tissue, laser reduction, and powered instrumentation. Navigating the literature,

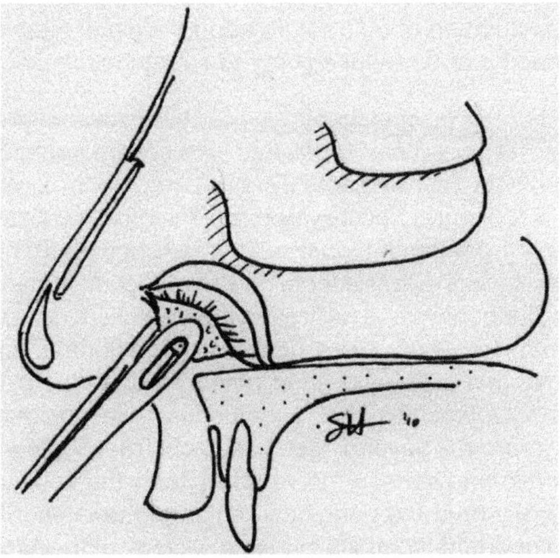

Fig. 4. Classic submucous resection of the lower turbinate.

one will find that submucous resection is used loosely and the specific technique may not be elucidated. The authors advise the judicious use of the term *submucous resection* and instead recommend naming and clearly describing the specific technique used. When referencing submucous resection of the inferior turbinate, this term should be reserved for the classic open technique.

Reduction of the submucous component of the inferior turbinate has a role in chronic nasal obstruction, rhinosinusitis, obstructive sleep apnea, and AR. The fundamental goal is to reduce bulky inflammatory tissue and perhaps turbinate bone, thereby enhancing nasal patency and improving the obstructive component. The overlying mucosa is maximally preserved, so as to not compromise ciliary function. Maintenance of surface epithelium is also necessary to reduce feared complications of crusting, synechiae, and osteitis that may result from bony exposure.[23]

Total inferior turbinectomy

As described by Passali and colleagues,[19] total inferior turbinectomy may result in significant adverse outcomes. In this regard, radical turbinectomy has largely fallen out of favor and is no longer routinely practiced. The development of empty nose syndrome is an iatrogenic disorder resulting from the loss of turbinate tissue.[29] Although the development of ENS is somewhat controversial and rare, it can be a devastating complication and its incidence is greatly reduced through conservative measures.[15,29] Therefore the authors recommend the cautious approach to inferior turbinate resection and advocate mucosal-sparing operations, which carry less risk for the development of ENS unless performed in an overly aggressive fashion.

Other techniques

Passàli and colleagues[19] compared classic submucosal resection of the inferior turbinate to various other modalities, including cryosurgery, laser cautery, and radical turbinectomy, over a 4-year follow-up period. Turbinectomy had the greatest effect on reducing nasal obstruction, but incurred adverse effects on mucociliary transport time and caused secondary hemorrhage. Submucous resection showed a lower incidence of bleeding and crusting, and the greatest improvement in mucociliary clearance and secretory IgA production, although patients had longer hospital stays compared with other groups. Additionally, when combined with lateralization outfracture, submucous resection had even further benefit, but the difference was not statistically significant. The addition of outfracture added minimal morbidity and time, and the authors recommend it as a useful adjunct to submucous resection alone.

Outcomes with submucous turbinectomy

Mori and colleagues[12] reported on 60 patients with severe perennial AR who underwent submucous turbinectomy. Subjects were followed up for 1 year and the authors evaluated changes in subjective nasal symptoms, rhinometry, nasal provocation, and immunohistochemistry from nasal biopsies. Results showed that submucous turbinectomy had statistically significant effects on the reduction of nasal discharge, stiffness, and sneezing. Eosinophils and infiltrating IgE cells were reduced in the turbinate tissue, although serum IgE levels were unaltered. Additionally, saccharin transport times were maintained primarily because of preservation of the overlying epithelium. These investigators hypothesized that submucous resection may be superior in reducing allergic symptoms beyond just nasal obstruction, possibly because of disruption of autonomic and sensory nerve fibers from the sphenopalatine foramen that travel submucosally or in the periosteal region of the inferior turbinate.[12] These nerves have shown important functions in the physiology of the nasal mucosa, microvascular circulation, and immunoglobulin production.[12,30]

Mori and colleagues[31] further reported on long-term outcomes over a 5-year follow-up period. The investigators noted a significant increase in total nasal airflow, a gradual reduction in the total nasal symptom score, and reduced nasal allergen responses over several years postoperatively after submucous resection of inferior turbinate tissue. At more than 3 years after surgery, 72.5% of patients were free of nasal allergic reactions. Moreover, quality of life was enhanced in this patient population, with 60% of patients noting excellent improvement in nasal allergic and 50% of patients maintaining a treatment-free disease state postoperatively. The authors identified a nerve fiber during endoscopic submucous resection that histochemical analysis suggested was a branch of the postnasal nerve. The authors believe that transection of this nerve may be responsible for the reduced sneezing and hypersecretion seen after submucous resection, as originally proposed in their previous study.[12]

Submucous electrocautery

Submucous electrocautery of the lamina propria after bony turbinate resection has shown promising reduction in symptoms with minimal crusting.[14] Ishida and colleagues[14,32] showed a significant reduction in anti-tryptase–positive mast cells after surgery, resulting in decreased histamine levels in nasal lavage. The authors advocate maximal preservation of overlying mucosa to aid with mucociliary transport, warming, and humidification of the nasal passages. The destruction of the lamina propria is perhaps the most important component of submucous resection. Preservation of normal nasal mucosa while adequately resecting submucosal tissue will maximize benefit to patients with AR.

Microdebrider turbinoplasty

Microdebrider turbinoplasty is a form of submucosal resection that uses a small stab or pocket-type submucosal incision, followed by resection of the cavernous tissue surrounding the bony turbinate (**Fig. 5**). Advantages include real-time suction with precise tissue removal, and this method has gained increasing popularity in recent years.[33] Chen and colleagues[34] compared submucosal resection with microdebrider-assisted turbinoplasty in 160 patients with perennial symptoms and turbinate hypertrophy. The study groups consisted of microdebrider-assisted turbinoplasty with lateral outfracture and submucous resection alone. Visual analog scales, saccharin transport testing, and anterior rhinomanometry were used to compare outcomes between the groups. The investigators noted an improvement in subjective complaints, nasal airflow, and mucociliary transport across both groups. They concluded that microdebrider turbinoplasty is equally as effective as submucous resection in these assessment

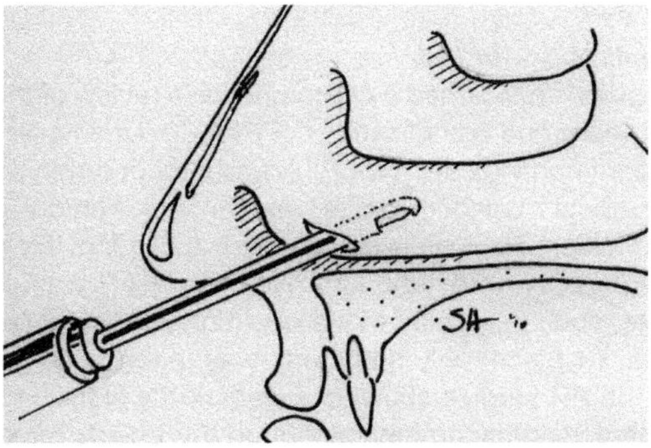

Fig. 5. Microdebrider-assisted turbinoplasty.

dimensions up to a 3-year follow-up period. Their data suggest improved mucociliary time with microdebrider technique compared with submucous resection, likely because of less trauma to overlying mucosa. The authors advocate microdebrider turbinoplasty as an effective method for turbinate reduction in AR, but unlike in submucous resection, bone is not removed, which may be problematic in patients with thick or calcified bony turbinates.

Summary: submucous resection of inferior turbinate

Submucous resection of the inferior turbinate has been shown to provide beneficial effects to patients with AR and is generally well tolerated with few long-term side effects. Despite the various terms used within the realm of submucous resection, the basic principles of augmenting the nasal airway through reduction of lower turbinate tissue remain the same. Regardless of the specific method used, respect for the superficial mucosal layer and conservative technique are vital to optimize outcomes. However, excessive or overzealous submucous resection of turbinate tissue may potentially lead to paradoxic nasal obstruction, the hallmark of empty nose syndrome, and the senior author has seen this complication from submucous resection.

Radiofrequency Ablation and Coblation Turbinoplasty

Radiofrequency ablation (RFA) has been well established as a means to achieve volume reduction of tissue of the upper airway. This technology has been applied to oropharyngeal, tongue base, and palatal tissue to alleviate obstructive symptoms in patients.[35] Radiofrequency reduction has also found a place in the treatment of nasal obstruction A probe is inserted directly into the inferior turbinate and is used to deliver a low-frequency energy, which induces ionic agitation of tissues.[23] A thermal effect occurs from elevated temperature, resulting in postoperative wound contracture and fibrosis.[23] The energy is apparently limited to the submucosa, which preserves the surface epithelium and, therefore, ciliary function.[36]

Coagulative necrosis is the first step in the process of tissue destruction by RFA, and the effects of scar contracture and tissue retraction occur later in the wound healing process. Over time, portions of the fibrotic scar undergo resorption and the submucosal scar will adhere to the bony periosteum, both reducing turbinate bulk while rendering it less susceptible to edema and engorgement.[36,37] The output frequency of most RFA devices and generators varies from 100 to 4,000 kHz, and the relationship between frequency and extent of the thermal lesion produced is not yet clear.[36] Coblation technology, which relies on electrodissection by molecular activation, is generally grouped as a subset within RFA and similarly targets the submucosal layers.[36,38]

Outcomes and complications of RFA

Hytönen and colleagues[36] performed a comprehensive review of the literature in 2009 to study the effectiveness and complications of RFA on patients with nasal symptomatology. The most common indication for RFA was inferior turbinate hypertrophy that was refractory to medical management. AR was an inclusion criterion in 6 of the 35 reviewed studies. Multiple devices were studied, including the coblation system. The outcome of RFA on symptomatic improvement in AR was primarily based on subjective measures, such as quality of life questionnaires and patient or physician visual analog scales. Of these, only one study was placebo-controlled and double-blinded.[18] Overall, the AR studies showed a statistically significant effect on symptoms and, in one case, rhinomanometry confirmed this effect.[39] In general, subjective improvement of nasal patency peaked around 3 weeks after treatment. When compared with other methods of turbinoplasty, RFA reduced nasal obstruction in a statistically significant manner, although microdebrider-assisted turbinoplasty showed superior results in reducing nasal volume and nasal blockage.[36,40] In the comparative studies, RFA had fewer side effects.

RFA is generally well tolerated across both pediatric and adult populations. Hytönen and colleagues[36] noted the absence of significant complications related to RFA across the 35 studies they reviewed. The most common complaint was pain during and after the procedure, and in some cases the treatment was terminated because of intraoperative pain.[41] RFA is often performed in the outpatient or clinical office setting; therefore, appropriate local or block anesthetic is imperative in minimizing intraoperative discomfort. Bleeding, crusting, and postoperative edema are also possible adverse effects, and some authors have noted the presence of localized infections.[42]

In the first long-term study of its kind, Lin and colleagues[16] recently published on 101 patients undergoing RFA turbinoplasty for the treatment of AR refractory to medical therapy. Patients were followed up to at least 5 years postoperatively. Both global patient questionnaires and visual analog scales were used to evaluate the efficacy of RFA in this series. Response rates at 6 months and 5 years were 77.3% and 60.5%, respectively, and statistically significant improvement in nasal obstruction, rhinorrhea, sneezing, itchy nose, and itchy eyes was noted. RFA alone produced no improvement in 17 patients, who subsequently underwent additional turbinate procedures, such as laser ablation or submucosal resection. The authors hypothesized that the reduction in ocular symptoms in their study, approximately 43%, may be from an RFA mediated inhibitory effect on the local immune response or naso-ocular reflex; however, further research is necessary to elucidate potential mechanisms. The authors acknowledge the lack of a control group, the need for objective measures to verify the subjective results, and a substantial number of patients lost to follow-up.

Garzaro and colleagues[43] recently published objective data on the effects of RFA on olfactory function on 40 patients with both allergic and nonallergic rhinitis presenting with nasal obstruction caused by inferior turbinate hypertrophy. Anterior rhinomanometry, subjective questionnaire, and odor identification, discrimination, and thresholds were used in this series. Although no correlation between allergy and the improvement of olfactory function was found, the authors showed statistically significant improvements in basal nasal resistance 2 months after surgery, and net improvement in the sum of odor thresholds, discrimination, and identification. Improvements in olfactory function may be related to the surgical modification of airspaces medial to the inferior turbinate or volume changes of the inferior meatus, which are induced by RFA.[44] Further research in the realm of olfactory function after RFA therapy is needed.

Coblation

A technique that has garnered increasing popularity in recent years is coblation, which exists within the umbrella of RFA. The coblation technology exploits molecular ionization to achieve low-temperature disintegration of tissues, with minimal damage to surrounding structures.[38] Fundamentally, this technology should incur less pain and is therefore especially popular in the pediatric population. Siméon and colleagues[38] investigated the efficacy of the Coblator (Arthocare Corporation) radiofrequency device on nine patients with AR with a mean age of 12.7 years. In this study, assessment consisted of rhinomanometry, visual analog scales, and quality of life questionnaires. Favorable and statistically significant decreases in binasal resistance, pruritus, sneezing, hyposmia, and rhinorrhea were observed and sustained at 6-month follow-up. The authors noted that coblation turbinoplasty did not abolish rhinitis but rather assisted in the efficacy of topical corticosteroids. Additionally, although this study did not specifically focus on pulmonary disease associated with AR, most patients showed some concomitant pulmonary improvement, possibly related to normalization of nasal airflow from the Coblator device.[38]

Summary: RFA and coblation

RFA and coblation have shown promising results. The procedures are well tolerated with minimal adverse effects, including less likelihood of empty nose syndrome, and can be performed safely in an outpatient clinical or in-office setting. Coblation, in particular, heralds less pain and may have expanded implications for the pediatric population. The main disadvantage of RFA technology relates to a lack of well planned, double-blind, placebo-controlled randomized trials to better elucidate causal relationships.[36] Additionally, longer patient follow-up, further objective assessment, and side-by-side comparison of various devices to evaluate cost-effectiveness and general efficacy are needed.

Septoplasty in Allergic Rhinitis

Septoplasty has long existed as a means to treat symptomatic nasal obstruction. However, the role of septoplasty in nasal obstruction associated with AR is poorly understood. A paucity of literature has investigated septoplasty alone as a means to improve nasal patency in AR, largely because the nasal septum is not believed to be a major contributor to the disease process or to nasal obstruction seen in AR. Compared with the nasal septum, the inferior turbinate has a more central role in symptomatology. The septum does not experience the extent of dynamic changes as turbinate tissue, including engorgement, mucosal edema, and glandular hyperplasia. The septum is also thought to have a lesser contribution to allergen deposition and mucociliary clearance. Historically, some authors have even cited AR as a relative contraindication to septal surgery, primarily because of the lack of significant improvement in nasal obstruction.[45,46] Structural support and regulation of airflow are key functions of the nasal septum. In many cases, anatomic deformities, such as bony spurs or cartilaginous deviation, may affect the normal laminar airflow in the nasal fossae and may worsen subjective nasal obstruction in patients with AR (**Fig. 6**). Most often, septoplasty is combined with turbinoplasty or endoscopic sinus surgery,

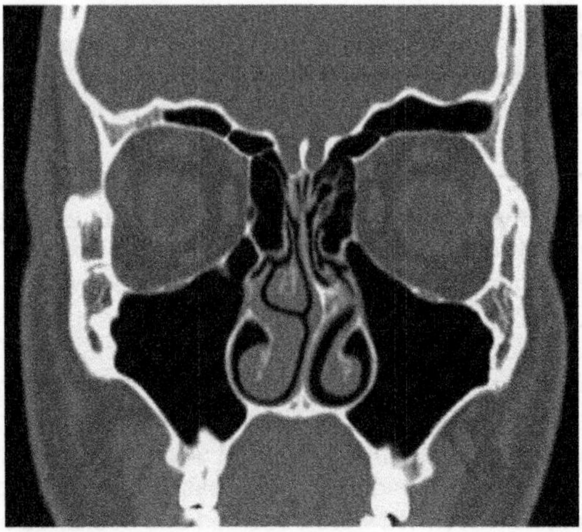

Fig. 6. Obstructive septal spur of the left nasal fossa.

especially when obvious anatomic septal deformity or obstruction exists.[36] Septoplasty may be undertaken to improve function and quality of life in patients afflicted with AR, although it is rarely used alone as primary surgical therapy.

In 1988, Fjermedal and colleagues[46] compared septal submucous resection with septoplasty in 478 patients. Of this group, 72 patients had AR based on either skin prick or serum IgE values. The authors noted that improvements in nasal patency and air passage were comparable between the allergic and nonallergic patients, whereas rhinorrhea remained unchanged from the preoperative state. With regard to patient satisfaction, the investigators found that patients with AR were significantly less satisfied than their nonallergic counterparts.[46] The authors concluded that patients with AR may undergo septal surgery on general lines, but did not advocate for AR as an absolute indication for septoplasty.

A 2009 study by Karatzanis and colleagues[47] confirmed these findings. In this study, 176 patients underwent septoplasty and all patients were evaluated using both anterior rhinomanometry and subjective questionnaires. Patients with AR with nasal septal deviation and those with nasal septal deviation alone were compared. The authors found that after septoplasty, subjective improvement in breathing was present in both groups but was significantly higher in patients without AR. Anterior rhinomanometry showed improvement in nasal airflow also in both groups, but the result was substantially higher in the group that had nasal septal deviation only. The authors therefore recommend a cautious approach to the management of nasal septal deviation in AR, because these patients are less likely to be satisfied after surgery than nonallergic patients.[47]

A recent study by Topal and colleagues[48] investigated the risk of septal perforation in patients with AR after septoplasty. The loss of epithelial integrity of nasal mucosa, chronic use of intranasal steroids, and increased mucosal fragility from chronic inflammation may predispose these patients to septal perforation.[48,49] The authors address the important question of whether septal procedures may increase the risk of nasal septal perforations in this patient population. In this study, septoplasty as described by Cottle and colleagues[50] was performed on 352 patients, 70 of whom had AR. The study group did not undergo concomitant turbinate or endoscopic procedures. The nonallergic and allergic groups had septal perforation rates of 1.4% and 0.7%, respectively. No statistical significance was found between the groups, and the authors concluded that septoplasty for AR does not impart a higher risk for nasal septal perforation.

Septoplasty has shown a beneficial effect on nasal obstruction in general, and may improve subjective nasal patency, especially when fixed anatomic obstruction of the septum is present. However, its role in the treatment of AR as a sole surgical modality is not convincing, although it may be a useful adjunct to turbinoplasty in the presence of an obvious and contributing obstructive component of the nasal septum. Additionally, the otolaryngologist should bear in mind that patient satisfaction after septoplasty may not be as substantial in allergic patients as in their nonallergic counterparts. Therefore, the authors recommend the judicious use of septoplasty in allergic patients.

Endoscopic Sinus Surgery and Vidian Neurectomy

Endoscopic sinus surgery has gradually evolved as one of the most common otolaryngologic procedures for the treatment of nasal obstruction caused by chronic sinusitis, paranasal and sinus polyposis, and allergic fungal sinusitis. Although endoscopic sinus surgery does not have a direct role in treating AR, it is of indirect benefit in patients with AR who also have chronic rhinosinusitis or polyposis. The main goal of endoscopic surgery is to maximize nasal patency and to alleviate the effects of edematous ostia leading to chronic sinusitis. Polyp disease that obstructs the ostiomeatal complex or nasal fossa should also be addressed, and surgical reduction of polyposis will assist with medical therapy and topical intranasal corticosteroids. Allergic fungal disease that is unresponsive to medical management is another indication for endoscopic sinus surgery, and mechanical debridement and removal of inspissated secretions and allergic mucin may be necessary. In these patients, maximizing medical management is of central importance in conjunction with endoscopic sinus procedures. Additionally, endoscopic interventions may be combined with turbinoplasty to provide relief to more refractory or advanced cases of AR, in which turbinoplasty alone may be inadequate.

Vidian neurectomy

Vidian neurectomy is of historical importance and is briefly mentioned. Originally described by Golding-Wood in 1961,[51] vidian neurectomy involves transection of the efferent pathway of the parasympathetic reflex, and a variety of methods have been described.[52] The vidian nerve gains contributions from the superficial and greater petrosal nerves and the pericarotid sympathetic plexus before joining the sphenopalatine ganglion. Injury to the sensory nerve fibers reduces hyperreactivity of the nasal reflex, effectively reducing sneezing and nasal hypersecretion.[51] Although historically effective, vidian neurectomy has largely fallen out of favor because of adverse outcomes. The most frequent and long-term side effect of vidian neurectomy is loss of lacrimation, or keratoconjunctivitis sicca, which mandates the use of artificial tear substitution.[51] This effect can be severely disabling and bothersome to patients, especially in warm weather climates. Abducens paralysis or other eye movement disorders and postoperative hemorrhaging have also been described.[53] Advances in both medical and surgical therapy have largely replaced the classic vidian neurectomy. Research into alternatives, such as selective ganglion ligation or endoscopic posterior neurectomy, is underway but further studies are needed to elucidate their role.[23,31,51] Presently, vidian neurectomy is seldom a treatment for AR and, when used, is a last resort after other surgical therapies have failed and the patient is adequately apprised of potential side effects.

SUMMARY: SURGERY FOR AR

AR is a very common condition, and the complaint of nasal obstruction can significantly affect the quality of life in patients. The surgical goal in AR is to augment the nasal airway through reducing turbinate tissue or obstructive components, such as septal spurs or polyposis. The inferior turbinate has proven to be the most important contributor to nasal obstruction and dynamic compliance of the nasal fossa in patients with AR. A variety of procedures for the surgical reduction of lower turbinate tissue have been described, although no single operation has been defined as the gold standard. Meticulous surgical technique, respect of tissue planes, and conservative reduction of lower turbinate tissue to help reduce adverse outcomes such as empty nose syndrome are crucial in maximizing surgical outcomes and improving symptoms.

REFERENCES

1. Krause HF. Allergy and chronic rhinosinusitis. Otolaryngol Head Neck Surg 2003; 128(1):14–6.
2. Trevino R, Gordon B. Allergic rhinosinusitis. Ear Nose Throat J 1993;72:116–29.
3. Beasley R, Keil U, Von Mutius E, et al. The international study of asthma and allergies in childhood (ISSAC) steering committee. Worldwide variation in prevalence

of asthma, allergic rhinoconjunctivitis, and atopic eczema: ISSAC. Lancet 1998; 351:1225–32.
4. Wright AL, Holberg CJ, Martinez FD, et al. Epidemiology of physician-diagnosed allergic rhinitis in childhood. Pediatrics 1994;94:895–901.
5. Nathan RA, Meltzer EO, Derebery, et al. The prevalence of nasal symptoms attributed to allergies in the United States: findings from the burden of rhinitis in an America survey. Allergy Asthma Proc 2008;29:600–8.
6. Ray NF, Baraniuk JN, Thamer M, et al. Direct expenditures for the treatment of allergic rhinoconjunctivitis in 1996, including the contributions of related airway illnesses. J Allergy Clin Immunol 1999;103:401–7.
7. Wayoff M, Moneret Vautrin DA. How and why the nose runs. J Allergy Clin Immunol 1991;87:457–67.
8. Siracusa A, Desrosiers M, Marabini A. Epidemiology of occupational rhinitis: prevalence, aetiology and determinants. Clin Exp Allergy 2000;30(11):1519–34.
9. Frew AJ. Advances in environmental and occupational diseases 2003. J Allergy Clin Immunol 2004;113(6):1161–6.
10. Iwasaki M, Saito K, Takemura M, et al. TNF-alpha contributes to the development of allergic rhinitis in mice. J Allergy Clin Immunol 2003;112(1):134–40.
11. Hansen I, Klimek L, Mosges R, et al. Mediators of inflammation in the early and the late phase of allergic rhinitis. Curr Opin Allergy Clin Immunol 2004;4(3):159–63.
12. Mori S, Fujieda S, Igarashi M, et al. Submucous turbinectomy decreases not only nasal stiffness but also sneezing and rhinorrhea in patients with perennial allergic rhinitis. Clin Exp Allergy 1999;29(11):1542–8.
13. Millas I, Liquidato BM, Dolci JE, et al. Histological analysis of the distribution pattern of glandular tissue in normal inferior nasal turbinates. Braz J Otorhinolaryngol 2009;75(4):507–10.
14. Ishida H, Yoshida T, Hasegawa T, et al. Submucous electrocautery following submucous resection of turbinate bone–a rationale of surgical treatment for allergic rhinitis. Auris Nasus Larynx 2003;30(2):147–52.
15. Houser SM. Surgical treatment for empty nose syndrome. Arch Otolaryngol Head Neck Surg 2007;133(9):858–63.
16. Lin HC, Lin PW, Friedman M, et al. Long-term results of radiofrequency turbinoplasty for allergic rhinitis refractory to medical therapy. Arch Otolaryngol Head Neck Surg 2010;136(9):892–5.
17. Aksoy F, Yıldırım YS, Veyseller B, et al. Midterm outcomes of outfracture of the inferior turbinate. Otolaryngol Head Neck Surg 2010;143(4):579–84.
18. Powell NB, Zonato AI, Weaver EM, et al. Radiofrequency treatment of turbinate hypertrophy in subjects using continuous positive airway pressure: a randomized, double-blind, placebo-controlled clinical pilot trial. Laryngoscope 2001;111: 1783–90.
19. Passàli D, Lauriello M, Anselmi M, et al. Treatment of hypertrophy of the inferior turbinate: long-term results in 382 patients randomly assigned to therapy. Ann Otol Rhinol Laryngol 1999;108(6):569–75.
20. O'Flynn PE, Milford CA, Mackay IS. Multiple submucosal out-fractures of interior turbinates. J Laryngol Otol 1990;104(3):239–40.
21. Janda P, Sroka R, Baumgartner R, et al. Laser treatment of hyperplastic inferior turbinates: a review. Lasers Surg Med 2001;28:404–13.
22. Wolfson S, Wolfson LR, Kaplan I. CO2 laser inferior turbinectomy: a new surgical approach. J Clin Laser Med Surg 1996;13:81–3.
23. Chang CW, Ries WR. Surgical treatment of the inferior turbinate: new techniques. Curr Opin Otolaryngol Head Neck Surg 2004;12(1):53–7.

24. Elwany S, Abel Salaam S. Laser surgery for allergic rhinitis: the effect on seromucinous glands. Otolaryngol Head Neck Surg 1999;120(5):742–4.
25. Fukutake T, Kumazawa T, Nakamura A. Laser surgery for allergic rhinitis. AORN J 1987;46(4):756–61.
26. Caffier PP, Scherer H, Neumann K, et al. Diode laser treatment in therapy-resistant allergic rhinitis: impact on nasal obstruction and associated symptoms. Lasers Med Sci 2011;26(1):57–67.
27. Takeno S, Osada R, Ishino T, et al. Laser surgery of the inferior turbinate for allergic rhinitis with seasonal exacerbation: an acoustic rhinometry study. Ann Otol Rhinol Laryngol 2003;112(5):455–60.
28. Supiyaphun P, Aramwatanapong P, Kerekhanjanarong V, et al. KTP laser inferior turbinoplasty: an alternative procedure to treat the nasal obstruction. Auris Nasus Larynx 2003;30(1):59–64.
29. Chhabra N, Houser SM. The diagnosis and management of empty nose syndrome. Otolaryngol Clin North Am 2009;42(2):311–30.
30. Fujieda S, Waschek JA, Zhang K, et al. Vasoactive intestinal peptide induces S/S switch circular DNA in human B cells. J Clin Invest 1996;98:1527–32.
31. Mori S, Fujieda S, Yamada T, et al. Long-term effect of submucous turbinectomy in patients with perennial allergic rhinitis. Laryngoscope 2002;112(5):865–9.
32. Ishida H. Electrocoagulation of the lamina propria following submucosal resection of the inferior turbinate bone for patients with nasal allergies. JJS HNS 1996;6:77–85.
33. Davis WE, Nishioka GJ. Endoscopic partial inferior turbinectomy using a power microcutting instrument. Ear Nose Throat J 1996;75:49–50.
34. Chen YL, Tan CT, Huang HM. Long-term efficacy of microdebrider-assisted inferior turbinoplasty with lateralization for hypertrophic inferior turbinates in patients with perennial allergic rhinitis. Laryngoscope 2008;118(7):1270–4.
35. Blumen MB, Dahan S, Fleury B, et al. Radiofrequency ablation for the treatment of mild to moderate obstructive sleep apnea. Laryngoscope 2002;112:2086–92.
36. Hytönen ML, Bäck LJ, Malmivaara AV, et al. Radiofrequency thermal ablation for patients with nasal symptoms: a systematic review of effectiveness and complications. Eur Arch Otorhinolaryngol 2009;266(8):1257–66.
37. Li KK, Powell NB, Riley RW, et al. Radiofrequency volumetric tissue reduction for treatment of turbinate hypertrophy: a pilot study. Otolaryngol Head Neck Surg 1998;119(6):569–73.
38. Siméon R, Soufflet B, Souchal Delacour I. Coblation turbinate reduction in childhood allergic rhinitis. Eur Ann Otorhinolaryngol Head Neck Dis 2010;127(2):77–82.
39. Oyake D, Ochi K, Takatsu M, et al. Clinical effect of bipolar radiofrequency thermotherapy on allergic rhinitis. Nippon Jibiinkoka Gakkai Kaiho 2004;107(7):695–701 [in Japanese].
40. Lee JY, Lee JD. Comparative study on the long-term effectiveness between coblation and microdebrider-assisted partial turbinoplasty. Laryngoscope 2006;116(5):729–34.
41. Coste A, Yona L, Blumen M, et al. Radiofrequency is a safe and effective treatment of turbinate hypertrophy. Laryngoscope 2001;111(5):894–9.
42. Madani M. Complications of laser-assisted uvulopalatopharyngoplasty and radiofrequency treatments of snoring and chronic nasal congestion: a 10-year review of 5,600 patients. J Oral Maxillofac Surg 2004;62(11):1351–62.
43. Garzaro M, Pezzoli M, Pecorari G, et al. Radiofrequency inferior turbinate reduction: an evaluation of olfactory and respiratory function. Otolaryngol Head Neck Surg 2010;143(3):348–52.

44. Leopold DA. The relationship between nasal anatomy and human olfaction. Laryngoscope 1988;98:1232–8.
45. Stoksted P, Gutierrez C. The nasal passage following rhinoplastic surgery. J Laryngol Otol 1983;97(1):49–54.
46. Fjermedal O, Saunte C, Pedersen S. Septoplasty and/or submucous resection? 5 years nasal septum operations. J Laryngol Otol 1988;102(9):796–8.
47. Karatzanis AD, Fragiadakis G, Moshandrea J, et al. Septoplasty outcome in patients with and without allergic rhinitis. Rhinology 2009;47(4):444–9.
48. Topal O, Celik SB, Erbek S, et al. Risk of nasal septal perforation following septoplasty in patients with allergic rhinitis. Eur Arch Otorhinolaryngol 2011;268(2): 231–3.
49. Amin K, Rinne J, Haahtela T, et al. Inflammatory cell and epithelial characteristics of perennial allergic and nonallergic rhinitis with a symptom history of 1 to 3 years' duration. J Allergy Clin Immunol 2001;107:249–57.
50. Cottle MH, Loring RM. Newer concepts of septum surgery: present status. Eye Ear Nose Throat Mon 1948;27:403–6.
51. Golding-Wood PH. Observation of petrosal and vidian neurectomy in chronic vasomotor rhinitis. J Laryngol Otol 1961;75:232–47.
52. Konno A. Historical, pathophysiological, and therapeutic aspects of vidian neurectomy. Curr Allergy Asthma Rep 2010;10(2):105–12.
53. Sadanaga M. Clinical evaluation of vidian neurectomy for nasal allergy. Auris Nasus Larynx 1989;16(Suppl 1):S53–7.

Inhalant Allergies in Children

James W. Mims, MD[a,*], Maria C. Veling, MD[b]

KEYWORDS

• Pediatric allergy • Allergies in children • Allergic rhinitis
• Childhood asthma • Otitis • Inhalant allergy

Most otolaryngologists see pediatric patients and treat disorders associated with chronic upper respiratory inflammation (rhinitis, otitis, pharyngitis, and laryngitis) as a routine part of their practice. In 2009, otolaryngologists were surveyed by telephone as part of the Pediatric Allergies in America Survey. Otolaryngologists estimated that they saw 43 patients aged 4 to 17 years per week and that 41% were diagnosed with AR.[1] Pillsbury and colleagues[2] noted that AR was the most common International Classification of Diseases-9 code used by otolaryngologists in a workforce study conducted in 2000. Because allergy is a common contributor of upper airway inflammation, a working knowledge of pediatric allergy is beneficial in the evaluation and treatment of children presenting to otolaryngologists. Upper and lower airway inflammation is linked epidemiologically and physiologically.[3] Therefore, considering and appropriately identifying coexisting lower respiratory inflammation (eg, asthma) is also logical. Identifying asthma in otolaryngology patients is especially compelling because unmanaged asthma impairs quality of life and can be fatal. It is also likely that asthma is underdiagnosed and undertreated.[4] This article informs the otolaryngologist about the development, manifestations, and treatment of allergy in pediatric patients.

GENETICS

Atopy is the predisposition to develop allergic diseases. The phenotype of allergy seems to have a complicated and variable genetic contribution. Gene–environment interactions have been identified,[5] and add another layer of variability to the development of allergic disease. There is no single genetic test to identify if an individual is likely to be atopic. Genetic studies looking at single nucleotide polymorphism have

The authors have nothing to disclose.

[a] Department of Otolaryngology, Medical Center Boulevard, Wake Forest University School of Medicine, Winston-Salem, NC 27157, USA
[b] Division of Otolaryngology, Department of Otolaryngology, University of Kentucky Medical Center, 800 Rose Street C-236, Lexington, KY 40536–0293, USA
* Corresponding author.
E-mail address: wmims@wfubmc.edu

Otolaryngol Clin N Am 44 (2011) 797–814
doi:10.1016/j.otc.2011.03.013 oto.theclinics.com

focused primarily on allergic inflammatory cells and mediators. Although hundreds of associations have been identified, each alone tends to be difficult to reproduce or represents only a small percentage of allergic individuals.[6] Large genome-wide association studies use a hypothesis-independent strategy to identify which genes are statistically different between an affected and nonaffected population. In asthma, genome-wide association studies have identified a small number of genes, such as ORMDL3,[7,8] of which the functions remain unclear. Currently, the allergy phenotype probably represents multiple and variable combinations of genetic predispositions many of which require a specific environmental interaction to be manifested. So far, the genes identified suggest alterations in both innate and adaptive immunity play a significant role in allergic disease.[9]

As suggested by the complicated genetics, family history of allergy is a risk factor, but inheritance does not follow a simple pattern. For AR, family history of atopy is one of several risk factors that include cigarette exposure; higher socioeconomic class; first-born or only child; and elevated total IgE (>100 IU/L) before age 6 years.[10] In the Danish twin study of asthma by Skadhauge and coworkers,[11] the proban-wise concordance of monozygotic males to develop asthma was 0.51 (0.39–0.63), whereas dizygotic opposite sex twins was only 0.07 (0.03–0.11). Another study showed that of those with one asthmatic parent, 26% developed asthma. Of note, maternal history was more predictive.[12] Although not definitive, asking about allergies in first-degree relatives is useful in the evaluation of a child with chronic upper or lower respiratory inflammation.

IN UTERO

There have been multiple studies investigating if variables in pregnancy affect the later development of allergies including the time of year the child is born, maternal diet, or route of delivery. One study suggested that North American children born in the late fall have a higher risk of developing asthma.[13] This is attributed to the role of winter respiratory viruses, such as respiratory syncytial virus, occurring in the first few months of life increasing the risk of asthma. However, the authors are not aware of any recommendations advising timing of pregnancy based on allergy risk because studies are conflicting and the overall evidence insufficient. Restricting maternal diet in pregnancy from proallergic foods has been shown not to affect the development of atopy in the child.[14] Some studies have shown some protection from atopy in children delivered vaginally compared with those delivered by cesarean section.[15] The affect is attributed to the "hygiene hypothesis," which is discussed later. IgE in cord blood has also been of interest. Nonspecific IgE is produced in utero starting around 11 weeks gestation, but specific IgE is first identified after birth. Initial reports of IgE levels in cord blood predicting atopy have not been supported in later prospective studies.[16]

Difficulties in identifying children at high risk for allergy beyond parental allergic history complicates research aimed at attempting to prevent the development of allergic disease.

INFANCY: 0 TO 2 YEARS

Although inhalant allergy is not prevalent during the first 2 years of life, there are clues in infancy as to the risk of later developing inhalant allergic disease. Knowledge of these risk factors can be useful when trying to determine if an older child's rhinitis may be allergic. Many studies have also examined if there are ways to prevent or reduce the development of allergic disease in children. A basic knowledge of the infant's developing immune system places the risk factors context.

In the atopic child, the bias of the immune system toward an allergic response is at least partially influenced by lymphocytes. Attention has been focused on T-helper cell lymphocytes because they direct much of the immunologic response to antigens. Stimulated T-helper lymphocytes produce different cytokine profiles that are broadly classified as Th1 or Th2 (a Th3 phenotype has also been described).[17,18] Th1 cytokines primarily influence the immune system to act against bacteria and include interleukin (IL)-2 and interferon-γ. Th2 cytokines direct activity more appropriate toward parasites. The Th2 influence toward IgE and eosinophils also occurs in allergic inflammation. Th2 cytokines include IL-4, IL-5, and IL-13. At birth, T-helper lymphocytes are Th2 biased (or allergy biased), and as the immune system develops the T-helper cells change to a Th1 bias. The "hygiene hypothesis" suggests that challenges to the immune system early in life facilitate the shift to a Th1 bias, which protects against allergy. Infections early in life,[19] or increased risk of infections represented by exposure to siblings or by early entry into daycare,[20] have been associated with a decreased risk of later developing allergic disease. Some studies of T lymphocytes from infants at high risk for atopy have shown not only bias toward Th2, but also a decreased production of both Th1 and Th2 cytokines. It may be that the greater reduction of stimulated Th1 cytokines accounts for most of the imbalance compared with controls.[21] Paradoxically, as infancy has become more sanitized in developed countries, atopy has become more prevalent. The reason for the increase in allergy is likely to be more complicated than the "hygiene hypothesis" alone and multiple competing theories from changes in exposures, to nutrition, to air pollution exist.

Manifestations of allergy in infancy include food allergy and atopic dermatitis, which are both risk factors for the later development of inhalant allergy. Food allergy is commonly seen in infants and is frequently the first identifier of the atopic child.[22] Ten percent of 1 year olds have an elevated IgE to a food, most commonly milk or egg.[23] Infants with milk or egg food allergy are at increased risk for developing AR and asthma.[23,24] Atopic dermatitis is another marker of atopy in infancy. Atopic dermatitis in infancy frequently presents as pruritic eczema of the cheeks and flexural surfaces of the elbows and knees. Infants with atopic dermatitis have a 30% risk of developing asthma and a 35% risk of developing AR.[25,26]

Early sensitization to inhalant allergies in infancy occurs, but infrequently. Herr and colleagues[27] used a standardized questionnaire in 1850 infants at their 18th-month examination to identify children with AR-like symptoms defined as runny nose, blocked nose, and sneezing apart from a cold. Of the 1850 infants, 9.1% were found to have AR-like symptoms. All children were then assessed with a specific inhalant IgE screen, total IgE, and eosinophilia. There was no difference in eosinophilia or total IgE in the "AR-like symptoms" group compared with the "no AR-like symptoms" group. Inhalant-specific IgE was elevated in 5.5% with AR-like symptoms versus 2.7% (P = .04) of those without symptoms. However, the Allergic Rhinitis and its Impact on Asthma (ARIA) guidelines include both specific IgE sensitization and symptoms in the definition of AR.[28] Only 9 of the 1850 children had both AR-like symptoms and elevated inhalant-specific IgE. In comparison, there were 43 of 1850 infants with elevated inhalant-specific IgE that were identified in the "no AR-like symptoms group." This suggests that AR is rare at 18 months of age and that screening infants for elevated specific IgE would lack specificity in identifying infants with clinical symptoms. Of interest, five of the nine infants with both AR-like symptoms and inhalant-specific IgE elevation were sensitized to dust mite.[28] Although AR is uncommon in infancy, viral rhinitis is prevalent. Children less than 6 years old average six to eight "colds" annually with symptoms lasting 10–14 days.[29] Rhinovirus accounted for 46% of childhood upper respiratory infections in one study.[30] Distinguishing between AR and viral rhinitis is clinically significant because a physician might reasonably treat an infant with AR with antihistamines, but antihistamines have been demonstrated as ineffective compared with placebo in viral rhinitis.[31]

Lower respiratory inflammation in infants has a similar clinical dilemma in differentiating viral bronchiolitis from asthma. Viral bronchiolitis (wheezing and tachypnea) accounts for outpatient visits in 15% of infants and 3% are hospitalized.[32] The common causes include respiratory syncytial virus, rhinovirus, metapneumovirus, and coronaviruses. Viral-triggered asthma and bronchiolitis are difficult to distinguish from each other, but viral-triggered asthma tends to occur in children who have multiple wheezing episodes, are older than 2 years, and have a family history of atopy.[33] Once children are older than 2 years, an association between viral-induced wheezing and asthma risks (elevation in inhalant-specific IgE, maternal asthma history) becomes significant.[34] The clinical distinction between bronchiolitis and asthma affects pharmacologic treatment. Although bronchodilators and corticosteroids are mainstays of asthma treatment, neither bronchodilators[35,36] nor corticosteroids[37] have been shown to be effective in uncomplicated viral bronchiolitis (discussed later).

Attenuating the development of allergy through environmental manipulation has not been very successful. A substantial number of studies have investigated restriction of food antigens or environmental controls to prevent inhalant sensitization, but these have yielded conflicting and often paradoxic results.

Because food allergy is frequently the first allergic manifestation in the atopic child and the prevalence of food allergy is increasing, multiple studies have investigated if restricting allergenic foods (eg, peanut products) from the infant's diet would reduce the development of allergic disease. Dietary avoidance of highly allergenic foods was supported by a 1990 study of 1200 infants that correlated the number of solid foods introduced by age 4 months with eczema at age 10 years.[38] However, dietary antigen avoidance has not proved to be effective in most studies and a 2008 review in *Pediatrics* states, "for infants at high risk of developing atopic disease, there is evidence that exclusive breastfeeding for at least 4 months compared with feeding intact cow milk protein formula decreases the cumulative incidence of atopic dermatitis and cow milk allergy in the first 2 years of life."[39] Beyond this, whether exposure to antigenic foods early in life promotes sensitization or tolerance is unclear.

The effect of breastfeeding in the development of asthma is controversial and studies conflict.[39] In a large cohort, breastfeeding seemed to reduce wheezing episodes in children less than 4 years, but in infants who had a family history of maternal asthma breastfeeding increased the risk of developing asthma after age 6 years.[39,40] However, a 2009 ISAAC II study of 54,000 children found no association between breastfeeding and allergy.[41] This type of disparity between study results is common in research examining the development of atopic diseases, but perhaps not unexpected given allergy's complicated genetics and multiple environmental influences.

Preventing the development of inhalant allergies with environmental modifications has also yielded inconsistent results. Studies have looked at whether cat exposure in infancy might increase the risk of allergic sensitization to cat. In Sweden, most children with allergic asthma are sensitized to cat. Unexpectedly, a large study reported that having a cat in the home during infancy was associated with a decreased risk of developing asthma.[42] However, the influence of cat exposure seems to be opposite in high-risk groups. In a high-risk population defined by maternal asthma, having a cat in the home during infancy was associated with an increased risk of asthma.[43] Attempts to reduce house dust mite exposure to prevent atopic disease in high-risk infants have yielded mixed results.[44,45] In the Manchester Asthma and Allergy Study wheezing was reduced with early intervention against dust mites.[44] The Isle of Wight study also found dust mite precautions reduced the development of allergy and asthma.[46–48] However, three other large studies showed no effect: the PIAMA study in the Netherlands,[49] the SPACE study in Europe,[45] and the CAPS study in Australia.[50]

Effective interventions to prevent development of allergic disease seem to vary by geographic location, ethnicity, socioeconomic class, and risk factors. Genetic tests may one day identify populations where allergic risk and effective prevention strategies are better matched.

Although preventing allergy through environmental control has shown mixed results, two controlled studies have shown that treating young children who have atopic dermatitis with antihistamines decreases the risk of developing asthma. Bustos and colleagues[51] treated children with atopic dermatitis, age 1 to 36 months, with daily antihistamine in a randomized, placebo-controlled trial. They reported 25% fewer diagnoses of asthma in the antihistamine group. The ETAC study treated 817 atopic dermatitis infants with either placebo or cetirizine. Fifty percent developed asthma in the control group, but 25% less in the cetirizine group when they had sensitization to dust or grass.[52]

Infants with food allergy or atopic dermatitis are at risk for later developing inhalant allergies, but inhalant allergies are uncommon in infancy. Successful prevention of inhalant allergy has remained elusive, but treating atopic dermatitis with antihistamines may have a modest but significant benefit. Asking about a family history of allergies, food allergy, and atopic dermatitis is likely helpful when considering if allergies contribute to upper or lower respiratory inflammation encountered in the older child.

CHILDHOOD: 2 TO 17 YEARS

Inhalant allergy sensitivities generally develop after the third birthday.[23] There is rarely a need to test for allergies in children less than 4 years of age. Total and specific IgE increases rapidly in children from 3 to 6 years and peaks in the teenage years.[23] Prevalence and spectrum of inhalant IgE sensitization increase with age. Allergies in children play a well-defined role in nasal and conjunctival inflammation. However, the role of allergy in adenoid hypertrophy and eustachian tube function is less clear. For this section, allergic disease is separated by the different anatomic sites.

Upper Airway Inflammation and Allergies

Allergic rhinitis

AR is defined by the ARIA guidelines of 2008 as a chronic disorder of the upper airways that is induced by IgE-mediated inflammation after exposure of the nasal membranes in sensitized patients to a specific allergen.[27] The symptoms include nasal congestion, rhinorrhea, sneezing, nasal itching, and postnasal drainage.

AR has been traditionally categorized as seasonal or perennial depending on allergen sensitivity. The more recent ARIA guidelines of the World Health Organization include a classification that uses duration of symptoms and impact on quality-of-life parameters.[53] The duration of symptoms is either "intermittent" (symptoms for <4 days per week or for a duration of <4 weeks per year) or "persistent" (symptoms that occur >4 days per week and are present for >4 weeks per year). The effect on quality of life is subdivided into either "mild disease" (no impairment of daily activities, no sleep interruption, and no troublesome symptoms) or "moderate to severe disease" (one or more of the previously mentioned symptoms). Other guidelines (and the Food and Drug Administration [FDA]) divide AR into seasonal and perennial.[54]

AR is estimated to affect 60 million people in the United States, and its prevalence is increasing.[55] The prevalence of AR in children is possibly as high as 40%,[56] making it the most common chronic disease in the pediatric population. However, whether AR is self-described, physician diagnosed, or includes allergy testing affects the reported incidence and prevalence.[27] Additionally, there is profound geographic variability.[57] Most individuals develop symptoms of AR before 20 years of age, with 40% of patients becoming symptomatic by age 6 years. In adults diagnosed with AR, 40% have perennial AR and 20% have seasonal AR; an additional 40% have perennial AR with seasonal flare-ups.[10]

The recently published Pediatric Allergies in America Survey suggests that children are more likely to have seasonal allergies compared with perennial AR.[1] The most common triggers of nasal symptoms in the allergic children were pollen, dust, and animal dander. The single most frequently experienced nasal allergy symptom reported by parents was nasal congestion (52%), which was said to occur either every day (25%) or most days (27%) each week during their children's worst month for allergy symptoms. In addition to parental responses, the children 10 to 17 years of age were asked which nasal allergy symptoms they experienced every day or most days during their worst allergy month in the past year. Nasal congestion or stuffed-up nose (39%), repeated sneezing (36%), runny nose (35%), and watering eyes (20%) were frequently reported as occurring either every day or on most days of the worst month.[1]

Although AR is not life-threatening, it can be associated with significant morbidity through loss of productivity,[58] cognitive functioning,[59] missed school,[60] and impaired quality of life.[61] Many of these health-related quality-of-life issues seem to stem in part from sleep disturbances associated with AR.[62] In addition to impaired quality of life that AR elicits in patients, it can have a substantial economic impact including both direct costs to patients and indirect costs that include patient absenteeism and inefficient performance at school.[60] Walker and colleagues[63] compared national examination test performance in winter (practice) and summer (final) in grass-allergic and nonallergic students. Compared with controls, grass-allergic students were found to have a significantly increased risk to unexpectedly fail a test section in the summer (grass pollen season) that they had previously passed in the winter.

The diagnosis of AR in children is based on clinical evaluation and allergy testing. Allergy testing in the absence of clinical likelihood of allergic disease yields unacceptable false-positive rates illustrated by a positive skin prick test in 53.9% of 10,509 Americans randomly sampled in Third National Health and Nutrition Survey.[64]

The differential diagnosis of AR in children differs from adults. Children are more likely to have adenoid hypertrophy, nasal foreign body, or choanal atresia contributing to their nasal obstruction than adults. Polyps, deviated septum, and neoplasia are more likely causes of nasal obstruction in adults than children.

Treatment of AR in children is similar to adults.[27] Environmental control, pharmacologic therapy, and desensitization are the three main options for treating AR.

Although counseling about environmental control of AR is recommended, clinical efficacy in controlled studies is often disappointing. Terreehorst and colleagues[65] performed a randomized placebo-control trial of dust mite mattress covers in 279 subjects allergic to dust mite. Although they did demonstrate decrease in dust mite counts, no clinical improvement in AR was detected between the groups. A recent Cochrane review suggested an extensive bedroom-based program including acaracides may "be of some benefit" in AR symptoms.[66]

Pharmacotherapy for AR consists of antihistamines, decongestants, intranasal corticosteroids, and leukotriene antagonists. The use of first-generation antihistamines should be limited in children because of drowsiness, impaired learning,[67] and paradoxical hyperactivity. Pediatric formulations of second-generation antihistamines are found in **Table 1**, and although appropriate for allergy they have not shown benefit in viral rhinitis or otitis media. Topical antihistamines have indications starting at age 5 years for azelastine and age 6 years for olopatadine but compliance in children can be hampered by taste in the authors' experience. Decongestants and over-the-counter cough and cold preparations are not currently recommended in children under 2 years of age because of lack of proved efficacy and an association with rare cardiac fatalities in infants.[68,69]

Intranasal corticosteroids are indicated down to age 2 years. Concerns of reduced growth and adrenal axis suppression have led to differences in the lowest indicated age listed for different steroid molecules (**Table 2**). Paired papers published in *Pediatrics* in 2000 measured a 0.9-cm reduction in annual height gained with intranasal beclomethasone[70] and no difference in height with intranasal mometasone.[71] The FDA has recommended using the lowest effective dose and monitoring growth in children when prescribing intranasal steroids. Nasal steroids seem to reduce adenoid size and can be considered for moderate adenoid hypertrophy. However, it is unclear how long the nasal steroids have to be maintained to sustain the reduced adenoid size.[72] Other allergy medications for children include pseudoephedrine, chromolyn, ipatropium, and montelukast (**Table 3**). Montelukast is indicated for perennial AR in children down to age 6 months and may also have a beneficial effect on lower respiratory inflammation.

Desensitization by subcutaneous immunotherapy in children has been shown to be effective.[73,74] Risk, time, and expense of subcutaneous immunotherapy needs to be carefully matched to severity and ability to control allergic disease. Desensitization is unique in its beneficial effect on allergies after the treatment is discontinued, its affect on reducing additional sensitizations, and reduction in the development of allergic asthma.[73] Data on sublingual immunotherapy in children have been less convincing than adults. Roder and colleagues[74] published a systematic review of sublingual immunotherapy in children that identified seven high methodologic studies of which only one of seven showed efficacy. However, in 2009 and 2010 three large studies showed statistical results for sublingual immunotherapy for grass (**Table 4**).[75–77] Each of these three studies showed similar percentages of symptom

Table 1
Second-generation antihistamines available for children in 2010

Second Generation Antihistamine	Formulations	Dose by Age
Cetirizine	5 mg/5 mL, 5- or 10-mg tablets	2–5 y, 2.5–5 mg 6–10 y, 5–10 mg
Fexofenadine	6 mg/mL, 30 ODT, 30, 60, 180	2–11 y, 30 mg/5mL bid ≥12 y, 60 mg bid or 180 mg qd
Loradatine	1 mg/mL, 5-mg chewable, 10 ODT	2–5 y, 5 mg daily (1 mg/mL) ≥6 y, 10 mg daily
Levocetirizine	2.5 mg/5 mL, 5-mg tablets	2–5 y, 1.25 po q AM 6–11, 2.5 mg po q AM >12 y, 2.5 to 5 mg po q AM
Desoradatine	0.5 mg/mL	6–11 mo, 1 mg daily 1–5 y, 1.25 mg 6–11 y, 2.5 mg daily >12 y, 5 mg po qd

Table 2
Intranasal corticosteroids by age of FDA approval

Ages by FDA Approval	Intranasal Corticosteroid
Age 2 y and older	Mometasone Fluticasone furoate
Age 4 y and older	Fluticasone prorionate
Age 6 y and older	Budesonide Triamcinolone Flunisolide Beclomethasone

improvement, strong placebo effects in the control groups, and promising safety profiles. Sublingual immunotherapy has not yet been FDA approved April 2011.

Allergic conjunctivitis

Although ocular disease is not part of the respiratory system, the overlap between AR and allergic conjunctivitis is so great that it is often considered one disease: rhinoconjunctivitis. Bielory[78] summarizes several epidemiologic studies to estimate that there is 80% overlap, with 10% having AR alone and 10% having allergic conjunctivitis alone. The large ISAAC studies looked at rhinoconjunctivitis as single diagnosis and reported symptoms in 8.5% of 6 to 7 year olds and 14.6% in 13 to 14 year olds.[57,79] As such, children with AR should be assessed for allergic conjunctivitis and topical antihistamine or cromolyn eye drops considered.

Allergy and ear disease

The relationship between otitis media and allergy has been the focus of several studies with a discrepancy of findings[80] suggesting either large regional differences or bias in associating otitis and allergic disease. The relationship between allergy and otitis media likely varies with the age of the children studied. In the authors' experience, inhalant allergy plays a smaller role in acute recurrent otitis media during infancy compared with chronic otitis media with effusion in 5- or 6-year-old children, especially when there is no infant history of eustachian tube dysfunction.

There is very little evidence that acute recurrent otitis media in infancy is associated with inhalant allergies. In 3549 case-controlled pairs, no increased risk of AR at age 6

Table 3
Nonsteroidal, nonantihistamine allergy medications by age and dose

Other Allergy Medications	Dose by Age
Pseudoephedrine	2–5 y, 15 mg q 6 h 6–12 y, 30 mg q 6 h
Cromolyn nasal spray (over the counter)	2 y and older
Ipratropium nasal spray	0.03% of 0.06%, 2 sprays q nostril 2–4 times per d 5 y and older for SAR
Montelukast	6–23 mo, 4 mg qd, granules 2–5 y, 4 mg qd, granules or chewables 6–14 y, 5 mg qd, chewables PAR age $\geq$6 mo Asthma age $\geq$12 mo SAR age $\geq$2 y

Abbreviations: Asthma, asthma maintenance; PAR, perennial allergic rhinitis; SAR, seasonal allergic rhinitis.

Table 4
Mean reduction in symptom scores of three grass sublingual preparations in three recent double-blind placebo-controlled trials

Grass SLIT in Children Mean % Reduction of Symptoms: Active Versus Placebo			
Whan et al[77]	2009	20 μg × 5	28%
Bufe et al[76]	2009	15 μg Phlp5	27%
Halken et al[75]	2010	20 μg × 5	28%

years was detected for acute otitis media (odds ratio [OR], 0.98; $P = .72$) or chronic otitis media (OR, 1.05; $P = .84$) diagnosed before age 1 year.[81] However, the Melbourne Atopy Cohort Study of 448 children identified at high risk by having an atopic first-degree relative found an association with asthma. They showed that of the 59% who had at least one episode of acute otitis media when less than 2 years old there was a small to moderate increased risk for physician-diagnosed asthma at age 6 years (relative risk, 1.3; 95% confidence interval, 1.15–1.81).[82]

Allergic rhinitis may occur more frequently in children with chronic otitis media with effusion,[80] but common pharmacologic therapy for AR (antihistamines, decongestants, and nasal steroids) has not been shown to be effective.[83] One study found 89% of children aged 3–8 years with "glue ear" also had AR diagnosed by symptoms and either nasal eosinophilia or a positive skin prick test[84]; however, some of these children may have had nonallergic rhinitis with eosinophil syndrome and there may have been a referral bias. In contrast, another study showed a lower but statistically significant association of 16.3% versus 5.5% between chronic otitis media with effusion and AR defined by nasal symptoms independent of a "cold" and positive skin prick test compared with a control group. Interestingly, 16.3% would not be characterized as an elevated rate of AR in some epidemiologic studies of children.[56] This underscores how regional differences, age of subjects, and different definitions of AR make comparing outcomes across studies difficult. The American Academy of Otolaryngology Head and Neck Surgery's 2004 practice guidelines for chronic otitis media with effusion specifically made no recommendation about allergies as a causal agent or effective treatment of chronic otitis media with effusion because of insufficient evidence.[83]

Adenoid hypertrophy and allergies

The relationship between adenoid hypertrophy and AR is also unclear and there is little evidence linking adenoid hypertrophy with allergy. Nuhoglu and coworkers[85] compared adenoid size in AR and non-AR, finding that non-AR was more significantly associated with adenoid hypertrophy in a retrospective study of 108 children ($P = .0001$). Marchisio and colleagues[86] found that the poor correlation between adenoid size and clinical nasal obstruction was worse in allergic children, presumably because of turbinate hypertrophy playing a larger role. However, adenoids from atopic children may be different pathologically and have showed increased IgE-positive macrophages and plasma cells compared with controls.[87] If turbinate hypertrophy is more frequently the cause of nasal obstruction in allergic children relative to adenoid hypertrophy, nasal steroid sprays or other management of the child's allergies should be carefully considered in the treatment of their nasal obstruction.

Lower Airway Inflammation in the Allergic Child

Although there are many causes of inflammation in the lower airway including infections, asthma is the archetypal disease of chronic lower respiratory inflammation in the allergic child. However, not all asthmatic children have allergies. Like many other complex chronic diseases, asthma is a single name for a spectrum of disease. Hundreds of genes likely influence the pathogenesis of asthma, many of which are influenced by environmental interactions.[88] Asthma varies clinically in onset, severity, triggers, and response to therapy. Asthma comprises a range of heterogeneous phenotypes that differ and overlap in presentation. Although we may be on the cusp of tailoring the diagnosis and treatment of asthma using genetic markers, in 2011 asthma is approached clinically by selecting treatment based primarily on severity and triggers (eg, exercise-induced asthma or allergic asthma).

Awareness of asthma is important for otolaryngologists because of the epidemiologic link between chronic upper and lower airway inflammation.[27] Asthma is underdiagnosed, impairs quality of life, and even mild persistent asthma is potentially life threatening.[4] The ability to identify asthma, initiate treatment, and ensure appropriate continued care should be the goal of every specialist who cares for children that are known to be at increased risk of this common disease.

Asthma is influenced by both genetic and environmental factors. Family and twin studies have indicated that genetics play an important role in the development of allergy and asthma. Twin studies suggest that approximately 60% of asthma susceptibility is caused by genetic factors, with indicators of allergic sensitization, such as serum IgE levels, also demonstrating heritability.[89] Genome-wide linkage studies and case-control studies have identified 18 genomic regions and more than 100 genes associated with allergy and asthma.[9] Recently, the gene ORMDL3 has been identified as exhibiting a highly significantly association with asthma, a finding that has been replicated in several populations.[90]

Although genetic predisposition is clearly evident, environmental factors also play a large role in asthma susceptibility and are likely to underlie the increases that have occurred in recent decades.[91] Observations of migrating populations and of Germany after unification have strongly supported the role of local environmental factors in determining the degree of expression of asthma within genetically similar populations.[92]

During early childhood, certain viruses have been associated with the development of the asthmatic phenotype. In a landmark 2008 study, Jackson and colleagues[93] showed that wheezing with rhinovirus at age 3 years was more predictive of asthma at age 6 years (OR, 25.6) than aeroallergen sensitization (OR, 3.4). Respiratory syncytial virus, rhinovirus, influenza, and parainfluenza are among viral pathogens associated with wheezing in the first few years of life.[94]

In contrast, exposure of an infant to a substantial number of infections, as suggested by the hygiene hypothesis, is seen as protective against the development of the asthma phenotype.[95] Although this theory has been supported by some studies of allergy prevalence,[96] it has been partially refuted by recent studies of asthma prevalence suggesting that although large family size (more than four children) is associated with a decreased risk of asthma, birth order is not involved.[97]

Wheezing and asthma are not synonymous in children. Although some 50% of preschool children have wheezing with viral respiratory infections, only 10% to 15% have a diagnosis of asthma by the time they reach school age.[98] Wheezing in early infancy and childhood has been divided into three courses: (1) transient wheezing, (2) persistent wheezing, and (3) late-onset wheezing.[99]

Transient wheezing in early infancy has been well characterized, with decreased airflow rates on pulmonary function testing at birth, onset of wheezing within the first year, and resolution by mid-childhood with no lasting effects on pulmonary function.[98] Transient wheezing is the most prevalent form of early wheezing and accounts for 60% of the children who wheeze in infancy. It has no significant relationship to atopy but maternal smoking during pregnancy has been identified as a variable significantly associated with this phenotype.[100] It is suspected that these children have smaller airways, which seems to be associated with maternal smoking, and as they grow the episodic narrowing of the already small airway by viral-induced inflammation becomes asymptomatic.[98]

Children with persistent wheezing can be subdivided into nonatopic and atopic. Nonatopic persistent wheezing comprises 20% of wheezy children under the age of three years and is associated with the first episode of wheezing occurring less than 1 year of age.[98] It is believed that this phenotype may be caused by an alteration in the regulation of airway tone leading to viral-induced wheeze.[101] The atopic persistent wheezing phenotype is found in 20% of children who wheeze during the first 3 years of life and symptoms typically present after age 1 year. Risk factors associated with atopic wheeze include male gender, parental asthma, atopic dermatitis, eosinophilia at 9 months, and a history of wheezing with lower respiratory tract infections.[101] This phenotype is also associated with early sensitization to food or inhalant allergens[102] and reduced lung function at age 6 years (compared with children with no history of wheezing with lower respiratory illnesses).[98]

Late-onset wheezing (wheezing absent before age 3 years, but present at age 6 years) seems to represent another phenotype. These children are more likely to be male, have mothers with asthma, be sensitized to allergens, and have early rhinitis than children who never wheezed. Late-onset wheezing represented 15% of children in one cohort.[98]

Wheezing may also have less common noninflammatory causes, such as an airway foreign body, subglottic cyst, hemangioma, or vascular ring.

The most common cause of asthma symptoms in children less than 5 years old is viral infections. There is no single test or risk factor that predicts who will progress to asthma. Instead, a predictive index may be used based on the cohort data that separated transient wheezing from persistent and late-onset wheezing. Castro-Rodriguez and colleagues[103] created a predictive index for ages 2 to 3 years that conferred a 76% chance of asthma by age 6 and a greater than 95% chance of not having asthma by age 6 if negative. Guilbert and colleagues[104] modified these criteria for the PEAK study for clinical use. The index used in the PEAK study was recommended by the 2007 National Institutes of Health (NIH) asthma guidelines and is as follows: children between ages 2 and 4 years who have had more than three episodes of wheezing (one physician diagnosed) within 1 year and who have met either one major criteria (parental asthma, physician-diagnosed atopic dermatitis, or inhalant allergen sensitization) or two minor criteria (wheezing unrelated to colds, food sensitization, or eosinophilia >4%). Children positive for this index had fewer asthma exacerbations and decreased burden of disease if treated with inhaled corticosteroids compared with placebo, but early inhaled corticosteroids failed to prevent asthma development.[105]

Because atopic children with rhinitis are well represented in otolaryngology clinics and at increased risk for asthma, asking about recurrent wheezing and considering treatment in children who meet the index's criteria would benefit these patients. A check list is provided in **Table 5**. Other important risks for childhood asthma include sensitization to the smaller inhalant allergens by age 6 to 8 years and maternal history of asthma. Smaller inhalant allergen travel preferentially to the lungs by virtue of their size and include cat, alternaria, dust mite, and cockroach.

The 2007 NIH asthma guidelines divides asthma into age groups of 0 to 4 years, 5 to 11 years, and older than age 12 years. Asthma is classified into intermittent and persistent disease. Persistent asthma is stratified into mild, moderate, and severe. Children can be classified based on frequency of wheezing, night time awakenings, frequency

Table 5
Asthma risk checklist for pediatric otolaryngology patients with rhinitis or allergies

Yes	No	Question
		Has your child had greater than four episodes of wheezing in the last year?
		Has a physician diagnosed wheezing in your child in the last year?
		Did your child have wheezing in absence of a "cold" in the last year?
		Has the child's father ever been diagnosed with asthma?
		Has the child's mother ever been diagnosed with asthma?
		Has your child ever been diagnosed with atopic dermatitis?
		Does your child have a food allergy or did they have a food allergy?
		Has your child tested positive for allergies?
		Does your child use an inhaler or nebulizer sometimes?
		Did your child wake up with coughing or difficulty breathing in the last month when they did not have a "cold"?
		Does your child wheeze or become abnormally short of breath with exercise?

of inhaled β2 agonist use, and exacerbations lasting greater than a day. Once classified, simple charts recommend the initial treatment for each age group.[4] Asthma is a heterogeneous disease and response to treatment needs to be assessed. In most children, optimally managed asthma should result in no missed school, rare use of rescue inhalers, no emergency room visits, and no hospitalizations. Treating asthma also reduces asthma mortality. The number of corticosteroid inhalers used annually is inversely proportionally to the chance of death in those with asthma.[106] The 2007 NIH Asthma Guidelines, including charts for classifying severity, stepwise approach to management, and recommendations for altering therapy based on standardized assessment of the control of asthma control, are available free online. The NIH Asthma Guidelines are written to improve the diagnosis and management of asthma by primary care physicians and can be easily incorporated by otolaryngologists.

SUMMARY

Children with rhinosinusitis and rhinoconjunctivitis are at risk for inhalant allergies. Allergies often contribute to upper and lower chronic respiratory inflammation. This population of children is likely well represented among otolaryngology patients. Inhalant allergies are uncommon in infancy, but food allergy, atopic dermatitis, and allergic disease in a first-degree relative are important risk factors. The differential diagnosis and treatment of AR and allergic asthma are different in children than adults and change with the age of the child. The prevalence of viral rhinitis and viral bronchiolitis should be carefully considered in young children suspected of inhalant allergies.

Inhalant allergies play a significant role in rhinitis and the associated conditions of allergic conjunctivitis and asthma, but it is less clear how inhalant allergies affect other upper respiratory conditions, such as eustachian tube dysfunction and adenoid hypertrophy. Familiarity with the diagnosis and treatment of pediatric inhalant allergy offers an opportunity substantially to improve the quality of life of allergic children.

REFERENCES

1. Meltzer EO, Blaiss MS, Derebery MJ, et al. Burden of allergic rhinitis: results from the pediatric allergies in America survey. J Allergy Clin Immunol 2009;124(Suppl 3):S43–70.

2. Pillsbury HCIII, Cannon CR, Sedory Holzer SE, et al. The workforce in otolaryngology-head and neck surgery: moving into the next millennium. Otolaryngol Head Neck Surg 2000;123(3):341–56.
3. Krouse JH. The unified airway: conceptual framework. Otolaryngol Clin North Am 2008;41(2):257–66.
4. NIH Guidelines for the diagnosis and management of asthma–2007 (EPR-3) 2007. Available at: http://www.nhlbi.nih.gov/guidelines/asthma/index.htm. Accessed November 2, 2010.
5. Zambelli-Weiner A, Ehrlich E, Stockton ML, et al. Evaluation of the CD14/-260 polymorphism and house dust endotoxin exposure in the Barbados Asthma Genetics Study. J Allergy Clin Immunol 2005;115(6):1203–9.
6. Ober C, Hoffjan S. Asthma genetics 2006: the long and winding road to gene discovery. Genes Immun 2006;7(2):95–100.
7. Breslow DK, Collins SR, Bodenmiller B, et al. Orm family proteins mediate sphingolipid homeostasis. Nature 2010;463(7284):1048–53.
8. Moffatt MF, Kabesch M, Liang L, et al. Genetic variants regulating ORMDL3 expression contribute to the risk of childhood asthma. Nature 2007;448(7152):470–3.
9. Holloway JW, Yang IA, Holgate ST. Genetics of allergic disease. J Allergy Clin Immunol 2010;125(Suppl 2):S81–94.
10. Skoner DP. Allergic rhinitis: definition, epidemiology, pathophysiology, detection, and diagnosis. J Allergy Clin Immunol 2001;108(Suppl 1):S2–8.
11. Skadhauge LR, Christensen K, Kyvik KO, et al. Genetic and environmental influence on asthma: a population-based study of 11,688 Danish twin pairs. Eur Respir J 1999;13(1):8–14.
12. Burrows B, Martinez FD, Halonen M, et al. Association of asthma with serum IgE levels and skin-test reactivity to allergens. N Engl J Med 1989;320(5):271–7.
13. Wu P, Dupont WD, Griffin MR, et al. Evidence of a causal role of winter virus infection during infancy in early childhood asthma. Am J Respir Crit Care Med 2008;178(11):1123–9.
14. Kramer MS, Kakuma R. Maternal dietary antigen avoidance during pregnancy or lactation, or both, for preventing or treating atopic disease in the child. Cochrane Database Syst Rev 2006;3:CD000133.
15. Pistiner M, Gold DR, Abdulkerim H, et al. Birth by cesarean section, allergic rhinitis, and allergic sensitization among children with a parental history of atopy. J Allergy Clin Immunol 2008;122(2):274–9.
16. Sybilski AJ, Doboszynska A, Samolinski B. Prediction of atopy in the first year of life using cord blood IgE levels and family history. Eur J Med Res 2009;14(Suppl 4):227–32.
17. Kay AB. Allergy and allergic diseases. First of two parts. N Engl J Med 2001;344(1):30–7.
18. Kay AB. Allergy and allergic diseases. Second of two parts. N Engl J Med 2001;344(2):109–13.
19. Bach JF. The effect of infections on susceptibility to autoimmune and allergic diseases. N Engl J Med 2002;347(12):911–20.
20. Kramer U, Heinrich J, Wjst M, et al. Age of entry to day nursery and allergy in later childhood. Lancet 1999;353(9151):450–4.
21. Holt PG, Clough JB, Holt BJ, et al. Genetic 'risk' for atopy is associated with delayed postnatal maturation of T-cell competence. Clin Exp Allergy 1992;22(12):1093–9.
22. Wang J, Visness CM, Sampson HA. Food allergen sensitization in inner-city children with asthma. J Allergy Clin Immunol 2005;115(5):1076–80.

23. Kulig M, Bergmann R, Klettke U, et al. Natural course of sensitization to food and inhalant allergens during the first 6 years of life. J Allergy Clin Immunol 1999; 103(6):1173–9.
24. Tariq SM, Matthews SM, Hakim EA, et al. Egg allergy in infancy predicts respiratory allergic disease by 4 years of age. Pediatr Allergy Immunol 2000;11(3):162–7.
25. Lammintausta K, Kalimo K, Raitala R, et al. Prognosis of atopic dermatitis. A prospective study in early adulthood. Int J Dermatol 1991;30(8):563–8.
26. Illi S, von Mutius E, Lau S, et al. The natural course of atopic dermatitis from birth to age 7 years and the association with asthma. J Allergy Clin Immunol 2004; 113(5):925–31.
27. Herr M, Clarisse B, Nikasinovic L, et al. Does allergic rhinitis exist in infancy? Findings from the PARIS birth cohort. Allergy 2011;66(2):214–21.
28. Bousquet J, Khaltaev N, Cruz AA, et al. Allergic Rhinitis and its Impact on Asthma (ARIA) 2008 update (in collaboration with the World Health Organization, GA(2)LEN and AllerGen). Allergy 2008;63(Suppl 86):8–160.
29. Heikkinen T, Jarvinen A. The common cold. Lancet 2003;361(9351):51–9.
30. Pappas DE, Hendley JO, Hayden FG, et al. Symptom profile of common colds in school-aged children. Pediatr Infect Dis J 2008;27(1):8–11.
31. Smith MB, Feldman W. Over-the-counter cold medications. A critical review of clinical trials between 1950 and 1991. JAMA 1993;269(17):2258–63.
32. Shay DK, Holman RC, Newman RD, et al. Bronchiolitis-associated hospitalizations among US children, 1980–1996. JAMA 1999;282(15):1440–6.
33. Landau LI. Bronchiolitis and asthma: are they related? Thorax 1994;49(4): 293–6.
34. Duff AL, Pomeranz ES, Gelber LE, et al. Risk factors for acute wheezing in infants and children: viruses, passive smoke, and IgE antibodies to inhalant allergens. Pediatrics 1993;92(4):535–40.
35. King VJ, Viswanathan M, Bordley WC, et al. Pharmacologic treatment of bronchiolitis in infants and children: a systematic review. Arch Pediatr Adolesc Med 2004;158(2):127–37.
36. Gadomski AM, Bhasale AL. Bronchodilators for bronchiolitis. Cochrane Database Syst Rev 2006;3:CD001266.
37. Patel H, Platt R, Lozano JM, et al. Glucocorticoids for acute viral bronchiolitis in infants and young children. Cochrane Database Syst Rev 2004;3: CD004878.
38. Fergusson DM, Horwood LJ, Shannon FT. Early solid feeding and recurrent childhood eczema: a 10-year longitudinal study. Pediatrics 1990;86(4):541–6.
39. Greer FR, Sicherer SH, Burks AW. Effects of early nutritional interventions on the development of atopic disease in infants and children: the role of maternal dietary restriction, breastfeeding, timing of introduction of complementary foods, and hydrolyzed formulas. Pediatrics 2008;121(1):183–91.
40. Sears MR, Greene JM, Willan AR, et al. Long-term relation between breastfeeding and development of atopy and asthma in children and young adults: a longitudinal study. Lancet 2002;360(9337):901–7.
41. Nagel G, Buchele G, Weinmayr G, et al. Effect of breastfeeding on asthma, lung function and bronchial hyperreactivity in ISAAC Phase II. Eur Respir J 2009; 33(5):993–1002.
42. Hesselmar B, Aberg N, Aberg B, et al. Does early exposure to cat or dog protect against later allergy development? Clin Exp Allergy 1999;29(5):611–7.
43. Celedon JC, Litonjua AA, Ryan L, et al. Exposure to cat allergen, maternal history of asthma, and wheezing in first 5 years of life. Lancet 2002;360(9335):781–2.

44. Custovic A, Simpson BM, Simpson A, et al. Effect of environmental manipulation in pregnancy and early life on respiratory symptoms and atopy during first year of life: a randomised trial. Lancet 2001;358(9277):188–93.
45. Horak F Jr, Matthews S, Ihorst G, et al. Effect of mite-impermeable mattress encasings and an educational package on the development of allergies in a multinational randomized, controlled birth-cohort study–24 months results of the Study of Prevention of Allergy in Children in Europe. Clin Exp Allergy 2004;34(8):1220–5.
46. Hide DW, Matthews S, Matthews L, et al. Effect of allergen avoidance in infancy on allergic manifestations at age two years. J Allergy Clin Immunol 1994;93(5):842–6.
47. Hide DW, Matthews S, Tariq S, et al. Allergen avoidance in infancy and allergy at 4 years of age. Allergy 1996;51(2):89–93.
48. Arshad SH, Bateman B, Matthews SM. Primary prevention of asthma and atopy during childhood by allergen avoidance in infancy: a randomised controlled study. Thorax 2003;58(6):489–93.
49. Koopman LP, van Strien RT, Kerkhof M, et al. Placebo-controlled trial of house dust mite-impermeable mattress covers: effect on symptoms in early childhood. Am J Respir Crit Care Med 2002;166(3):307–13.
50. Mihrshahi S, Peat JK, Marks GB, et al. Eighteen-month outcomes of house dust mite avoidance and dietary fatty acid modification in the Childhood Asthma Prevention Study (CAPS). J Allergy Clin Immunol 2003;111(1):162–8.
51. Bustos GJ, Bustos D, Romero O. Prevention of asthma with ketotifen in preasthmatic children: a three-year follow-up study. Clin Exp Allergy 1995;25(6):568–73.
52. Warner JO. A double-blinded, randomized, placebo-controlled trial of cetirizine in preventing the onset of asthma in children with atopic dermatitis: 18 months' treatment and 18 months' posttreatment follow-up. J Allergy Clin Immunol 2001; 108(6):929–37.
53. Bousquet J, Van Cauwenberge P, Khaltaev N. Allergic rhinitis and its impact on asthma. J Allergy Clin Immunol 2001;108(Suppl 5):S147–334.
54. Dykewicz MS, Fineman S, Skoner DP, et al. Diagnosis and management of rhinitis: complete guidelines of the Joint Task Force on Practice Parameters in Allergy, Asthma and Immunology. American Academy of Allergy, Asthma, and Immunology. Ann Allergy Asthma Immunol 1998;81(5 Pt 2):478–518.
55. Settipane RA. Rhinitis: a dose of epidemiological reality. Allergy Asthma Proc 2003;24(3):147–54.
56. Wright AL, Holberg CJ, Martinez FD, et al. Epidemiology of physician-diagnosed allergic rhinitis in childhood. Pediatrics 1994;94(6 Pt 1):895–901.
57. Fok AO, Wong GW. What have we learnt from ISAAC phase III in the Asia-Pacific rim? Curr Opin Allergy Clin Immunol 2009;9(2):116–22.
58. Hemp P. Presenteeism: at work–but out of it. Harv Bus Rev 2004;82(10):49–58, 155.
59. Wilken JA, Berkowitz R, Kane R. Decrements in vigilance and cognitive functioning associated with ragweed-induced allergic rhinitis. Ann Allergy Asthma Immunol 2002;89(4):372–80.
60. Smith DH, Malone DC, Lawson KA, et al. A national estimate of the economic costs of asthma. Am J Respir Crit Care Med 1997;156(3 Pt 1):787–93.
61. Blaiss MS. Allergic rhinoconjunctivitis: burden of disease. Allergy Asthma Proc 2007;28(4):393–7.
62. Nathan RA. The burden of allergic rhinitis. Allergy Asthma Proc 2007;28(1):3–9.
63. Walker S, Khan-Wasti S, Fletcher M, et al. Seasonal allergic rhinitis is associated with a detrimental effect on examination performance in United Kingdom teenagers: case-control study. J Allergy Clin Immunol 2007;120(2):381–7.

64. Arbes SJ Jr, Gergen PJ, Elliott L, et al. Prevalences of positive skin test responses to 10 common allergens in the US population: results from the third National Health and Nutrition Examination Survey. J Allergy Clin Immunol 2005;116(2):377–83.
65. Terreehorst I, Hak E, Oosting AJ, et al. Evaluation of impermeable covers for bedding in patients with allergic rhinitis. N Engl J Med 2003;349(3):237–46.
66. Sheikh A, Hurwitz B, Nurmatov U, et al. House dust mite avoidance measures for perennial allergic rhinitis. Cochrane Database Syst Rev 2010;7:CD001563.
67. Vuurman EF, van Veggel LM, Sanders RL, et al. Effects of semprex-D and diphenhydramine on learning in young adults with seasonal allergic rhinitis. Ann Allergy Asthma Immunol 1996;76(3):247–52.
68. Bell EA, Tunkel DE. Over-the-counter cough and cold medications in children: are they helpful? Otolaryngol Head Neck Surg 2010;142(5):647–50.
69. Sharfstein JM, North M, Serwint JR. Over the counter but no longer under the radar–pediatric cough and cold medications. N Engl J Med 2007;357(23):2321–4.
70. Skoner DP, Rachelefsky GS, Meltzer EO, et al. Detection of growth suppression in children during treatment with intranasal beclomethasone dipropionate. Pediatrics 2000;105(2):E23.
71. Schenkel EJ, Skoner DP, Bronsky EA, et al. Absence of growth retardation in children with perennial allergic rhinitis after one year of treatment with mometasone furoate aqueous nasal spray. Pediatrics 2000;105(2):E22.
72. Chadha NK, Zhang L, Mendoza-Sassi RA, et al. Using nasal steroids to treat nasal obstruction caused by adenoid hypertrophy: does it work? Otolaryngol Head Neck Surg 2009;140(2):139–47.
73. Halken S, Lau S, Valovirta E. New visions in specific immunotherapy in children: an iPAC summary and future trends. Pediatr Allergy Immunol 2008;19(Suppl 19): 60–70.
74. Roder E, Berger MY, de Groot H, et al. Immunotherapy in children and adolescents with allergic rhinoconjunctivitis: a systematic review. Pediatr Allergy Immunol 2008;19(3):197–207.
75. Halken S, Agertoft L, Seidenberg J, et al. Five-grass pollen 300IR SLIT tablets: efficacy and safety in children and adolescents. Pediatr Allergy Immunol 2010; 21(6):970–6.
76. Bufe A, Eberle P, Franke-Beckmann E, et al. Safety and efficacy in children of an SQ-standardized grass allergen tablet for sublingual immunotherapy. J Allergy Clin Immunol 2009;123(1):167–73.
77. Wahn U, Tabar A, Kuna P, et al. Efficacy and safety of 5-grass-pollen sublingual immunotherapy tablets in pediatric allergic rhinoconjunctivitis. J Allergy Clin Immunol 2009;123(1):160–6.
78. Bielory L. Allergic conjunctivitis and the impact of allergic rhinitis. Curr Allergy Asthma Rep 2010;10(2):122–34.
79. Bjorksten B, Clayton T, Ellwood P, et al. Worldwide time trends for symptoms of rhinitis and conjunctivitis: phase III of the international study of asthma and allergies in childhood. Pediatr Allergy Immunol 2008;19(2):110–24.
80. Luong A, Roland PS. The link between allergic rhinitis and chronic otitis media with effusion in atopic patients. Otolaryngol Clin North Am 2008;41(2):311–23.
81. Bremner SA, Carey IM, DeWilde S, et al. Original article: Infections presenting for clinical care in early life and later risk of hay fever in two UK birth cohorts. Allergy 2008;63(3):274–83.
82. Thomson JA, Widjaja C, Darmaputra AA, et al. Early childhood infections and immunisation and the development of allergic disease in particular asthma in

a high-risk cohort: a prospective study of allergy-prone children from birth to six years. Pediatr Allergy Immunol 2010;21(7):1076–85.
83. Rosenfeld RM, Culpepper L, Doyle KJ, et al. Clinical practice guideline: otitis media with effusion. Otolaryngol Head Neck Surg 2004;130(Suppl 5):S95–118.
84. Alles R, Parikh A, Hawk L, et al. The prevalence of atopic disorders in children with chronic otitis media with effusion. Pediatr Allergy Immunol 2001;12(2):102–6.
85. Nuhoglu C, Nuhoglu Y, Bankaoglu M, et al. A retrospective analysis of adenoidal size in children with allergic rhinitis and nonallergic idiopathic rhinitis. Asian Pac J Allergy Immunol 2010;28(2–3):136–40.
86. Marchisio P, Torretta S, Capaccio P, et al. Clinical assessment of adenoidal obstruction based on the nasal obstruction index is no longer useful in children. Otolaryngol Head Neck Surg 2010;142(2):237–41.
87. Papatziamos G, Van Hage-Hamsten M, Lundahl J, et al. IgE-positive plasma cells are present in adenoids of atopic children. Acta Otolaryngol 2006;126(2):180–5.
88. Holloway JW, Arshad SH, Holgate ST. Using genetics to predict the natural history of asthma? J Allergy Clin Immunol 2010;126(2):200–9 [quiz: 210–1].
89. Los H, Postmus PE, Boomsma DI. Asthma genetics and intermediate phenotypes: a review from twin studies. Twin Res 2001;4(2):81–93.
90. Tavendale R, Macgregor DF, Mukhopadhyay S, et al. A polymorphism controlling ORMDL3 expression is associated with asthma that is poorly controlled by current medications. J Allergy Clin Immunol 2008;121(4):860–3.
91. Eder W, Ege MJ, von Mutius E. The asthma epidemic. N Engl J Med 2006;355(21):2226–35.
92. von Mutius E, Martinez FD, Fritzsch C, et al. Prevalence of asthma and atopy in two areas of West and East Germany. Am J Respir Crit Care Med 1994;149(2 Pt 1):358–64.
93. Jackson DJ, Gangnon RE, Evans MD, et al. Wheezing rhinovirus illnesses in early life predict asthma development in high-risk children. Am J Respir Crit Care Med 2008;178(7):667–72.
94. Heymann PW, Carper HT, Murphy DD, et al. Viral infections in relation to age, atopy, and season of admission among children hospitalized for wheezing. J Allergy Clin Immunol 2004;114(2):239–47.
95. Schaub B, Lauener R, von Mutius E. The many faces of the hygiene hypothesis. J Allergy Clin Immunol 2006;117(5):969–77 [quiz: 978].
96. Kinra S, Davey Smith G, Jeffreys M, et al. Association between sibship size and allergic diseases in the Glasgow Alumni Study. Thorax 2006;61(1):48–53.
97. Goldberg S, Israeli E, Schwartz S, et al. Asthma prevalence, family size, and birth order. Chest 2007;131(6):1747–52.
98. Martinez FD, Wright AL, Taussig LM, et al. Asthma and wheezing in the first six years of life. The Group Health Medical Associates. N Engl J Med 1995;332(3):133–8.
99. Lowe LA, Simpson A, Woodcock A, et al. Wheeze phenotypes and lung function in preschool children. Am J Respir Crit Care Med 2005;171(3):231–7.
100. Rusconi F, Galassi C, Corbo GM, et al. Risk factors for early, persistent, and late-onset wheezing in young children. SIDRIA Collaborative Group. Am J Respir Crit Care Med 1999;160(5 Pt 1):1617–22.
101. Martinez F, Godfrey S. Wheezing disorders in the preschool child: pathogenesis and management. New York: Martin Dunitz; 2003.

102. Guilbert TW, Morgan WJ, Zeiger RS, et al. Atopic characteristics of children with recurrent wheezing at high risk for the development of childhood asthma. J Allergy Clin Immunol 2004;114(6):1282–7.
103. Castro-Rodriguez JA, Holberg CJ, Wright AL, et al. A clinical index to define risk of asthma in young children with recurrent wheezing. Am J Respir Crit Care Med 2000;162(4 Pt 1):1403–6.
104. Guilbert TW, Morgan WJ, Krawiec M, et al. The prevention of early asthma in kids study: design, rationale and methods for the Childhood Asthma Research and Education network. Control Clin Trials 2004;25(3):286–310.
105. Guilbert TW, Morgan WJ, Zeiger RS, et al. Long-term inhaled corticosteroids in preschool children at high risk for asthma. N Engl J Med 2006;354(19):1985–97.
106. Suissa S, Ernst P. Inhaled corticosteroids: impact on asthma morbidity and mortality. J Allergy Clin Immunol 2001;107(6):937–44.

Food Allergy in Adults and Children

Elizabeth J. Mahoney, MD[a,*], Maria C. Veling, MD[b], James W. Mims, MD[c]

KEYWORDS

• Food allergy • IgE • Peanut allergy • Oral food challenge

Food allergies are immunologically mediated phenomena that may involve immediate or delayed symptoms and result in both acute and chronic disease. Food allergies not only affect quality of life, but can be potentially fatal. Diagnosis currently relies on a careful history and an appreciation of epidemiologic aspects of the disorder; the role and limitation of simple diagnostic tests; and if needed, the use of an oral food challenge to confirm allergy or tolerance.

Although an understanding of food allergies has increased in the past decade, knowledge about the epidemiology and causes of food allergy remains limited. In general, it is recognized that food allergy represents an abnormal response of the mucosal immune system to antigens delivered through the oral route. The mucosal immune system regularly encounters enormous quantities of antigen and must suppress immune reactivity to food and harmless foreign organisms. Even though intact foreign food antigens routinely penetrate the gastrointestinal (GI) tract, they infrequently induce clinical symptoms because tolerance develops in most individuals.

To help differentiate food allergies from adverse food reactions, the recently published *Guidelines for the Diagnosis and Management of Food Allergy* by the National Institutes of Health (NIH) have recommended that the term "food allergy" be used to describe an adverse health effect arising from a specific immune response that occurs reproducibly on exposure to a given food. The guidelines further define a "food" as any substance that is intended for human consumption including chewing gum, drinks, food additives, and dietary supplements. Substances used only as drugs, tobacco products, and cosmetics that may be ingested are not included.[1]

"Food allergens" are defined as those specific components of food or ingredients within food (typically proteins, but sometimes also chemical haptens) that are

The authors have no conflicts of interest or financial affiliations to disclose.

[a] Department of Otolaryngology-Head and Neck Surgery, Boston University Medical Center, 4th floor, FGH Building, 820 Harrison Avenue, Boston, MA 02118, USA

[b] Division of Otolaryngology, Department of Otolaryngology, University of Kentucky Medical Center, 800 Rose Street C-236 Lexington, KY 40536–0293, USA

[c] Department of Otolaryngology, Medical Center Boulevard, Wake Forest University School of Medicine, Winston-Salem, NC 27157, USA

* Corresponding author.

E-mail address: elizabeth.mahoney@bmc.org

Otolaryngol Clin N Am 44 (2011) 815–833
doi:10.1016/j.otc.2011.03.014
oto.theclinics.com

recognized by allergen-specific immune cells and elicit specific immunologic reactions resulting in characteristic symptoms. Foods or food components that elicit reproducible adverse reactions but do not have established immunologic mechanisms are not considered food allergens.[1]

It is conceptually helpful to categorize food-induced allergic disorders based on immunopathology among those that are IgE-mediated, non–IgE-mediated, mixed IgE- and non–IgE-mediated, and cell-mediated.[1] IgE-mediated reactions are characterized by immediate allergic reactions, which can involve the skin; respiratory tract; GI tract; or generalized reactions, such as anaphylaxis. In most of these patients, serum food-specific IgE antibodies can be measured that, in conjunction with specific signs and symptoms on exposure to the specific food, confirm the IgE-mediated pattern of the reaction. Symptoms of IgE-mediated food allergy typically occur within minutes to hours of the ingested food.

Non–IgE-mediated GI diseases are often classified as dietary protein enteropathies. Dietary protein enterocolitis and celiac disease are the most common forms. Celiac disease is characterized by villous atrophy, crypt hyperplasia, increased intraepithelial lymphocytes, and a mixed inflammatory infiltrate. Dietary protein enterocolitis and enteropathy are typically caused by cow's milk or soy protein and cause variable small or large bowel injury associated with nonspecific villous atrophy and inflammation.

Mixed IgE and non-IgE mediated disorders include the eosinophilic gastroenteropathies of eosinophilic protocolitis, eosinophilic gastroenteritis, and eosinophilic esophagitis. These diseases are characterized by infiltration of the GI tract with eosinophils with an absence of other inflammatory cells. The eosinophils may infiltrate the mucosa, the muscular layer, and the serosa.[2]

Cell-mediated skin reactions to foods include contact dermatitis and dermatitis herpetiforme. Atopic dermatitis is considered a mixed IgE and cell-mediated reaction that can be triggered by ingestion of foods to which the patient is sensitized. Several studies involving standardized exposure to food by double-blind, placebo-controlled food challenges (DBPCFC) have carefully characterized these manifestations of food allergy occurring in up to 40% of children with moderate to severe atopic dermatitis.[3]

An understanding of these categories of food-induced allergic disorders is important for the otolaryngologist because many patients with upper airway inflammatory disease are atopic and at increased risk for having concomitant food allergy. Food allergy seems to be increasing and the otolaryngologist is likely to encounter an increasing number of patients with various manifestations of food allergy. Thus, an awareness of basic definitions, categories of food allergy and clinical manifestations, and familiarity with diagnostic testing and treatment strategies for food allergy, will engender quality comprehensive patient care. This article provides a review of the epidemiology, pathophysiology, clinical manifestations, diagnosis, and treatment of food allergy focusing primarily on IgE-mediated disease.

EPIDEMIOLOGY

Knowledge of the epidemiology of food allergy is essential in directing the otolaryngologist's evaluation of a patient with possible food allergy. Interestingly, the prevalence of food allergies is greatest in the first few years of life, affecting about 6% of infants less than 3 years of age[4] and decreasing over the first two decades. Although genetic risk factors are not solely responsible for the incidence of food allergy, there are genetic predisposing factors for its development, just as there are genetic factors that predispose toward other atopic diseases.

In the case of peanut allergy, a child has a seven-fold increase in the risk of peanut allergy if he or she has a parent or sibling with peanut allergy.[5] It has been shown that in monozygotic twins, a child has a 64% likelihood of peanut allergy if his or her twin sibling has peanut allergy. This indicates a strong genetic contribution to peanut allergy.[6]

The expression of genetic predisposition seems to be influenced by environmental factors, such as molecular characteristics of the food antigen and the timing and route of exposure. Evidence supporting the hypothesis that the timing of exposure to foods is important includes a recent study showing Israeli Jewish children of school age (consumption of peanut at ages 8–14 months was 7.1 g) had peanut allergy rates of 0.17%, compared with Jewish children in the United Kingdom (consumption of peanut at ages 8–14 months was 0 g) where the rate of peanut allergy was 10-fold higher (1.85%).[7] This study supports the theory that early oral exposure to peanut might promote tolerance, and that perhaps in the absence of oral tolerance sensitization occurs.

There is a well-documented association between food allergy and other atopic diseases.[8] Highlighting the importance of food allergy to the otolaryngologist, there is a strong association between food allergy and allergic rhinitis noted in the literature. Bozkurt and coworkers[9] showed that food allergy was the most common coexisting atopic condition in adult rhinitis patients. In a recent study by Sahin-Yilmaz and colleagues[10] aimed at evaluating the prevalence of IgE-mediated food allergy among adults with allergic rhinitis, a 23.4% prevalence of peanut sensitization was observed.

There is also a well-documented link between the presence of early eczema in childhood and the development of food allergy. About 33% of children with infantile eczema have IgE-mediated food allergy.[11] Eczema severity in the first year of life is associated with the development of egg, milk, and peanut allergies. The presence of eczema in the first 6 months of life was associated with an increased risk of peanut allergy, and this risk increased with more severe eczema.[12] More recently, a study of 2184 infants showed that the risk of egg, milk, or peanut allergy was approximately twice as high if eczema was present in the first 6 months of life compared with the second 6 months of life.[13]

Food allergy rates vary by age, local diet, and many other factors. The prevalence of food allergy is difficult to establish because of the lack of studies applying reliable diagnostic methodologies, inconsistencies in reporting, and variations in the definition of food allergy. Despite these challenges to accurate epidemiology, most studies suggest individual food allergies have increased over the last decade, and there clearly is the impression that new food allergies are increasing in prevalence, particularly kiwi allergy[14] and sesame seed allergy.[15]

A 2008 Centers for Disease Control and Prevention report indicated an 18% increase in childhood food allergy from 1997 to 2007, with an estimated 3.9% of children currently affected.[16] Recent studies focusing on peanut indicate that the prevalence rates in children have increased, essentially doubling, and exceed 1% of school-aged children.[17]

Although an allergy could be triggered by virtually any food, a small number of foods account for most food allergies. In young children the most common causal foods are cow's milk (2.5%); egg (1.3%); peanut (0.8%); wheat (0.4%); soy (0.4%); tree nuts (0.2%); fish (0.1%); and shellfish (0.1%).[18] Historically, studies indicated that childhood food allergies typically resolve by age 5 years, but more recent studies reveal that rates of resolution may be significantly slower. Although this may be affected by selection bias (because of the referral patterns to academic centers, which may draw patients with more severe and persistent disease), recent studies show resolution for cow's milk allergy at 79% by age 16 years[19] and for egg allergy at 68% by 16 years.[20] In contrast to milk and egg allergy, only 20% of children develop tolerance to peanut[21] and less than 10% outgrow allergy to tree nuts.[22]

Accordingly, adults are more likely to have allergies to shellfish (2%); peanut (0.6%); tree nuts (0.5%); and fish (0.4%).[18] The clinician must also consider a variety of adverse reactions to foods that are not food allergies. Although up to 25% of adults report symptoms that may be related to certain foods, the prevalence of food allergies among adults is less than 3%, making self-reporting of food allergy highly inaccurate. It is estimated that more than 20% of adults and children alter their diets based on these perceptions.[23]

Adverse food reactions that are not classified as food allergies include host-specific metabolic disorders, such as lactose intolerance, galactosemia, and alcohol intolerance. Individuals may also experience a response to a pharmacologically active component in food, such as caffeine. Other examples include tyramine in aged cheeses triggering migraine headaches and histaminic chemicals in the spoiled dark meat of certain fish resulting in scombroid poisoning. Toxin-mediated reactions (food poisoning) also cause food-induced symptoms.[18]

Another challenge in determining the existence of food allergy relates to the diagnostic tools available. Simply establishing the presence of allergen-specific IgE (sensitization), whether measured in vivo (skin testing) or in vitro (IgE testing), does not independently indicate clinically relevant disease. Because sensitization may be symptomatic (as in food allergy) or asymptomatic, the latest food allergy guidelines recommend that both the presence of sensitization and the development of specific signs and symptoms on exposure to that food be present for a diagnosis of IgE-mediated food allergy.[1]

IMMUNOLOGY AND PATHOPHYSIOLOGY

In considering food allergy, the clinician must first determine whether the adverse reaction to food is immunologic in nature. There exist many adverse reactions to foods that are not classified as food allergies because they lack an immunologic basis. For the purposes of this review of food allergy immunology and pathophysiology, the definition of food allergy outlined by the expert panel in the NIH 2010 *Guidelines for the Diagnosis and Management of Food Allergy* is used. Again, the panel defines as food allergy an "adverse health effect arising from a specific immune response that occurs reproducibly on exposure to a given food."[1]

Host factors, including both innate and adaptive immunity, are thought to contribute to the development of food allergy. Nonhost factors, such as dosing and frequency of exposure, may also play a role in the pathophysiology of food allergy.

Food allergy represents an abrogation of normal oral tolerance. The GI mucosa encounters large quantities of non–self antigen. While processing and absorbing nutrients, the GI immune system is also determining which non–self antigens are harmful. GI innate immune factors include the physical barrier of the gut, intestinal enzymes, and pH maintenance, and natural killer cells, macrophages, and toll-like receptors. Adaptive factors include lymphocytes, Peyer patches, specific IgA, and cytokines that drive a specific response to antigen. Developmental immaturity of these various components, particularly altered intestinal permeability, poorly maintained gut pH, and immature secretory IgA, have all been highlighted as possible factors in the development of sensitization and food allergy in early childhood.

Several cell types have been identified as playing an important role in developing oral tolerance. Suppressor $CD8^+$ cells and natural killer cells have been shown to be mediators of tolerance. Additionally, several groupings of regulatory $CD4^+$ T cells, including TH3 cells, TR1 cells, and $CD4^+$ and $CD25^+$ cells, seem to play an important role in intestinal immunity.[24]

Nonhost factors, or antigen-related factors, including the dose, frequency, and form of the antigen, may affect the balance of antigen sensitization or tolerance. It has been theorized that high-dose antigen challenges result in a state of lymphocyte anergy, promoting tolerance. Investigation of low-dose antigen challenges suggests a role for regulatory T cells inducing a state of tolerance. The properties of the antigen also seem to play a role in tolerance induction. Antigen qualities that may affect sensitization include solubility, cross reactivity with pollen, and extraintestinal exposure.

Murine studies[25] and evidence from human epidemiologic studies[12] indicate that such allergens as egg and peanut might evade oral tolerance by initial sensitizing exposure through the skin. Interestingly, symptoms of peanut allergy have been noted to occur on the first known peanut exposure in an estimated 75% of patients,[26] supporting the theory that the initial sensitizing exposure may actually bypass the gut. The argument that epicutaneous exposure contributes to the development of allergy, particularly peanut allergy, has been supported by the correlation of peanut allergy with exposure to topical application of oils containing peanut protein.[12] These investigations into alternate routes of sensitization remain ongoing areas of research. Defects of the skin barrier, as seen in atopic dermatitis, have been suggested to allow easier extraintestinal sensitization, which bypasses oral tolerance.

Additional host-related factors include genetics, age, and host flora. Murine models have demonstrated support for genetic influence on the development of food allergy.[27] Studies in human subjects have been more elusive, partially because of difficulties in experimental design. Age has also been identified as a factor that may contribute to oral tolerance. Eastham and coworkers[28] showed stronger immunologic reactions to dietary antigens in infants 3 months and younger and attributed this phenomena to immature gut permeability. Host flora also seem to contribute to oral tolerance development. The importance of commensal flora has been supported by the finding that administering lactobacillus to cow's milk–allergic children with atopic dermatitis improved their eczema.[29]

With an understanding of the basic immunology and pathophysiology of food allergy, the clinician must next focus attention on the variable manifestations of food allergy. There are several frameworks for categorizing the clinical manifestations of food allergy. Food allergy can be categorized based on pathophysiologic mechanisms, specifically IgE-mediated and non–IgE-mediated disorders. Food allergies may also be categorized by severity. Finally, an alternate means of conceptualizing food allergy focuses attention on the primary system involved. Although these groupings are commonly used in the literature, there is no agreed on uniform classification. Despite limitations, a systems-based approach is used for the purposes of this article.

CLINICAL MANIFESTATIONS

The clinical picture of food allergy can be quite varied making the diagnosis of food allergy challenging. The clinician must exclude adverse reactions to food that are not true food allergies. Examples of these include lactose intolerance; scombroid poisoning; and pharmacologic reactions to components in food, such as tyramine or caffeine. Once such adverse reactions are considered and excluded, the diagnosis of food allergy continues to be challenging because the clinical manifestations can be so varied.

Food-induced Anaphylaxis

Perhaps most familiar for the otolaryngologist is the IgE-mediated clinical presentation of anaphylaxis, which can be associated with food ingestion. Consideration of food allergy in the evaluation of any anaphylactic event is important because food allergy has been recognized as the leading cause of outpatient anaphylaxis in most surveys.[30] Failure to recognize a food as an anaphylactic trigger may result in serious morbidity and mortality.

Typically occurring in close temporal proximity to a food ingestion, food-induced anaphylaxis is IgE-mediated and affects multiple organ systems. There are no universally accepted diagnostic criteria or reliable biomarkers to facilitate the diagnosis of anaphylaxis. Cutaneous manifestations are common, occurring in 80% of individuals with anaphylaxis, and may include acute-onset urticaria or angioedema. Respiratory compromise with dyspnea or wheezing and cardiovascular manifestations including hypotension and tachycardia may also occur. There are rare reports of isolated hypotension as the primary manifestation of anaphylaxis, yet cardiovascular symptoms occur less frequently in food-induced anaphylaxis.[31]

Familiarity with the manifestations of anaphylaxis and recognition of the appropriate trigger are essential in caring for the food-allergic patient. Food-induced anaphylaxis can be life-threatening; however, it is a treatable and largely preventable manifestation of allergic disease. Most patients with food-induced anaphylaxis are aware of their food allergies,[32] which highlights the importance of patient education and avoidance once the diagnosis is established.

Cutaneous Food Hypersensitivities

Reactions involving the skin or mucus membranes are among some of the most common manifestations of food allergy. Acute urticaria and angioedema can be IgE mediated and are sometimes related to food allergy. Atopic dermatitis is also associated with food allergy, and its pathophysiology is more complex. A mixed reaction including both cellular and IgE-mediated responses to foods induces atopic dermatitis. The role of food allergy in the pathophysiology of atopic dermatitis continues to be controversial[33]; however, there does seem to be induction of urticarial lesions and itching associated with ingestion of specific food allergens, particularly in infants and young children.[34]

GI Food Hypersensitivities

A broad spectrum of GI food hypersensitivities has been described and there is some overlap between these various conditions. Oral allergy syndrome most commonly affects patients who are allergic to cross reactive inhalant allergens. An IgE-mediated allergic reaction, oral allergy syndrome is characterized by itching or swelling of the mucus membranes of the oral cavity and is usually associated with ingestion of plant proteins, which cross react with inhalant allergens. Common examples include patients with birch allergy may have symptoms after ingesting apples, pears, or hazelnuts; similarly, patients with ragweed allergy may have oral allergy symptoms after ingestion of fresh melon.

Immediate GI hypersensitivity, or GI anaphylaxis, is also IgE-mediated and presents with symptoms of nausea, vomiting, and abdominal pain. Most commonly, acute vomiting occurs rapidly with exposure to the food trigger.[1]

Eosinophilic esophagitis seems to be mediated by both IgE and non-IgE mechanisms and is characterized by eosinophilic inflammation of the esophagus. In infants and young children, the clinical presentation can be quite varied and may include weight loss, vomiting, reflux symptoms, or failure to thrive. Adults tend to present with such symptoms as esophageal food impaction and dysphagia. Diagnosis is made by biopsy and the exact role of food allergy in its pathogenesis remains unclear.[35]

Eosinophilic gastroenteritis is also mediated by both IgE and non-IgE mechanisms and is characterized by eosinophilic infiltration of localized or widespread lengths of the GI tract. Clinical manifestations correlate with the location and extent of eosinophilic infiltration but range from abdominal pain, vomiting, diarrhea, and blood in the stool. Presentation in infants may actually be pyloric outlet obstruction with projectile vomiting. Although commonly associated with food allergy, the true role of food allergy in its pathogenesis remains unclear as is also the case in eosinophilic esophagitis.[36]

Food protein-induced proctocolitis typically appears in early infancy and is characterized by gross or microscopic blood in the stool. Unique from other disorders, infants are otherwise healthy and asymptomatic. This clinical entity seems to be associated with non-IgE mechanisms because IgE to specific foods is most typically absent. A causal relationship is inferred from a typical history related to specific exposures. It is thought to be related to ingestion of milk or soy proteins transmitted either via formula or maternal breast milk. Unfortunately, there are no specific diagnostic tests for this clinical entity.[37]

Food protein-induced enterocolitis syndrome is similarly a non–IgE-mediated food hypersensitivity reaction characterized most typically by vomiting and diarrhea leading to dehydration in infants. The pathophysiology is believed to be a cell-mediated reaction to cow's milk or soy proteins. A similar syndrome is described in adults, which is most commonly associated with shellfish ingestion.[37]

Respiratory Food Hypersensitivities

Although food allergy can induce acute respiratory symptoms associated with anaphylaxis, isolated respiratory manifestations of food allergy are uncommon. Both allergic rhinitis (upper airway) and asthma (lower airway) can be exacerbated by food allergy. It has been well documented that worsening of chronic asthma can occur after the ingestion of particular foods in sensitized subjects and food allergy has been noted to be an independent risk factor for severe life-threatening asthma.[38,39]

DIAGNOSIS

The diagnosis of food allergy begins with a thorough history and physical examination. In initiating the evaluation of a patient who may have food allergy, the clinician should aim to ascertain potential causative foods, the typical timing of the reaction, and reaction consistency. The history may also provide supportive evidence for the allergic mechanism (IgE-mediated or non–IgE-mediated). Importantly, the newly published NIH *Guidelines for the Diagnosis and Management of Food Allergy* clearly outline that, although medical history is useful for directing the evaluation of the food-allergic patient, depending on the history alone lacks sufficient sensitivity and specificity definitively to diagnose food allergy.[1] In terms of physical examination, there are no objective findings that are diagnostic of food allergy; nevertheless, noting findings that are supportive of atopic disease, such as dermatitis or urticaria, may prove helpful in the clinician's evaluation.

The selection of tests aimed at diagnosis of food allergy depends on the history that has been ascertained. It is not advisable to test large general panels of food allergens because this may yield many false-positives and result in more, rather than less, diagnostic confusion. Furthermore, there is no justification for food allergy "screening" that is not predicated on relevant history. Thus, the history should direct testing for potentially causative foods, and test selection may also be influenced by the clinician's suspicion for allergic mechanism. Although there are numerous tests that have been used for diagnosing food allergy, the most commonly studied are skin prick testing (SPT), food allergen-specific serum IgE (sIgE), and atopy patch testing (APT). SPT and sIgE tests tend to be used in suspected IgE-mediated disorders, whereas APT is increasingly studied in patients with mixed or non-IgE allergic mechanisms, such as atopic dermatitis and allergic eosinophilic esophagitis. In evaluating the sensitivity and specificity of these tests, the DBPCFC remains the gold standard.[40]

Skin Prick Test

SPT provides a safe and rapid means to assist in the identification of sensitization. A negative SPT can be quite valuable for the clinician because a negative SPT response confirms the absence of IgE-mediated sensitivity (negative predictive accuracy >90%); however, a positive SPT does not confirm that the tested food is causal.[41] Unfortunately, SPTs have a low positive predictive value and low specificity for making the diagnosis of food allergy. A positive SPT is only a measure of sensitization, and the NIH Guidelines are clear to delineate that a positive SPT alone cannot be considered diagnostic of food allergy.

As with most diagnostic tests, interpretation of the SPT requires the clinician to combine clinical features and history with test results. For example, a positive SPT in the setting of a recent clear history of allergic reaction to the tested food may be adequate for the clinician to advise strict avoidance of the suspicious food. Also, studies have shown that the larger the wheal size provoked, the more likely the food allergen is of clinical relevance.[42] This fact may also aid in the clinician's interpretation of the significance of a positive SPT. Efforts have been made to define the diagnostic accuracy of different wheal sizes for different foods; however, these have been done in very selective study populations and certainly additional studies are necessary.

Food Allergen-specific sIgE

Similar to the SPT, food allergen-specific sIgE testing is valuable for assessing patients for whom there is suspicion for an IgE-mediated allergic mechanism because both testing modalities require the presence of allergen-specific antibodies. Much like a positive SPT, a positive in vitro test simply indicates sensitization to a particular food and may not correlate with clinical food allergy confirmed by a food challenge. Much like increasing diagnostic accuracy associated with increasing wheal size when evaluating the positive predictive value of a SPT, studies have shown that the greater the levels of sIgE, the higher the probability that the positive test is of true clinical relevance. These values are sometimes referred to as "diagnostic values" and are outlined in **Table 1**. It is important to understand that these values, for the most part, have been derived in patient populations with suspicious clinical histories for food allergy and should not be extrapolated to the general population; nevertheless, they provide some guidance in the interpretation of sIgE tests.[36] Unfortunately an undetectable level of sIgE may still be associated with clinical reaction, including anaphylaxis, in 10% to 25% of cases and should be followed with an oral food challenge test.[43]

There are specific situations in which an sIgE test may be preferred over a SPT. For example, in patients with severe skin disease or dermatographism, sIgE may be preferable over SPT. When antihistamines cannot be discontinued or where medical conditions preclude skin testing (ie, pregnancy, β-blockade), serum testing may be preferable.

Table 1
Predictive value of food allergen-specific IgE levels 95% predictive level

Allergen	kU/L	Positive Predictive Value
Egg	7	98
Milk	15	95
Peanut	14	100
Fish	20	100
Tree nuts	15	95
Soybean	30	73
Wheat	26	74

Data from Sampson HA. Update on food allergy. J Allergy Clin Immunol 2004;113(5):805–19.

Atopy Patch Tests

Although not as well-studied as the SPT or sIgE tests, the APT holds promise for evaluation of food allergy that occurs in a delayed or non–IgE-mediated fashion. The difference between the APT and a traditional patch test is that the APT uses food allergens that are typically only used for assessing IgE-mediated reactions. There are not standardized reagents or methodology for this testing modality, and the sensitivity and specificity of the test varies among studies.[44] Because of the insufficient evidence to support the use of APT, the NIH Guidelines suggest that the APT currently not be used to make a definitive diagnosis of food allergy.

Elimination Diets

The 2010 NIH Guidelines acknowledge that there is little support in the literature for the use of dietary elimination trials or food diaries. Despite this, it is clear that there are unique situations where an elimination diet may be the preferred diagnostic test or minimize the morbidity in the diagnostic process. Particularly in evaluating patients with probable non–IgE-mediated disorders, such as eosinophilic esophagitis or proctocolitis, elimination of one or two specific foods from the diet may be helpful in establishing a diagnosis of food allergy. In these particular situations, there are no diagnostic laboratory tests and oral food challenges may actually induce significant morbidity. For this reason, many clinicians use a dietary elimination diet to establish a diagnosis when there is clearing of symptoms with elimination of a particular food. The elimination diet has the added advantage of being simultaneously therapeutic. One caveat to consider, however, when implementing an elimination diet is the fact that dietary elimination of multiple foods has been reported to cause severe malnutrition and the approach of eliminating multiple staples from an individual's diet should be avoided.[45]

Oral Food Challenges

The DBPCFC remains the gold standard in diagnosing food allergy. Clearly, the DBPCFC has the advantage of being a blinded in vivo test of food allergy; however, there are obvious disadvantages. DBPCFCs are quite expensive; labor-intensive; and although helpful experimentally, difficult to execute in clinical practice. All oral food challenges carry the added risk of severe allergic reaction because of the in vivo nature of the test.

Because of these limitations, most oral challenges executed in patient care settings are single-blind or open. Any oral food challenge carries the risk of anaphylaxis or severe allergic reaction, so these tests should be performed in settings prepared to manage such allergic emergencies. There is currently no standardized protocol for performing or interpreting oral food challenges.[1]

Unproved Food-testing Procedures

A variety of different testing modalities have been used historically in the assessment of food allergy. The 2010 NIH guidelines discourage the use of the following tests for the routine evaluation of food allergy because of lack of standardization and low quality of evidence: basophil histamine release and activation, lymphocyte stimulation, and allergen-specific IgG and IgG4.[1] The use of IgG and IgG4 testing deserves specific mention because many commercial laboratories promote this modality of testing as an alternate means of identifying food allergy. Rather than indicating imminent food allergy, it seems that IgG4 actually provides evidence of exposure to food components and can, therefore, be found in a large number of healthy asymptomatic individuals. IgG4 has been noted to increase as some patients develop oral tolerance to specific foods; however, many of these studies are contradictory. For example, Ahrens and coworkers[46] recently studied the role of IgG and IgG4 levels in the diagnosis of hen's egg allergy and showed that levels of IgG and IgG4 were not significantly different among sensitized and tolerant, sensitized and allergic, and nonsensitized subjects. In addition to discouraging the use of allergen-specific IgG and IgG4 as a diagnostic testing modality, the expert panel also recommends that intradermal testing, a core component of the provocation-neutralization food testing technique, should not be used in the diagnosis of food allergy. Certainly, the topic of unproved food allergy testing methodology remains an area of controversy and additional studies are warranted.

TREATMENT FOR FOOD ALLERGIES

Once the diagnosis of food allergy is established, the patient care focus must shift to treatment strategies. Although the diagnosis of food allergy is grouped by clinical presentation, treatment is categorized by whether the food allergy is IgE-mediated or non–IgE-mediated.

Treatment of IgE-mediated Food Allergy

Current treatment for IgE-mediated food allergy consists of avoidance and preparation for accidental ingestion.[47] Successful avoidance requires knowing which foods contain the allergic ingredient, common sources of accidental ingestion, and possible cross reactivities for that allergen. Preparation for accidental ingestion should include an action plan for anaphylaxis; access to epinephrine; and medical alert information (eg, bracelet).

Knowing which foods to avoid in the food-allergic patient is easier in theory than practice. One of the reasons the Food and Drug Administration requires that the ingredients are listed on the label of foods is to facilitate avoidance by food-allergic individuals. In 2006, the Food and Drug Administration required clearer labeling specifically for food allergy (eg, milk rather than casein). However, daily encounters with foods in restaurants and social events require more knowledge than reading labels alone. Fortunately, there are good resources for the food-allergic patient and their families. Meeting with a nutritionist may be helpful. However, in a recent survey pediatric dieticians rated themselves as "moderate" in educating families about food allergies, and 75% categorized their instruction in food allergy as "self-educated."[48] **Table 2** lists

Table 2
Resources for the food allergic patient

Food Allergy and Anaphylaxis Network	www.foodallergy.org
Anaphylaxis Campaign	www.anaphylaxis.org.uk
National Institute of Allergy and Infectious Disease	http://www.niaid.nih.gov/topics/foodallergy/Pages/default.aspx
FDA	http://www.fda.gov/Food/ResourcesForYou/Consumers/SelectedHealthTopics/ucm119075.htm
Mayo Clinic	http://www.mayoclinic.com/health/food-allergy/DS00082

several quality patient resources available on the Internet for the food-allergic patient and their family.

Accidental ingestions of allergic foods happen on average every 3 years.[49] Common causes are foods prepared outside the home[50]; restaurants (specifically Asian restaurants)[51]; and desserts.[50,51] Based on fatality papers, the authors warn peanut- and tree nut–allergic families of the "Three Cs: Candy, Cookies, and Cake."[50] In children, foods eaten outside their routine at birthday parties, friends' homes, or vacation may pose increased risk.

When an individual has been diagnosed with an IgE-mediated food allergy, two practical concerns arise: with what other foods are that patient likely to cross-react, and are they at risk to develop sensitizations to other highly allergenic foods.

Cross reactivity occurs when the epitope that binds IgE comes from a different source. Tree nut allergy provides an example of how knowledge of cross reactivity is important. An individual may have a reaction to walnut and test positive for walnut; should they avoid other tree nuts? Because there is a significant clinical cross reactivity between tree nuts, most recommend that all tree nuts should be avoided. Balancing safety against the inconvenience of unnecessary restrictions can be clinically challenging. At present, it is difficult to predict an individual's cross reactivity definitively and relying on epidemiologic data is necessary. Curiously, in vitro cross reactivity and clinical cross reactivity are frequently discordant.[47] For example, wheat exhibits significant in vitro cross reactivity with other grains, but clinically other grains are generally tolerated in the wheat-allergic individual.[47] A list of clinically significant food cross reactivities is provided in **Table 3**.

Table 3
Clinical food allergen cross reactivities

Cow's milk	Goat's milk 90% Beef 10%
Hen's egg	Turkey, duck, goose egg
Soy	Clinical cross reactivities with other legumes uncommon
Peanut	Other legumes generally tolerated (5% clinical intolerance)
Fish	Significant cross reactivity between species (74%)
Tree nut	High cross reactivity with other tree nuts
Crustaceans	Between crustaceans considerable cross reactivity Mollusks less well defined
Wheat	In vitro cross reactivity not reflected clinically

Data from Chapman JA, Bernstein IL, Lee RE, et al. Food allergy: a practice parameter. Ann Allergy Asthma Immun 2006;96:S1–68.

Name: ______________________ **D.O.B.:** __/__/__

Allergy to: ______________________

Weight: ______ lbs. **Asthma:** ☐ Yes (higher risk for a severe reaction) ☐ No

Place Student's Picture Here

Extremely reactive to the following foods: ______________________
THEREFORE:
☐ If checked, give epinephrine immediately for ANY symptoms if the allergen was *likely* eaten.
☐ If checked, give epinephrine immediately if the allergen was *definitely* eaten, even if no symptoms are noted.

Any SEVERE SYMPTOMS after suspected or known ingestion:

One or more of the following:
LUNG: Short of breath, wheeze, repetitive cough
HEART: Pale, blue, faint, weak pulse, dizzy, confused
THROAT: Tight, hoarse, trouble breathing/swallowing
MOUTH: Obstructive swelling (tongue and/or lips)
SKIN: Many hives over body

Or **combination** of symptoms from different body areas:
SKIN: Hives, itchy rashes, swelling (e.g., eyes, lips)
GUT: Vomiting, crampy pain

→

1. **INJECT EPINEPHRINE IMMEDIATELY**
2. Call 911
3. Begin monitoring (see box below)
4. Give additional medications:*
   -Antihistamine
   -Inhaler (bronchodilator) if asthma

*Antihistamines & inhalers/bronchodilators are not to be depended upon to treat a severe reaction (anaphylaxis). USE EPINEPHRINE.

MILD SYMPTOMS ONLY:

MOUTH: Itchy mouth
SKIN: A few hives around mouth/face, mild itch
GUT: Mild nausea/discomfort

→

1. **GIVE ANTIHISTAMINE**
2. Stay with student; alert healthcare professionals and parent
3. If symptoms progress (see above), USE EPINEPHRINE
4. Begin monitoring (see box below)

Medications/Doses

Epinephrine (brand and dose): ______________________
Antihistamine (brand and dose): ______________________
Other (e.g., inhaler-bronchodilator if asthmatic): ______________________

Monitoring

Stay with student; alert healthcare professionals and parent. Tell rescue squad epinephrine was given; request an ambulance with epinephrine. Note time when epinephrine was administered. A second dose of epinephrine can be given 5 minutes or more after the first if symptoms persist or recur. For a severe reaction, consider keeping student lying on back with legs raised. Treat student even if parents cannot be reached. See back/attached for auto-injection technique.

Parent/Guardian Signature ______ **Date** ______ **Physician/Healthcare Provider Signature** ______ **Date** ______

TURN FORM OVER **Form provided courtesy of FAAN (www.foodallergy.org) 7/2010**

Fig. 1. Sample of a food allergy action plan (*From* Food Allergy & Anaphylaxis Network. Food allergy action plan. Available at: http://www.foodallergy.org/page/food-allergy-action-plan1. Accessed November 21, 2010; with permission).

Cross sensitization or "co-allergy" refers to the risk of an allergic patient becoming sensitized to an allergenically distinct food. Should the peanut allergic patient avoid tree nuts? This is an area of controversy in the literature and recommendations vary with patient risk profile and allergen considered. "Co allergy" between peanut and tree nut was 2.5% in a telephone survey,[52] but 34% in a "selected atopic" population.[53] Children with egg allergy have a 30% risk of developing allergies to tree nuts, peanuts, or sesame.[54]

Sampson and coworkers[55] reported on 13 cases of fatal or near-fatal food anaphylaxis in children and adolescents finding 13 of 13 were asthmatic; 10 of 13 reacted to peanuts and tree nuts; and all of the cases involved candies, cookies, or pastries. Only

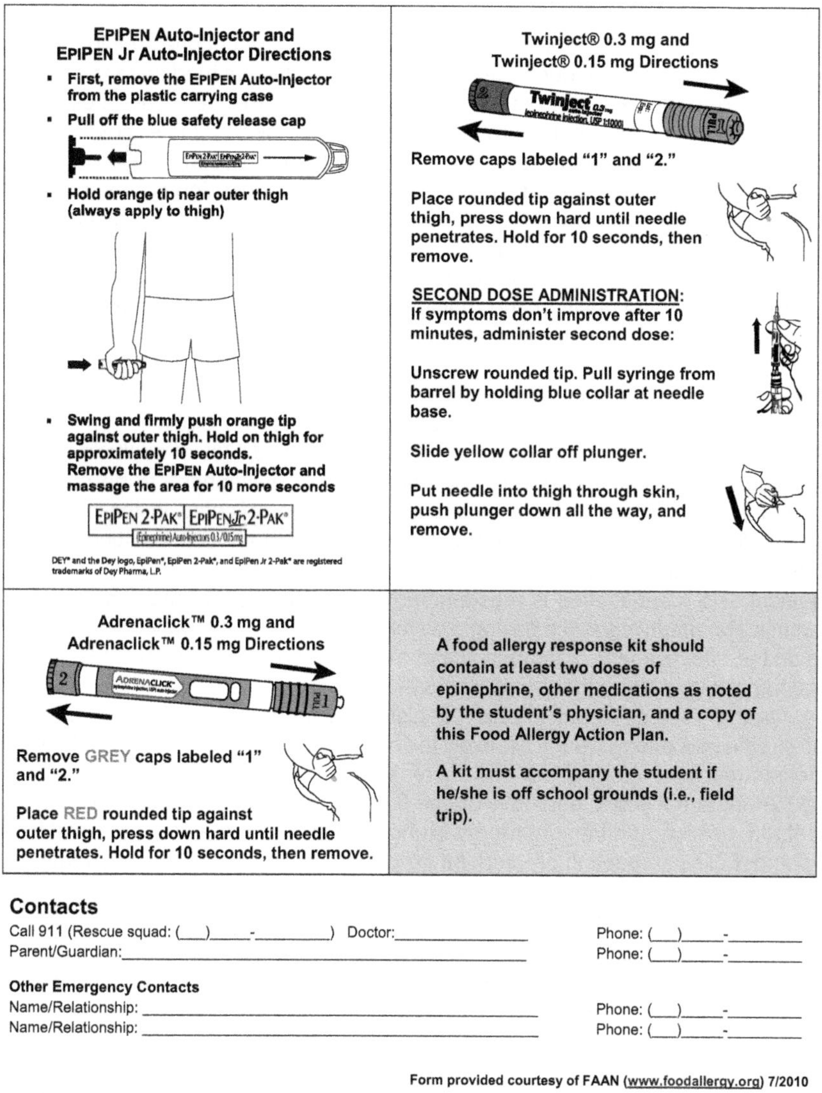

EPIPEN Auto-Injector and EPIPEN Jr Auto-Injector Directions

- First, remove the EPIPEN Auto-Injector from the plastic carrying case
- Pull off the blue safety release cap
- Hold orange tip near outer thigh (always apply to thigh)
- Swing and firmly push orange tip against outer thigh. Hold on thigh for approximately 10 seconds. Remove the EPIPEN Auto-Injector and massage the area for 10 more seconds

EPIPEN 2-PAK® EPIPEN Jr 2-PAK®

DEY® and the Dey logo, EpiPen®, EpiPen 2-Pak®, and EpiPen Jr 2-Pak® are registered trademarks of Dey Pharma, L.P.

Twinject® 0.3 mg and Twinject® 0.15 mg Directions

Remove caps labeled "1" and "2."

Place rounded tip against outer thigh, press down hard until needle penetrates. Hold for 10 seconds, then remove.

SECOND DOSE ADMINISTRATION:
If symptoms don't improve after 10 minutes, administer second dose:

Unscrew rounded tip. Pull syringe from barrel by holding blue collar at needle base.

Slide yellow collar off plunger.

Put needle into thigh through skin, push plunger down all the way, and remove.

Adrenaclick™ 0.3 mg and Adrenaclick™ 0.15 mg Directions

Remove GREY caps labeled "1" and "2."

Place RED rounded tip against outer thigh, press down hard until needle penetrates. Hold for 10 seconds, then remove.

A food allergy response kit should contain at least two doses of epinephrine, other medications as noted by the student's physician, and a copy of this Food Allergy Action Plan.

A kit must accompany the student if he/she is off school grounds (i.e., field trip).

Contacts

Call 911 (Rescue squad: (___)_____-_________) Doctor:_______________ Phone: (___)_____-_________
Parent/Guardian:_______________ Phone: (___)_____-_________

Other Emergency Contacts

Name/Relationship: _______________ Phone: (___)_____-_________
Name/Relationship: _______________ Phone: (___)_____-_________

Form provided courtesy of FAAN (www.foodallergy.org) 7/2010

Fig. 1. (*continued*)

two of the six who died received epinephrine in the first hour. Yunginger and colleagues[56] described six food anaphylaxis deaths and common themes included failure to use epinephrine (often treating with antihistamines alone) and failure to realize symptoms.

Accidental ingestion of a diagnosed allergic food is likely. Bock and Adkins reported that 50% of children with a known peanut allergy ingested peanut in a 3-year period and 75% had ingested peanut over 5 years.[49] As such, preparation for this foreseeable event is required. Adolescents and young adults warrant careful clinical attention because they statistically account for half to two thirds of the food allergy deaths.[32,57]

NIH Guidelines have recommended the use of "action plans" in the treatment of food anaphylaxis[1] and asthma attacks.[58] An action plan lists the symptoms expected and the recommended action that should be initiated **Fig. 1** shows a sample action plan[59] for an anaphylactic food reaction. Auto-injection epinephrine should be immediately available for food-induced anaphylaxis and additional medications should be individualized to the patient. Epinephrine is widely recommended[60] and delayed use of epinephrine is a common feature in anaphylaxis deaths.[50,55] Other considerations include antihistamines or inhaled β_2 agonists (if asthma coexists). The importance of educating all caregivers to administer medications is highlighted by reports of teachers injecting their own fingers when trying to administer epinephrine to students.[60] Epinephrine is not stable in heat (eg, inside a car in the summer) and has a limited shelf-life requiring attention to the expiration date. In anaphylaxis, laying the patient in a supine position and maintaining that position is also strongly recommended. Quickly sitting or standing after epinephrine in anaphylaxis has been associated with death.[61]

Immediate use of an epinephrine auto-injector is not a substitute for calling emergency services because the anaphylaxis may progress and biphasic reactions are well described.[62] It is not uncommon (12% of children and 17% of adults in an emergency department setting) for more than one dose of epinephrine to be required in food anaphylaxis,[63,64] and this contingency should be reflected in the action plan and prescriptions. The management of anaphylaxis in the hospital setting has been discussed in other articles.[60,65]

Medical alert identification is reasonable because the patient may not be able to communicate effectively while having a severe reaction or if the patient is young.[60,66] Data on the effectiveness or compliance of medical alert identification are limited, but it is recommended throughout the literature.

Counseling patients about the natural history of food allergies is advised. Young children with milk or egg allergy are likely to "out grow" the allergy. A prospective study demonstrated how tolerance to milk increases over early childhood: 50% at age 1 year, 70% at age 2 years, and 85% at age 3 years.[67] However, developing tolerance in seafood, peanut, and tree nut allergy is uncommon.[68] Whether an accidental ingestion without clinical reaction predicts future or continued tolerance is uncertain.

Treatment of Non–IgE-mediated Food Allergy

Scientific study of otolaryngologic manifestations of non–IgE-mediated food allergy is very limited. Historically, Rinkel[69] described observing "cyclical" food allergy and recommended a rotation diet. A PubMed search in November of 2010 of "Cyclical Food Allergy" yielded only one case report of cyclical emesis in a patient with ulcerative colitis.[70] Looking at treatments of two non–IgE-mediated food processes, eosinophilic esophatitis[71] and celiac disease,[72] suggests that avoidance may also be useful when non–IgE-mediated disease is suspected.

RESEARCH AND FUTURE DEVELOPMENTS IN FOOD ALLERGY

Subcutaneous immunotherapy for food has not been demonstrated as effective and is likely unsafe.[73,74] However, published research has shown some success with promoting oral tolerance in carefully administered research protocols. Jones and coworkers[75] reported a protocol for oral immunotherapy using peanut in which 27 peanut-allergic children developed tolerance to 3.9 g of peanut protein. They also demonstrated decreased peanut-specific IgE and increased specific IgG4. A recent letter by many of the oral immunotherapy researchers expressed their concern that oral immunotherapy for foods was not yet ready for clinical application outside of research trials.[76]

Many allergic foods have multiple allergic epitopes. Sensitized patients may vary as to which epitope or epitopes against which they produce IgE. Some research has investigated whether knowing which epitope the IgE binds could predict clinical outcomes, such as severity, cross reactivity, or future tolerance.[77,78] Microarray technology has made this line of investigation possible and this testing is sometimes called "component" IgE testing. Also, sIgE thresholds have traditionally been negative at less than 0.35 kIU; however, advances in diagnostics have made it possible to detect sIgE greater than 0.10 kIU. Some research has looked at the sIgE levels for food between 0.10 and 0.35 kIU as possibly predictive of food allergy. Codreanu and coworkers[79] recently compared those with clinical peanut allergy with controls using component specific IgE to Ara h 2 and Ara h 6 and the lower 0.10 kU/L positive threshold. They reported 98% sensitivity and 91% specificity. The data on this are still evolving and the Food and Drug Administration has not approved these tests for clinical use in the United States.

IgE signaling requires that two IgE molecules cross-link with the antigen. It is theorized that cross-linking is more likely to occur as a sIgE type comprises a higher percentage of the total IgE. Hamilton and coworkers[80] have shown that patients with a sIgE comprising 4% of their total IgE tend to be observed more frequently in allergens known to cause severe reactions (venoms and foods). More research on this is required before it is clinically applicable.

The NIH guidelines emphasize that many knowledge gaps pertaining to food allergy remain, and research about food allergy is ongoing. Many "best practice" recommendations made by the expert panel are limited by this low quality of evidence and certain practices are subject to change pending more rigorous research. It is clear on review of the current body of food allergy literature that evidence regarding epidemiology, diagnostic evaluation, and treatment of food allergy is limited by lack of uniformity in definitions and imperfect diagnostic testing modalities. Food allergy is a focus of much current study and it is expected that there will be more rapidly evolving evidence regarding food allergy in the very near future.

SUMMARY

A food allergy is defined as an immunologic phenomenon that occurs reproducibly on exposure to a given food and must be distinguished from food intolerances. The prevalence of food allergy is difficult to assess because of reporting inconsistencies; however, individual food allergy seems to be increasing. The clinician's knowledge of food allergy epidemiology can aid in the diagnostic evaluation. First, a small number of foods account for most food allergies. Also, childhood food allergy is characterized by allergies to hen's egg and cow's milk, whereas adult food allergy is characterized by more allergies to shellfish, peanut, tree nuts, and fish. Evidence-based testing modalities for IgE-mediated food allergy include SPT and food-allergen specific sIgE testing. The DBPCFC remains the gold standard for food allergy diagnosis. Research about the treatment of food allergy is ongoing; however, avoidance remains the mainstay of treatment at the present time.

REFERENCES

1. Guidelines for the diagnosis and management of food allergy. 2010. Available at: http://www.niaid.nih.gov/topics/foodallergy/clinical/Pages/default.aspx. Accessed November 14, 2010.
2. Klein NC, Hargrove RL, Sleisenger MH, et al. Eosinophilic gastroenteritis. Medicine (Baltimore) 1970;49(4):299–319.

3. Hill DJ, Hosking CS. Food allergy and atopic dermatitis in infancy: an epidemiologic study. Pediatr Allergy Immunol 2004;15(5):421–7.
4. Bock SA. Prospective appraisal of complaints of adverse reactions to foods in children during the first 3 years of life. Pediatrics 1987;79(5):683–8.
5. Hourihane JO, Dean TP, Warner JO. Peanut allergy in relation to heredity, maternal diet, and other atopic diseases: results of a questionnaire survey, skin prick testing, and food challenges. BMJ 1996;313(7056):518–21.
6. Sicherer SH, Furlong TJ, Maes HH, et al. Genetics of peanut allergy: a twin study. J Allergy Clin Immunol 2000;106(1 Pt 1):53–6.
7. Du Toit G, Katz Y, Sasieni P, et al. Early consumption of peanuts in infancy is associated with a low prevalence of peanut allergy. J Allergy Clin Immunol 2008; 122(5):984–91.
8. Mattila L, Kilpelainen M, Terho EO, et al. Food hypersensitivity among Finnish university students: association with atopic diseases. Clin Exp Allergy 2003; 33(5):600–6.
9. Bozkurt B, Karakaya G, Kalyoncu AF. Food hypersensitivity in patients with seasonal rhinitis in Ankara. Allergol Immunopathol (Madr) 2005;33(2):86–92.
10. Sahin-Yilmaz A, Nocon CC, Corey JP. Immunoglobulin E-mediated food allergies among adults with allergic rhinitis. Otolaryngol Head Neck Surg 2010;143(3): 379–85.
11. Eigenmann PA, Sicherer SH, Borkowski TA, et al. Prevalence of IgE-mediated food allergy among children with atopic dermatitis. Pediatrics 1998;101(3):E8.
12. Lack G, Fox D, Northstone K, et al. Factors associated with the development of peanut allergy in childhood. N Engl J Med 2003;348(11):977–85.
13. Hill DJ, Hosking CS, de Benedictis FM, et al. Confirmation of the association between high levels of immunoglobulin E food sensitization and eczema in infancy: an international study. Clin Exp Allergy 2008;38(1):161–8.
14. Lucas JS, Lewis SA, Hourihane JO. Kiwi fruit allergy: a review. Pediatr Allergy Immunol 2003;14(6):420–8.
15. Cohen A, Goldberg M, Levy B, et al. Sesame food allergy and sensitization in children: the natural history and long-term follow-up. Pediatr Allergy Immunol 2007;18(3):217–23.
16. Branum AM, Lukacs SL. Food allergy among U.S. children: trends in prevalence and hospitalizations. NCHS Data Brief 2008;(10):1–8.
17. Sicherer SH, Sampson HA. Peanut allergy: emerging concepts and approaches for an apparent epidemic. J Allergy Clin Immunol 2007;120(3):491–503 [quiz: 504].
18. Sicherer SH, Sampson HA. 9. Food allergy. J Allergy Clin Immunol 2006; 117(Suppl Mini-Primer 2):S470–5.
19. Skripak JM, Matsui EC, Mudd K, et al. The natural history of IgE-mediated cow's milk allergy. J Allergy Clin Immunol 2007;120(5):1172–7.
20. Savage JH, Matsui EC, Skripak JM, et al. The natural history of egg allergy. J Allergy Clin Immunol 2007;120(6):1413–7.
21. Skolnick HS, Conover-Walker MK, Koerner CB, et al. The natural history of peanut allergy. J Allergy Clin Immunol 2001;107(2):367–74.
22. Fleischer DM, Conover-Walker MK, Matsui EC, et al. The natural history of tree nut allergy. J Allergy Clin Immunol 2005;116(5):1087–93.
23. Rona RJ, Keil T, Summers C, et al. The prevalence of food allergy: a meta-analysis. J Allergy Clin Immunol 2007;120(3):638–46.
24. Chehade M, Mayer L. Oral tolerance and its relation to food hypersensitivities. J Allergy Clin Immunol 2005;115(1):3–12 [quiz: 13].

25. Hsieh KY, Tsai CC, Wu CH, et al. Epicutaneous exposure to protein antigen and food allergy. Clin Exp Allergy 2003;33(8):1067–75.
26. Burks AW. Peanut allergy. Lancet 2008;371(9623):1538–46.
27. Morafo V, Srivastava K, Huang CK, et al. Genetic susceptibility to food allergy is linked to differential TH2-TH1 responses in C3H/HeJ and BALB/c mice. J Allergy Clin Immunol 2003;111(5):1122–8.
28. Eastham EJ, Lichauco T, Grady MI, et al. Antigenicity of infant formulas: role of immature intestine on protein permeability. J Pediatr 1978;93(4):561–4.
29. Majamaa H, Isolauri E. Probiotics: a novel approach in the management of food allergy. J Allergy Clin Immunol 1997;99(2):179–85.
30. Wang J, Sampson HA. Food anaphylaxis. Clin Exp Allergy 2007;37(5): 651–60.
31. Cianferoni A, Novembre E, Mugnaini L, et al. Clinical features of acute anaphylaxis in patients admitted to a university hospital: an 11-year retrospective review (1985-1996). Ann Allergy Asthma Immunol 2001;87(1):27–32.
32. Bock SA, Munoz-Furlong A, Sampson HA. Fatalities due to anaphylactic reactions to foods. J Allergy Clin Immunol 2001;107(1):191–3.
33. Rowlands D, Tofte SJ, Hanifin JM. Does food allergy cause atopic dermatitis? food challenge testing to dissociate eczematous from immediate reactions. Dermatol Ther 2006;19(2):97–103.
34. Burks W. Skin manifestations of food allergy. Pediatrics 2003;111(6 Pt 3): 1617–24.
35. Furuta GT, Liacouras CA, Collins MH, et al. Eosinophilic esophagitis in children and adults: a systematic review and consensus recommendations for diagnosis and treatment. Gastroenterology 2007;133(4):1342–63.
36. Sampson HA. Update on food allergy. J Allergy Clin Immunol 2004;113(5):805–19 [quiz: 820].
37. Sicherer SH. Clinical aspects of gastrointestinal food allergy in childhood. Pediatrics 2003;111(6 Pt 3):1609–16.
38. Roberts G, Patel N, Levi-Schaffer F, et al. Food allergy as a risk factor for life-threatening asthma in childhood: a case-controlled study. J Allergy Clin Immunol 2003;112(1):168–74.
39. James JM. Respiratory manifestations of food allergy. Pediatrics 2003;111(6 Pt 3): 1625–30.
40. Chafen JJ, Newberry SJ, Riedl MA, et al. Diagnosing and managing common food allergies: a systematic review. JAMA 2010;303(18):1848–56.
41. Sicherer SH, Sampson HA. Food allergy. J Allergy Clin Immunol 2010;125(Suppl 2): S116–25.
42. Verstege A, Mehl A, Rolinck-Werninghaus C, et al. The predictive value of the skin prick test weal size for the outcome of oral food challenges. Clin Exp Allergy 2005;35(9):1220–6.
43. Sampson HA. Utility of food-specific IgE concentrations in predicting symptomatic food allergy. J Allergy Clin Immunol 2001;107(5):891–6.
44. Mehl A, Rolinck-Werninghaus C, Staden U, et al. The atopy patch test in the diagnostic workup of suspected food-related symptoms in children. J Allergy Clin Immunol 2006;118(4):923–9.
45. David TJ, Waddington E, Stanton RH. Nutritional hazards of elimination diets in children with atopic eczema. Arch Dis Child 1984;59(4):323–5.
46. Ahrens B, Lopes de Oliveira LC, Schulz G, et al. The role of hen's egg-specific IgE, IgG and IgG4 in the diagnostic procedure of hen's egg allergy. Allergy 2010;65(12):1554–7.

47. Food allergy: a practice parameter. Ann Allergy Asthma Immunol 2006;96(Suppl 2): S1–68.
48. Groetch ME, Christie L, Vargas PA, et al. Food allergy educational needs of pediatric dietitians: a survey by the Consortium of Food Allergy Research. J Nutr Educ Behav 2010;42(4):259–64.
49. Bock SA, Atkins FM. The natural history of peanut allergy. J Allergy Clin Immunol 1989;83(5):900–4.
50. Bock SA, Munoz-Furlong A, Sampson HA. Further fatalities caused by anaphylactic reactions to food, 2001–2006. J Allergy Clin Immunol 2007;119(4):1016–8.
51. Furlong TJ, DeSimone J, Sicherer SH. Peanut and tree nut allergic reactions in restaurants and other food establishments. J Allergy Clin Immunol 2001;108(5): 867–70.
52. Sicherer SH, Munoz-Furlong A, Burks AW, et al. Prevalence of peanut and tree nut allergy in the US determined by a random digit dial telephone survey. J Allergy Clin Immunol 1999;103(4):559–62.
53. Sicherer SH, Burks AW, Sampson HA. Clinical features of acute allergic reactions to peanut and tree nuts in children. Pediatrics 1998;102(1):e6.
54. Sampson HA. Clinical practice. Peanut allergy. N Engl J Med 2002;346(17): 1294–9.
55. Sampson HA, Mendelson L, Rosen JP. Fatal and near-fatal anaphylactic reactions to food in children and adolescents. N Engl J Med 1992;327(6):380–4.
56. Yunginger JW, Sweeney KG, Sturner WQ, et al. Fatal food-induced anaphylaxis. JAMA 1988;260(10):1450–2.
57. Pumphrey RS, Gowland MH. Further fatal allergic reactions to food in the United Kingdom, 1999–2006. J Allergy Clin Immunol 2007;119(4):1018–9.
58. NIH Guidelines for the Diagnosis and Management of Asthma – 2007 (EPR-3) 2007. Available at: http://www.nhlbi.nih.gov/guidelines/asthma/index.htm. Accessed November 2, 2010.
59. Food allergy action plan. Available at: http://www.foodallergy.org/page/food-allergy-action-plan. Accessed November 21, 2010.
60. Simons FE. Anaphylaxis. J Allergy Clin Immunol 2010;125(Suppl 2):S161–81.
61. Pumphrey RS. Fatal posture in anaphylactic shock. J Allergy Clin Immunol 2003; 112(2):451–2.
62. Ellis AK, Day JH. Incidence and characteristics of biphasic anaphylaxis: a prospective evaluation of 103 patients. Ann Allergy Asthma Immunol 2007; 98(1):64–9.
63. Rudders SA, Banerji A, Corel B, et al. Multicenter study of repeat epinephrine treatments for food-related anaphylaxis. Pediatrics 2010;125(4):e711–8.
64. Banerji A, Rudders SA, Corel B, et al. Repeat epinephrine treatments for food-related allergic reactions that present to the emergency department. Allergy Asthma Proc 2010;31(4):308–16.
65. Muraro A, Roberts G, Clark A, et al. The management of anaphylaxis in childhood: position paper of the European Academy of Allergology and Clinical Immunology. Allergy 2007;62(8):857–71.
66. Sampson HA, Munoz-Furlong A, Campbell RL, et al. Second symposium on the definition and management of anaphylaxis: summary report–Second National Institute of Allergy and Infectious Disease/Food Allergy and Anaphylaxis Network symposium. J Allergy Clin Immunol 2006;117(2):391–7.
67. Host A. Cow's milk protein allergy and intolerance in infancy. Some clinical, epidemiological and immunological aspects. Pediatr Allergy Immunol 1994; 5(Suppl 5):1–36.

68. S HA. Adverse reactions to food. In: Adkinson FN, Yunginger JW, Busse WW, et al, editors. Middleton's Allergy: Principles and Practice. 6th edition. Philadelphia: Mosby; 2003.
69. Rinkel HJ. Food allergy. Springfield (IL): Thomas; 1951.
70. Copeland BH, Aramide OO, Wehbe SA, et al. Eosinophilia in a patient with cyclical vomiting: a case report. Clin Mol Allergy 2004;2(1):7.
71. Blanchard C, Wang N, Rothenberg ME. Eosinophilic esophagitis: pathogenesis, genetics, and therapy. J Allergy Clin Immunol 2006;118(5):1054–9.
72. Rubio-Tapia A, Murray JA. Celiac disease. Curr Opin Gastroenterol 2010;26(2): 116–22.
73. Nelson HS, Lahr J, Rule R, et al. Treatment of anaphylactic sensitivity to peanuts by immunotherapy with injections of aqueous peanut extract. J Allergy Clin Immunol 1997;99(6 Pt 1):744–51.
74. Oppenheimer JJ, Nelson HS, Bock SA, et al. Treatment of peanut allergy with rush immunotherapy. J Allergy Clin Immunol 1992;90(2):256–62.
75. Jones SM, Pons L, Roberts JL, et al. Clinical efficacy and immune regulation with peanut oral immunotherapy. J Allergy Clin Immunol 2009;124(2):292–300.
76. Thyagarajan A, Varshney P, Jones SM, et al. Peanut oral immunotherapy is not ready for clinical use. J Allergy Clin Immunol 2010;126(1):31–2.
77. Goikoetxea MJ, Cabrera-Freitag P, Sanz ML, et al. The importance of in vitro component-resolved diagnosis in paediatric patients. Allergol Immunopathol (Madr) 2010;38(1):37–40.
78. Lin J, Sampson HA. The role of immunoglobulin E-binding epitopes in the characterization of food allergy. Curr Opin Allergy Clin Immunol 2009;9(4):357–63.
79. Codreanu F, Collignon O, Roitel O, et al. A novel immunoassay using recombinant allergens simplifies peanut allergy diagnosis. Int Arch Allergy Immunol 2010; 154(3):216–26.
80. Hamilton RG, MacGlashan DW Jr, Saini SS. IgE antibody-specific activity in human allergic disease. Immunol Res 2010;47(1–3):273–84.

Index

Note: Page numbers of article titles are in **boldface** type.

Otolaryngol Clin N Am 44 (2011) 835–843
doi:10.1016/S0030-6665(11)00079-X

C

D

E

L

M

Q

R

V

W